Pediatric Oncology

Kathy Pritchard-Jones • Jeffrey S. Dome
Editors

Renal Tumors of Childhood

Biology and Therapy

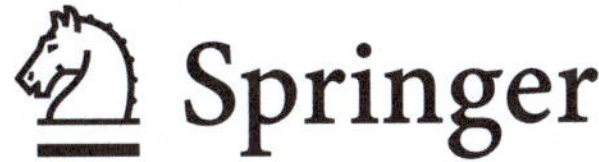

Editors
Kathy Pritchard-Jones
Department of Developmental Biology and Cancer
Institute of Child Health
University College London
London
UK

Jeffrey S. Dome
Children's National Medical Center
Center for Cancer and Blood Disorders
Washington, District of Columbia
USA

ISSN 1613-5318 ISSN 2191-0812 (electronic)
ISBN 978-3-662-51918-9 ISBN 978-3-662-44003-2 (eBook)
DOI 10.1007/978-3-662-44003-2
Springer Heidelberg New York Dordrecht London

Softcover reprint of the hardcover 1st edition 2014

Printed on acid-free paper

Springer is part of Springer Science+Business Media (www.springer.com)

Foreword

Astonishing progress has been made in pediatric oncology. More than 80 % of children with acute lymphocytic leukemia now survive; the disease was considered incurable a scant five or six decades ago [1]. Moreover, treatment intensity is now modified according to well-defined clinical and more sophisticated risk factors.

This progress has been mirrored in the solid malignant tumors of childhood, notably in the case of Wilms' tumor (WT). The long-term cure rate is in the 90 % range, therapy being modulated in strength according to accurately established clinical, pathologic, and molecular genetic characteristics [2].

Indeed, the evolution of pediatric oncology can be traced by following the advances made in WT management. The concept of coordinated care was first developed when surgeons collaborated with radiation therapists in the treatment of WT. These children were often irradiated preoperatively in European centers and routinely postoperatively across the Atlantic [3, 4]. Soon, the chemotherapist joined the multimodal team and cure rates climbed [5].

A very important part of this history is the fact that the emphases for decades have been placed not only on improving survival rates in WT patients, but also on reducing short- and long-term iatrogenic adversities. Steps were taken early to lessen the postirradiation growth disturbances first identified 100 years ago by Perthes [6]. In no other tumor has the adage "Cure is not enough" been followed more assiduously. Chapters 5 and 6 reviews these critical aspects of WT care.

Epidemiologists, pathologists, and clinical and molecular geneticists became involved as well. The contributions made by this rich admixture of talents are recounted in Chaps. 1–4 and 8–10.

The debate concerning post- or preoperative therapy – chemotherapy having supplanted radiation therapy in the latter case – continues today. The raw question "Which is better?" requires a Talmudic answer, "It depends …." The two editors of this volume are very prominent spokespersons for the two approaches. The merits and demerits of either method are detailed by them and their coauthors in Chaps. 5 and 6. Diagnostic uncertainty, an objection to preoperative therapy, has been reduced by major advances in imaging methods and techniques, as discussed in Chap. 8.

There remain unsolved problems that require attention, but in large measure, the heavy work has been done. It is unlikely that new classes of antimitotic agents or modifications of those existing will be introduced to reduce the mortality in problem cases. These include, for example, children with diffusely anaplastic WT or the very malignant rhabdoid tumor of the kidney. Therapeutic answers to these daunting challenges lie in the domain of molecularly specific agents. Research seeking such agents is actively under way, the bases for which are described in Chaps. 9 and 10. They deserve careful reading because they serve as blueprints for what is to come.

Thus, both the past and the future of the WT story are well covered in these pages, written by international authorities. All those interested in the malignant renal tumors of childhood will profit from reading their work.

While one can look back and marvel at the distance that has been covered, it clearly is not time to furl the sails. The longest stretches over difficult waters lead to children in underdeveloped societies. For them, early diagnosis and effective intervention are dreams seldom realized. An army of modern-day heroes of Herculean stamp is needed to attack the many-headed monsters that lie in wait. And such heroes exist, are willing, and are able to confront the hydra of poverty, ignorance, superstition, avarice, malnutrition, endemic disease, and isolation.

Major progress is being made by teams derived from local civic and medical authorities who work with supporting teams from more developed countries. As described in Chap. 15, the Burkitt lymphoma project in Malawi, pioneered by Professor Peter Hesseling of South Africa, is a heartening example of what can be done [7]. It was soon expanded to include the study of African Wilms' tumor patients and their treatment in that setting [8]. Another success story is of the MASCOTA program initiated in Nicaragua by Professor G. Masera. It has been widened and has transformed pediatric cancer care in the countries rimming the Caribbean Sea [9]. Many individuals, institutions, and national and international groups are now involved in such efforts. The International Society of Pediatric Oncology (SIOP), for example, has a longstanding committee of Pediatric Oncology in Developing Countries, chaired for decades by Professor Hans Peter Wagner of Switzerland.

Thus, the hardest problems remain, some affecting a small percentage of renal tumor patients, others affecting millions of children. There is no room for complacency. Hard sailing against strong headwinds over these and other roiled seas lies ahead.

Pennsylvania, USA Dr Giulio D'Angio

References

1 Jeha S, Pui CH (2009) Risk-adapted treatment of pediatric acute lynphoblastic leukemia. Hematol Oncol Clin North Am 23:973–990

2 Metzger ML, Dome JS (2005) Current therapy for Wilms tumor. 10:815–826

3 Schweisguth O, Bamberger J (1963) Nephroblastoma in children (In French). Ann Chir Infant 4:335–354

4 Gross RE, Neuhauser EBD (1950) Treatment of mixed tumors of the kidney in Childhood. Pediatrics 6:843–852

5 Farber S (1966) Chemotherapy in the treatment of leukemia and Wilms' tumor. JAMA 198:826–836

6 Perthes G (1903) Über den einfluss der Röntgen-strahlen auf epithelial Gewebe insbesondere auf das Carcinom. Archiv Für Klinische Chirurgie 971:955–982
7 Hesseling P, Broadbent R, Mansvelt E et al (2005) The 2000 Burkitt lymphoma trial in Malawi. Pediatr Blood Cancer 44:245–250
8 Wessels G, Hesseling PB, Van Ommeren KH, Boonstra V (1999) Nutrition, morbidity, and survival in South African children with Wilms' tumor. Pediatr Hematol Oncol 16:321–327
9 Masera G (2009) Bridging the childhood mortality gap between economically developed and low-income countries. J Pediatr Hematol Oncol 31:710–712

Contents

Epidemiology of Renal Tumors of Childhood

1

Charles A. Stiller and Andrew F. Olshan

Contents

C.A. Stiller (✉)
Childhood Cancer Research Group, Department of Paediatrics, University of Oxford, Oxford, UK
e-mail: charles.stiller@new.ox.ac.uk

A.F. Olshan
Gillings School of Global Public Health and Lineberger, Comprehensive Cancer Center, University of North Carolina, Chapel Hill, USA
e-mail: Andy_Olshan@UNC.edu

Abstract

Primary renal tumors, predominantly Wilms tumor, account for 4–7 % of all childhood cancers. The incidence of renal cancer among children and adolescents in industrialised countries is presented in detail. Worldwide variations in incidence, which are predominantly on ethnic rather than geographical lines, are discussed. The available information on the occurrence of non-malignant tumors is collated.

The wide range of syndromes, congenital anomalies and constitutional chromosomal abnormalities associated with Wilms tumor and other renal tumors is reviewed. Although associations have been reported with a diverse array of risk factors including lifestyle exposures, medical history, birth characteristics, and occupational and environmental exposures, there is no consistent pattern. Methodological issues and future directions in aetiological studies are discussed.

International survival from childhood renal tumors is documented, wherever possible, using population-based data. Five-year survival exceeds 80 % in high-income countries but is lower in other world regions. The chapter concludes with an epidemiological overview of long-term survival, subsequent malignancies and other late effects.

K. Pritchard-Jones, J.S. Dome (eds.), *Renal Tumors of Childhood: Biology and Therapy*, Pediatric Oncology, DOI 10.1007/978-3-662-44003-2_1,

Table 1.1 Numbers of registrations and annual incidence rates for malignant renal tumors in children. United Kingdom, 1996–2005

Diagnostic group/subgroup/ division (ICCC-3)		Registrations M	F	Total	Annual rates per million for age group (years) 0	1–4	5–9	10–14	Total ASR
VI	Renal tumors	429	462	891	17.9	19.4	4.4	1.3	9.2
(a)	Wilms tumor and other non-epithelial renal tumors	418	453	871	17.9	19.3	4.3	0.9	9.0
1	Wilms tumor	369	427	796	14.0	18.1	4.1	0.8	8.2
2	Rhabdoid renal tumor	19	13	32	2.9	0.4	0.0	0.0	0.4
3	Kidney sarcomas[a]	25	9	34	0.9	0.9	0.1	0.0	0.4
4	Peripheral primitive neuroectodermal tumor	5	4	9	0.1	0.0	0.1	0.1	0.1
(b)	Carcinomas	9	8	17	0.0	0.1	0.1	0.3	0.1
(c)	Unspecified	2	1	3	0.0	0.0	0.1	0.0	0.0
II (b–d)	Non-Hodgkin lymphomas	5	0	5	0.0	0.1	0.0	0.0	0.0
IV (a)	Neuroblastoma	7	7	14	0.4	0.3	0.0	0.0	0.2
IX	Soft tissue sarcomas	3	6	9	0.1	0.1	0.1	0.0	0.1
X (b)2	Malignant teratoma	1	0	1	0.0	0.0	0.0	0.0	0.0
	Total	445	475	920	18.5	20.1	4.6	1.3	9.5

Source: National Registry of Childhood Tumors
[a]All cases were clear cell sarcoma

1.1 Introduction

Primary malignant tumors of the kidney generally account for 4–7 % of cancers diagnosed in children under the age of 15 years in western industrialised countries and for less than 1 % of cancers in adolescents aged 15–19 years. Non-malignant renal tumors also occur, especially in infancy. This chapter begins with an overview of the incidence of childhood renal tumors. We then review aetiology and risk factors for these tumors including genetic associations, birth characteristics and childhood development, socio-economic factors and exogenous risk factors. We also examine survival from renal tumors and the factors that influence survival. The chapter concludes with long-term survival, subsequent malignancies, and other late effects from an epidemiological point of view.

1.2 Incidence

Malignant renal tumors constitute Group VI in the International Classification of Childhood Cancer, Third Edition (ICCC-3) (Steliarova-Foucher et al. 2005), in which tumors are grouped according to morphology as well as primary site. In addition, small numbers of tumors from other ICCC-3 groups can occur in the kidney. Table 1.1 shows the numbers of cases and incidence rates for malignant renal tumors diagnosed among children under 15 years of age in the United Kingdom during the 10-year period 1996–2005, based on data from the population-based National Registry of Childhood Tumors (NRCT). The total age-standardised rate (ASR), using the weights of the World Standard Population, was 9.5 per million child-years. The peak incidence, 23.5 per million, occurred at the age of 3 years; rates declined steadily with increasing age through the rest of childhood.

The great majority of tumors (97 %) were in ICCC-3 Group VI. Wilms tumor, or nephroblastoma, one of the characteristic embryonal tumors of childhood, was by far the most frequent histology, accounting for 87 % of tumors overall. The ASR was 8.2 per million, implying a risk of about 1 in 9,000 that a child will develop Wilms tumor in the first 15 years of life. Between the ages of 1 and 9 years, more than 90 % of tumors were Wilms, but

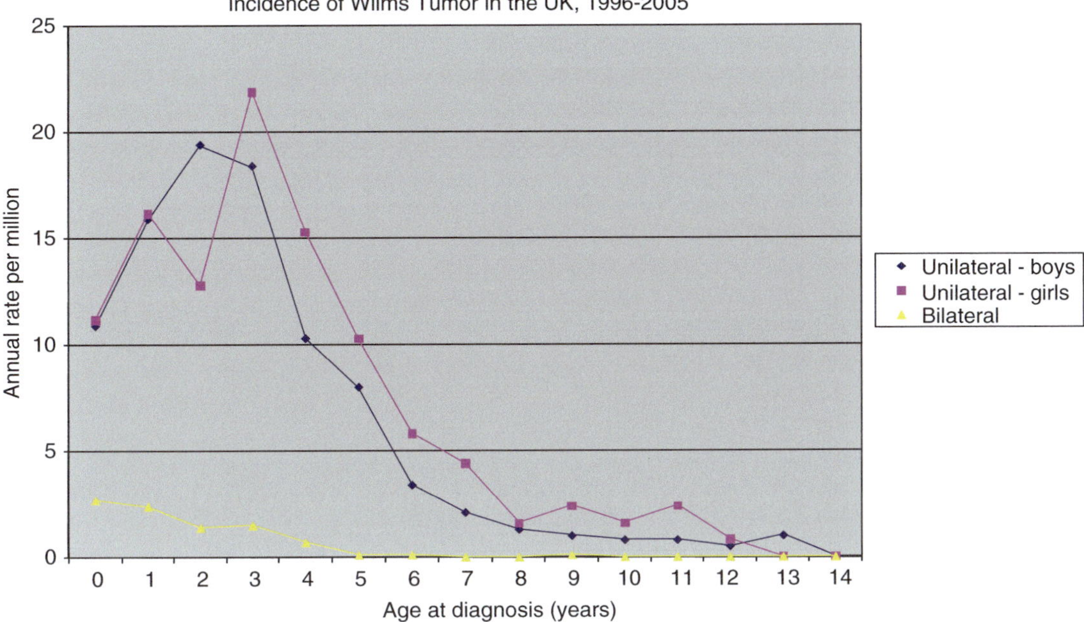

Fig. 1.1 Incidence of Wilms tumor by single year of age in the United Kingdom, 1996–2005 (Source: National Registry of Childhood Tumors)

only 76 % in the first year of life and 61 % at age 10–14 years. Of the 796 registered cases, 717 (90 %) were unilateral kidney tumors, 65 (8 %) were bilateral and 11 (1 %) were of unknown laterality; the remaining 3 cases were extrarenal. Infants aged under a year accounted for 11 % of unilateral and 29 % of bilateral cases. Figure 1.1 shows incidence by single year of age for unilateral Wilms tumor in boys and girls and for bilateral Wilms tumor in the two sexes combined. Peak incidence of unilateral disease was at age 3 years, whereas bilateral tumors were most frequent in the first 2 years of life. Unilateral tumors occurred slightly more often in girls, but there was a pronounced female excess of bilateral tumors, with 71 % of affected children being girls. Among children with unilateral tumors, girls tended to be older than boys at diagnosis.

The next most frequent categories were rhabdoid renal tumor and clear cell sarcoma, each with an overall incidence of 0.4 per million and accounting for 3–4 % of all tumors. Both were almost entirely tumors of early childhood. Clear cell sarcoma occurred at a fairly constant rate throughout the first 5 years of life, and 63 % of rhabdoid tumors were diagnosed in infants under 1 year of age. There was a marked excess of boys with clear cell sarcoma. Peripheral primitive neuroectodermal tumor (pPNET) accounted for only 1 % of all renal tumors and represented 5 % of all registrations for extraosseous Ewing sarcoma family tumors. Incidence may have been underestimated, however, since renal pPNET was first recognised as an entity in the mid-1990s (Rodriguez-Galindo et al. 1997) and only 2 of the 9 cases tabulated here were diagnosed before 2000. Carcinomas accounted for 1.7 % of all tumors, and their incidence increased with age. The 17 cases comprised 13 renal cell carcinomas, 2 medullary carcinomas, 1 oncocytic carcinoma and 1 neuroendocrine carcinoma.

Tumors in other ICCC-3 Groups accounted for only 3 % of the grand total. The most frequent type was neuroblastoma, cases of which were only included if the primary site was specified as intrarenal. The 14 registrations accounted for 1.5 % of all neuroblastomas registered over the 10-year period. There were nine soft tissue sarcomas: three desmoplastic small round cell tumors (DSRCT), one rhabdomyosarcoma and five unspecified sarcomas. They accounted for less than 1 % of all childhood soft tissue sarcomas registered over the same period but 17 % of DSRCT. NHL was restricted to cases where there was good evidence that the primary site was in the kidneys. The five registrations accounted for less

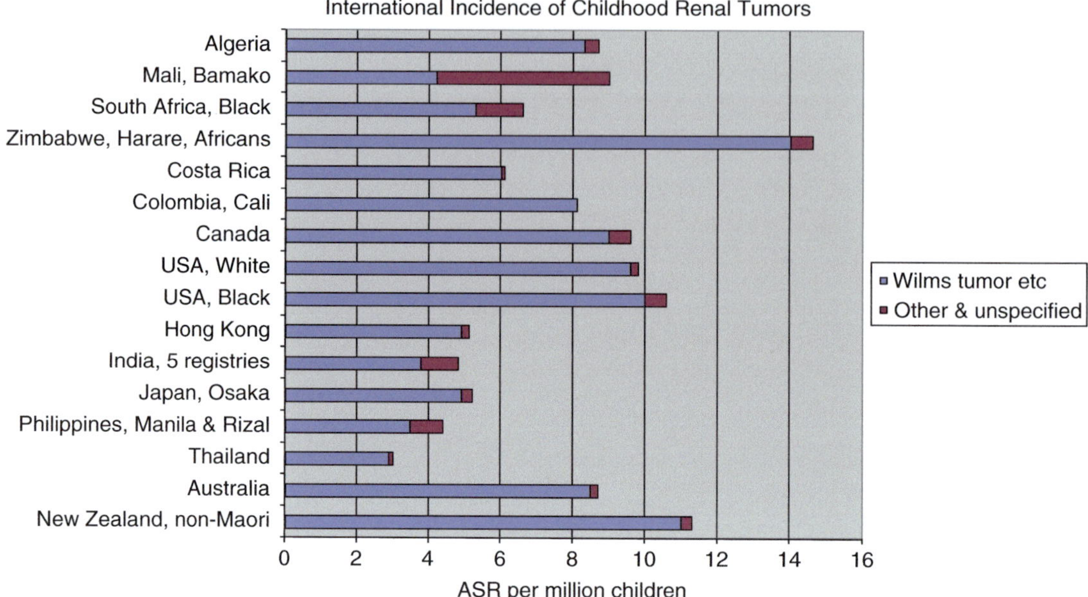

Fig. 1.2 International incidence of malignant renal tumors of childhood in 15 countries outside Europe. Age-standardised rates per million children under 15 years of age, using weights of the World Standard Population (Sources: *Cancer in Africa* (Parkin et al. 2003) and *International Incidence of Childhood Cancer, Volume II* (Parkin et al. 1998))

than 1 % of all childhood NHL; they comprised two lymphoblastic lymphomas, two Burkitt lymphomas and one post-transplant diffuse large B-cell lymphoma.

Incidence rates for malignant renal tumors in UK children are generally typical of those observed among mainly white populations in Europe (Pastore et al. 2006; Stiller 2007a) and the United States (Bernstein et al. 1999; Linabery and Ross 2008), though the excess of girls with bilateral Wilms tumor is unusual. Figure 1.2 shows ASRs for ICCC-3 Group VI (Renal tumors) and Subgroup VIa (Wilms tumor and other non-epithelial renal tumors) in population-based series from 15 countries outside Europe (Parkin et al. 1998, 2003). At one time, it was suggested that the incidence of Wilms tumor was similar in all populations (Innis 1972), but it has been clear for decades that its occurrence varies considerably between ethnic groups (Goodman et al. 1989; Stiller and Parkin 1990; Ducore et al. 2004). The highest rate was found in the African population of Harare, Zimbabwe. In the United States, incidence was slightly higher among Black children than among White children. A relative frequency study of children registered at paediatric oncology centres throughout the United Kingdom found that Wilms tumor was significantly more frequent among children of West Indian ethnic origin compared with White Caucasians (Stiller et al. 1991). The lowest rates have tended to be found in South and East Asia. In Japan, the deficit was less pronounced in the first year of life and there was a marked excess of boys (M/F=1.8). Lower incidence has also been found among children of East and South East Asian ethnicity in the United States (Goodman et al. 1989; Stiller and Parkin 1990; Ducore et al. 2004) and among South Asian children in the UK (Stiller et al. 1991; Cummins et al. 2001). In the National Wilms Tumor Study (NWTS) in North America, 17.5 % of Asian children had clear cell sarcoma or rhabdoid tumor, compared with 4.6–6.4 % of non-Hispanic white, Black and Hispanic children, consistent with a deficit of Wilms tumor but not of these other, rarer tumor types in populations of Asian origin (Breslow et al. 1994). It has been suggested that, in developing countries, girls with cancer are less likely than boys to be diagnosed, leading to underestimates of incidence for girls and for both sexes combined and to inflation of the ratio of male to female rates (Pearce and Parker 2001). There is little evidence, however, that this is the case for renal tumors, including Wilms tumor. In the combined data from 14 countries of sub-Saharan Africa in *Cancer in*

Africa (Parkin et al. 2003), the sex ratio was close to unity. In the Indian registries contributing to Fig. 1.2, the ASR for boys and girls were very similar both for Wilms tumor (3.9 and 3.8 per million respectively) and for all renal tumors (4.9 and 4.6 per million).

Several types of non-malignant renal tumors also occur in childhood. The most frequent is mesoblastic nephroma. The NRCT included 42 cases during 1996–2005, all but one of which were diagnosed in the first year of life. The recorded incidence was 5.9 per million at age 0 and a total ASR of 0.5 per million. These rates should be regarded as minimum estimates since non-malignant tumors are not always registered, especially if they are not seen by paediatric oncologists. Nevertheless, the incidence rate is similar to that of 0.4 per million estimated from three population-based series whose ascertainment was believed to be complete (Stiller 2008). There was a small excess of girls (M/F=0.83) among the NRCT cases, similar to that found in Wilms tumor. In national clinical trials from the United States and Germany, however, boys were about twice as frequently affected as girls (Howell et al. 1982; Furtwaengler et al. 2006).

Other non-malignant tumors are probably less completely registered than mesoblastic nephroma and are almost certainly rarer. Cystic partially differentiated nephroblastoma (CPDN) accounted for 0.5 % of 5,100 renal tumors in the NWTS (Blakely et al. 2003); most cases were diagnosed before the age of 2 years and there was a marked excess of boys (M/F=3.2). No cases of CPDN were found in the NRCT for 1996–2005, but it seems likely that historical registry data include a few cases coded as Wilms tumor, since CPDN did not acquire its own morphology code until the most recent edition of ICD-O. There were 10 registrations for cystic nephroma in the NRCT, of which 7 were diagnosed before the age of 2 years. The minimum estimate for the ASR was 0.1 per million. Various other benign renal tumors are seen in childhood, including oncocytoma, angiomyolipoma and leiomyoma, but they are all probably much rarer. There is no reliable, published information on the occurrence of non-malignant childhood renal tumors in different world regions or ethnic groups.

Renal cancer is even less frequent at age 15–19 that at age 10–14. In England during 1979–1997, the combined incidence of Wilms tumor and renal carcinoma was 0.6 per million person years; Wilms tumor accounted for 31 % of cases and carcinomas for 69 % (Birch et al. 2003). In a recent study, incidence of renal cancer at age 15–19 years was below 5 per million in all regions of the world, with no clear geographical variation (Stiller 2007b). Population-based data on morphology are rarely available for this age group, but carcinomas predominate in Europe and the United States (Stiller et al. 2006; Bernstein et al. 1999).

In common with most other childhood cancers, recorded incidence of renal tumors – predominantly Wilms tumor – increased during the last few decades of the twentieth century in the United Kingdom and elsewhere in Europe (Pastore et al. 2006; Stiller 2007a), though the rate of increase was well under 1 % per year. In the US SEER registries, there was little evidence for change in incidence among White children between 1975 and 1995 (Bernstein et al. 1999). Incidence among Black children, historically higher than among Whites, fell to the same as or less than that for White children in 1985–1995 in the SEER registries, but this pattern was not repeated in other US registries (Parkin et al. 1998), and in SEER data for 1992–2004, the incidence for Black children again exceeded that for Whites (Linabery and Ross 2008). During the latter period, there was a suggestion of decreasing incidence. The estimated rate of decrease, 2.1 % per year overall, was remarkably constant between males and females and between the Black and White ethnic groups, but the trend was statistically significant only for males (Linabery and Ross 2008).

1.3 Genetic Associations

That fact that incidence of Wilms tumor varies predominantly on ethnic rather than geographical lines is one of several pointers to a strong role for genetic predisposition in its aetiology. An unusually wide range of syndromes, congenital anomalies and constitutional chromosomal abnormalities has also been reported in conjunction with Wilms tumor. These have been documented in a comprehensive review which included an assessment of the evidence for an increased risk of Wilms tumor (Scott et al. 2006). The genetics of Wilms tumor and other childhood renal tumors are reviewed in detail in Chap. 2. We concentrate here on familial associations and on conditions for which there is definitely an increased risk or whose occurrence with Wilms tumors has been frequently reported. A summary of known genetic associations with other childhood renal tumors is also provided.

The first Wilms tumor gene to be discovered was WT1, which is located at 11p13 and is involved in three syndromes that carry a markedly raised risk of Wilms tumor. WAGR (Wilms tumor, aniridia, genitourinary abnormalities, mental retardation) syndrome is caused by constitutional microdeletions encompassing WT1 and the nearby gene PAX6. More than 30 % of children with WAGR syndrome develop Wilms tumor (Coppes et al. 1994), and it accounts for upwards of 0.75 % of all patients with Wilms tumor (Breslow et al. 2003). Aniridia is in fact caused by deletions or mutations of PAX6, which do not give rise to Wilms tumor, and only 30 % of individuals with aniridia also have deletions of WT1 (Muto et al. 2002). In a population-based record-linkage study in Denmark, the risk of Wilms tumor in children with sporadic aniridia was estimated as 4.5 %, 67 times that in the general population (Grønskov et al. 2001). Denys-Drash syndrome (Wilms tumor, nephropathy and genitourinary abnormalities) is caused by missense mutations in WT1. Wilms tumor occurs in over 90 % of cases of Denys-Drash syndrome (Coppes et al. 1994), and it accounts for 0.3–0.4 % of cases of Wilms tumor (Breslow et al. 2000). Frasier syndrome (nephropathy with gonadal dysgenesis and gonadoblastoma), which is caused by intron 9 splice mutations of WT1, is much rarer and carries a lower risk of Wilms tumor (Scott et al. 2006).

In a British national cohort study of persons with constitutional chromosome deletions, from which patients who underwent cytogenetic testing as a consequence of cancer diagnosis were excluded, the risk of renal cancer in subjects with 11p deletions was almost 2,000 times that in the general population (Swerdlow et al. 2008). All of the eight cases occurred before the age of 5 years and all but one had deletions encompassing 11p13.

Several childhood overgrowth syndromes have been associated with Wilms tumor. Phenotypic overlap between syndromes means that earlier reports linking Wilms tumor to a specific syndrome before its genetic basis was known may be unreliable. Beckwith-Wiedemann syndrome (BWS) is caused by dysregulation of various imprinted growth-regulating genes at 11p15 and carries an elevated risk of several cancers, mostly embryonal tumors. Wilms tumor is the most frequently reported, affecting 1–8 % of children in the largest series. The risk varies between epigenetic subgroups of BWS, some of which are not at increased risk of Wilms tumor (Scott et al. 2006). About 1 % of children with Wilms tumor have BWS (Porteus et al. 2000). Simpson-Golabi-Behmel syndrome is an X-linked overgrowth syndrome, with 70 % of cases caused by mutations or deletions of GPC3 at Xq26; Wilms tumor has been reported in 9 % of patients with GPC3 mutations (Scott et al. 2006). Perlman syndrome, an autosomal recessive condition of unknown cause, has very high infant mortality. Wilms tumor has been reported in one third of all cases and in more than half of those surviving the first month of life (Scott et al. 2006). Sotos syndrome was formerly believed to have a raised risk of cancer including Wilms tumor (Hersh et al. 1992). Since the establishment of haploinsufficiency of NSD1 on 5q35 as the cause of Sotos syndrome and the consequent advent of molecular diagnosis, it has been shown that the risk of Wilms tumor is very low (Tatton-Brown et al. 2005). Increased risk of Wilms tumor has been reported in isolated hemihypertrophy (IHH), with 3 % affected in one large prospective study (Hoyme et al. 1998). Interpretation is complicated by the facts that IHH can have a wide range of causes and is often so subtle as not to be diagnosed until tumor diagnosis or even later. It seems likely that children with IHH caused by 11p15 defects have a similar risk of Wilms tumor to those with BWS, but it is unclear whether other IHH patients are at increased risk (Scott et al. 2006).

Several other syndromes have an increased risk of Wilms tumor (Scott et al. 2006). In both mosaic variegated aneuploidy and Fanconi anaemia subgroup D1, the risk among reported cases is 20–25 %. In Bloom syndrome, hereditary hyperparathyroidism-jaw tumor syndrome and mulibrey nanism, the risk is probably below 5 %. There also appears to be an increased risk of Wilms tumor associated with three constitutional chromosomal abnormalities, namely, trisomy 18 (Edwards syndrome), trisomy 13 (Patau syndrome) and 2q37 deletion. The first two of these have very high infant mortality so, although their prevalence at birth is relatively high, they account for a very small proportion of all cases of Wilms tumor.

Turner syndrome was found in 4 (0.07 %) patients in the NWTS (Olson et al. 1995). Only one case of Wilms tumor occurred among nearly 1,000 individuals with Turner syndrome from national cohorts in Denmark and the United Kingdom (Hasle et al. 1996; Swerdlow et al. 2001), indicating that the risk may be similar to that in the general population.

Several specific congenital abnormalities have been suggested to carry a raised risk of Wilms tumor. There may be a small increased risk with horseshoe kidney, which was found in 0.4 % of children without chromosomal abnormalities in the NWTS, about 1.6 times the population frequency (Neville et al. 2002). An excess of cardiac defects has been reported in several unselected series of Wilms tumor, but it should be noted that these defects are also found in several syndromes that predispose to Wilms tumor (Scott et al. 2006). There is no evidence for a substantially raised risk of Wilms tumor in association with multicystic dysplastic kidney (Narchi 2005). A blinded case-control study did not support a previous suggestion of raised risk in association with cervical rib abnormalities (Merks et al. 2005). In an unselected series of 156 children with Wilms tumor at a single paediatric oncology centre, congenital abnormalities or syndromes were noted in 30 % (Ng et al. 2007), although some of the abnormalities would probably not have been detected without careful examination. The total included seven patients whose only abnormality was height/weight above the 95th centile, very close to the expected number of 7.8 such patients. A population-based study linking the national cancer registries and medical birth registries in Norway and Sweden found an overall excess risk of renal cancer of about 80 % in children with birth defects, which was largely attributable to excesses among children with urinary organ malformations or multiple defects (Bjørge et al. 2008).

A family history of Wilms tumor is present in 1–2 % of cases, but these pedigrees have many different causes (Scott et al. 2006). A few affected families are associated with syndromes described above. One familial Wilms tumor gene, FWT1, has been mapped to 17q21 and there is some evidence for another such gene, designated FWT2, on 19q13. Several Wilms tumor families exist that are not linked to any of the genes or syndromes discussed above, indicating that there are still further Wilms tumor genes to be discovered (Rapley et al. 2000). Wilms tumor is not a cardinal tumor for Li-Fraumeni syndrome, but it has been reported in several Li-Fraumeni and Li-Fraumeni-like families. Support for an association is provided by the fact that five of six TP53 mutations reported with Wilms tumor affect splicing, compared with only 4 % of all germline TP53 mutations (Scott et al. 2006). Excesses of various cancers have occasionally been reported in relatives of children with Wilms tumor, but there is little evidence of an overall increase in the risk of cancer among family members (Moutou et al. 1994; Olsen et al. 1995; Hemminki and Mutanen 2001; Felgenhauer et al. 2001).

In addition to the associations described above, germline mutations of WT1 occur in about 2 % of Wilms tumor patients without any underlying syndrome (Little et al. 2004), and constitutional 11p15 abnormalities occur in a further 3 % (Scott et al. 2008). At present, around 10 % of cases of Wilms tumors can be linked to identifiable constitutional genetic abnormalities; in about half of these cases, Wilms tumor is the sole clinical manifestation.

The variation in Wilms tumor incidence along ethnic rather than geographical lines also suggests that genetic predisposition is important in its aetiology. Wilms tumor is fairly often accompanied by perilobar and/or intralobar nephrogenic rests (Breslow et al. 2006). In a study of more than 5,000 children, 24 % of white American children in the NWTS also had perilobar nephrogenic rests, compared with 8 % of Asian-American children in the NWTS and 2 % of children from Japan (Fukuzawa et al. 2004). An absence of perilobar nephrogenic rests has also been reported among Wilms tumor patients in India (Mishra et al. 1998). These results suggest that at least some of the recorded deficit of Wilms tumor in Asian populations is real and might be attributable to relatively infrequent loss of IGF2 imprinting, a defect which is associated with perilobar nephrogenic rests (Fukuzawa et al. 2004). Since Wilms tumor with perilobar rests is more often seen in girls and in older children (Breslow et al. 2006), these results could also help to explain the preponderance of boys and young average age at diagnosis among Japanese Wilms tumor patients (Fukuzawa et al. 2004).

Rhabdoid tumor of the kidney, together with atypical teratoid/rhabdoid tumors of the CNS and rhabdoid tumors of other sites, occur in the rhabdoid tumor predisposition syndrome associated with germline mutation or deletion of SMARCB1 (also known as INI1, hSNF5 or BAF47) on chromosome 22q (Biegel et al. 1999; Biegel 2006).

The overall risk of renal cell carcinoma in patients with tuberous sclerosis is not raised, but it tends to be diagnosed earlier than in the general population (Crino et al. 2006). In a population-based German study, 2/49 cases (4 %) of childhood renal carcinoma occurred in patients with tuberous sclerosis (Selle et al. 2007). Renal clear-cell carcinoma is a frequent finding in von Hippel-Lindau syndrome but virtually never in childhood (Ong et al. 2007). Most patients with renal medullary carcinoma have sickle cell trait (Swartz et al. 2002).

There is clearly a strong tendency for cystic nephroma and pleuropulmonary blastoma to occur in members of the same family (Boman et al. 2006), but no risk estimates are available. Renal angiomyolipoma often occurs in tuberous sclerosis, especially in patients with mutations in the TSC2 gene (Au et al. 2007).

1.3.1 Epidemiologic Studies of Risk Factors for Wilms Tumor

In this section, we summarise the results from epidemiologic studies that have evaluated lifestyle, environmental and occupational, medical, reproductive, childhood and other factors in relation to the risk of Wilms tumor (Table 1.2). In addition, we discuss methodologic issues that may have had an impact on the study findings.

Most studies that have investigated risk factors for Wilms tumor have been case-control studies and have identified cases from local,

Table 1.2 Current epidemiologic evidence on causes of Wilms tumor

Exposure or characteristic	Comments
Known risk factors	
Race	Incidence in Asians is about half that in blacks and whites
Aniridia, genitourinary anomalies, WAGR syndrome (Wilms tumor, aniridia, genitourinary abnormalities, mental retardation), Beckwith-Wiedemann syndrome, Perlman syndrome, Denys-Drash syndrome, Simpson-Golabi-Behmel syndrome and certain other rare syndromes (see text)	Risk is increased in children with these congenital anomalies and genetic conditions
Factors for which evidence is inconsistent or limited	
Paternal occupation	An increased risk for fathers employed as a welder or mechanic has been reported in several studies. Paternal occupational exposure to hydrocarbons or metals had an elevated risk in some studies
Parental age	Increased parental age was associated with increased risk in some studies
Pregnancy complications	Hypertension during pregnancy was associated with an increased risk in several studies. Infections during pregnancy increased risk in some studies
High birth weight	Association with birth weight over 4,000 g has been reported in some studies

Table 1.2 (continued)

Exposure or characteristic	Comments
Gestational length	Lengths less than 37 weeks had elevated risks in several studies
Parental exposure to pesticides	Some studies found an increased risk for parental occupational or residential exposure to pesticides
Maternal consumption of coffee and tea during pregnancy	A few studies reported association with coffee and/or tea; others did not replicate this finding
Maternal hair dye use during pregnancy	Use was associated with risk in one study, but not in others
Maternal medication use during pregnancy	Studies reported associations with various drugs including hormones, vitamins, antibiotics, dipyrone, metoclopramide and pethrane anaesthesia during delivery. Most of these results were found in only a single study
Maternal occupation	One study found an association with job groupings that included hairdressers, electronic and clothing manufacturing workers, laboratory workers and dental assistants
Factors for which evidence is suggestive of no association, but not conclusive	
Parental cigarette smoking	Multiple negative studies
Maternal alcohol use during pregnancy	Only one study reported a positive association
History of miscarriage	Multiple negative studies

Updated from SEER Pediatric Monograph (Bernstein et al. 1999)

regional or national cancer registries, hospitals or clinical trials network. Controls have been identified from hospitals, birth files, telephone number random digit dialing or other cases of cancer. Maternal self-report was the most common source of exposure data. Other studies have been of a cohort design including vital records or other routinely collected data linkage.

All other types of childhood renal tumor are so rare that no epidemiological studies of their aetiology have been conducted.

1.4 Lifestyle Exposures

Parental smoking around or during pregnancy has been examined in case-control studies (Stjernfeldt et al. 1986; McKinney and Stiller 1986; Olshan et al. 1993; Schüz et al. 2001; Pang et al. 2003; Tsai et al. 2006). No pattern of elevated risk was reported for maternal or paternal smoking. All but one case-control study (Tsai et al. 2006) failed to find an association with maternal alcohol use during pregnancy (Olshan et al. 1993; Sharpe and Franco 1996; Schüz et al. 2001).

Maternal coffee or tea consumption during pregnancy has been linked with a twofold increased risk of Wilms tumor in one small case-control study (Bunin et al. 1987), but other studies failed to support this finding (Olshan et al. 1993; Schüz et al. 2001).

A small number of studies have investigated the relationship between parental medication use and risk of Wilms tumor. The findings have been mixed with some studies, but not all, reporting elevated odds ratios for maternal antibiotic use, vitamins and supplements (Olshan et al. 1993; Sharpe and Franco 1996; Schüz and Forman 2007). Oral contraceptive use has not been associated with an increased risk in most studies (Olshan et al. 1993; Sharpe and Franco 1996; Schüz et al. 2001).

A study published in 1987 (Bunin et al. 1987) first reported a potential association between maternal hair dye use and an increased risk of Wilms tumor. Subsequent studies failed to replicate this finding (Olshan et al. 1993; Sharpe and Franco 1996; Tsai et al. 2006).

1.5 Medical History

Pregnancy complications and conditions have been investigated in multiple studies. The risk related to a history of spontaneous abortion has been examined in three studies (Bunin et al. 1987; Schüz et al. 2001; Puumala et al. 2008). No pattern of elevated risk was reported. Hypertension during pregnancy has been associated with a moderately increased risk of Wilms tumor [odds ratios (OR) from 1.3 to 2.1] in multiple studies (Bunin et al. 1987; Lindblad et al. 1992; Puumala et al. 2008). However, studies that looked at the risk associated with hypertension medications, including diuretics, did not report any increase (Bunin et al. 1987; Olshan et al. 1993; Sharpe and Franco 1996; Schüz and Forman 2007). Self-reported infections during pregnancy, especially vaginal infections, were associated with an increased risk of Wilms tumor in two North American studies (Bunin et al. 1987; Daniels et al. 2008), but not in other studies (Lindblad et al. 1992; Olshan et al. 1993). A large North American case-control study reported modest associations for labour induction (OR = 1.4) and upper respiratory infection (OR = 1.5) (Daniels et al. 2008). Maternal diabetes before or during pregnancy was not related to the risk of Wilms tumor (Daniels et al. 2008; Puumala et al. 2008). Anaesthetic use during labour has been associated with an increased risk of Wilms tumor in Swedish and North American studies (Lindblad et al. 1992; Daniels et al. 2008). Maternal medical radiation during pregnancy was not associated with an elevated risk (Goel et al. 2009).

1.6 Birth Characteristics

Birth weight has been extensively studied as a risk factor for Wilms tumor. Birth weight was obtained from birth records or was self-reported by the mother. Low birth weight (<2,500 or 3,000 g) was not associated with an elevated risk in three studies (Olshan et al. 1993; Schüz et al. 2001; Puumala et al. 2008), although a North American study reported a weakly increased risk (OR = 1.3) for birth weight less than 2,500 g (Daniels et al. 2008). A recent analysis of linked birth and cancer files showed no elevated risk for low birth weight and Wilms tumor (Spector et al. 2009). High birth weight (>3,500 g or 4,000 g) was consistently associated with an increased risk (ORs = 1.3–5.1), with the more precise odds ratios from the larger studies ranging from 1.3 to 2.0 (Yeazel et al. 1997; Schüz and Forman 2007; Puumala et al. 2008; Daniels et al. 2008). In most studies that stratified by age at diagnosis, a stronger association was seen for high birth weight among children diagnosed at 2 years of age or older than for children diagnosed at less than 2 years of age. Analyses from the NWTS found that patients whose tumors had perilobar nephrogenic rests were heavier at birth (Breslow et al. 2006). This result was replicated in a North American case-control study in which the association for high birth weight was present only among children with perilobar nephrogenic rests (OR = 2.1) (Daniels et al. 2008).

Several studies reported an increased risk of Wilms tumor (ORs from 1.2 to 2.1) for births that had gestational lengths less than 37 weeks (Jepsen et al. 2004; Tsai et al. 2006; Daniels et al. 2008; Puumala et al. 2008). Birth order was inversely and weakly associated with the risk of Wilms tumor in several studies (Schüz et al. 2001; Daniels et al. 2008; Puumala et al. 2008; Laurvick et al. 2008). The analysis of more than 2,000 patients registered with the NWTS (Olson et al. 1993) found elevated incidence ratios for both increasing maternal and paternal age. Other studies have reported an association with a younger maternal age at birth (Schüz et al. 2001; Puumala et al. 2008) or with older maternal age (Tsai et al. 2006), or no association (Mogren et al. 1999; Sharpe et al. 1999; Yip et al. 2006).

Breastfeeding has been examined in a few case-control studies and in general no association was reported (Smulevich et al. 1999; Hardell and Dreifaldt 2001), although the large North American study reported that breastfeeding was associated with a 30 % reduced risk (Saddlemire et al. 2006).

1.7 Occupational and Environmental Exposures

Parental occupation, analysed by either job or industry classification or inferred exposure, has been examined as a risk factor in a series of epidemiologic studies since the 1970s (Kantor et al. 1979; Wilkins and Sinks 1984a, b; Bunin et al. 1989; Olshan et al. 1990; Sharpe et al. 1995; Fear et al. 1998, 2009).

When considering specific paternal occupations or occupational groups, associations have been reported including vehicle mechanics, auto body repairmen and welders (Olshan et al. 1990). Studies have reported an increased risk of Wilms tumor associated with paternal employment in occupations considered to have hydrocarbon or metal exposures (Kantor et al. 1979; Bunin et al. 1989), although other studies have not supported these findings (Fear et al. 2009). Studies have observed an increased risk with paternal occupational exposure to pesticides (Sharpe et al. 1995; Kristensen et al. 1996), although other studies have not reported similar findings (Schüz et al. 2001; Flower et al. 2004; Fear et al. 2009). A recent analysis of birth registration data for cases ($n=2{,}568$) from the NRCT and matched controls from the general population of Great Britain failed to replicate previous associations for paternal occupational exposure groups and Wilms tumor (Fear et al. 2009).

Fewer associations have been found for maternal occupational exposures. Bunin et al. (1989) reported associations with job clusters including hairdressers, electronic and clothing manufacturing workers, laboratory workers and dental assistants. This study also reported an association with personal hair dye use (Bunin et al. 1987). Other studies have not supported the association with hair dye use or maternal occupation as a hairdresser (Olshan et al. 1993; Tsai et al. 2006).

Maternal residential pesticide exposure before or during pregnancy has been found to have an elevated risk (ORs from 1.30 to 3.0) of Wilms tumor in offspring in multiple studies (Sharpe et al. 1995; Schüz et al. 2001; Tsai et al. 2006; Cooney et al. 2007). A geographic study in Texas failed to find an association between agricultural pesticide use and risk of Wilms tumor (Carozza et al. 2009).

1.8 Methodologic Issues and Future Studies

The epidemiologic evidence for an association between an array of lifestyle, environmental and other factors and the risk of Wilms tumor remains uncertain. There are multiple explanations for this lack of clarity. The epidemiologic approach to delineating the aetiology of Wilms tumor and other childhood cancers faces several challenges. The relative rarity of these diseases coupled with the potential biases owing to confounding, selection, and exposure misclassification are significant barriers to obtaining precise and valid estimates of an exposure effect. The rarity of Wilms tumor has meant that the case-control design is preferable (in most situations a comprehensive prospective cohort study is not possible). Most previous case-control studies with new data-collection components (e.g. maternal interview) have had a relatively limited sample size (<500 cases), too small to allow precise estimation of effects for less common exposures (e.g., individual medications) and interactions. A critical limitation is the measurement of exposure. Studies often have relied on maternal self-report, which is adequate for some factors but not for others, especially if the interview is many years after pregnancy. The additional motivation of case parents may also introduce some differential recall (recall bias) compared to mothers of usually healthy control children. The choice of control groups can be problematic with concerns about representativeness, adequate response rates and selection bias.

Some studies have overcome some of these challenges, for example, national registry linkage studies in Scandinavia, the United States, and Great Britain. These studies have been very helpful for commonly recorded demographic or other factors but often do not include sufficient information on other exposures of interest.

With these challenges in mind, future study designs will have to be creative and opportunistic. Studies with a linkage to clinical trials, such as the NWTS, with its routine collection of biologic data, may be informative especially when examining risks among biologic subgroups. For example, recent findings that nephrogenic rest type may define different aetiologic pathways may be a fruitful research avenue (Breslow et al. 2006). The ongoing determination of the molecular pathways for Wilms tumor may offer new markers for epidemiologic studies. The examination of the effect of common genetic variation (single nucleotide polymorphisms) and gene-exposure interaction can be more efficient through family-based designs (e.g., case-parent triads (Wilcox et al. 1998)) and affordable large-scale genotyping efforts. These designs do not require control groups, a particular challenge for past studies. Improvement in exposure measurement will be important, especially for complex environmental and other exposures. New methods such as the measurement of toxicants in newborn dried blood spots and other samples obtained during pregnancy or at birth may now be possible (Olshan 2007).

1.9 Survival

Wilms tumor, and renal tumors overall, have for several decades been among the childhood cancers with a relatively good prognosis. In Britain, five-year survival of children with renal cancer was 59 % for those diagnosed in 1971–1975 and 75 % for those diagnosed in 1976–1980 (Stiller 2007a). In recent population-based data from Europe and North America, 5-year survival has generally been over 85 % for Wilms tumor and over 80 % for all renal tumors combined (Pastore et al. 2006; Stiller 2007a; Gatta et al. 2009; Horner et al. 2009). Survival was somewhat lower in Japan until recently; in the Osaka Cancer Registry, five-year survival from childhood renal tumors diagnosed during 1985–1994 was 75 %, compared with 84 % in Britain and 90 % in the United States during similar periods (Ajiki et al. 2004). This was almost certainly due to poor outcome for children with stage III or IV disease, but population-based survival should have risen considerably since 1996 with the success of the first Japan Wilms Tumor Study (Oue et al. 2009). Recent population-based 5-year survival rates for renal clear cell sarcoma in Europe have been slightly lower than for Wilms tumor, around 65–75 % (Pastore et al. 2006; Stiller 2007a). Rhabdoid renal tumor still has a very poor prognosis, with 5-year survival of 20–25 % (Pastore et al. 2006; Stiller 2007a).

Population-based survival data for childhood cancer are seldom available from lower-income countries. For renal tumors, as for other diagnostic groups, survival has tended to be lower than in western industrialised countries. In Cuba, the 5-year survival for renal tumors diagnosed in 1988–1989 was 62 % (Boschmonar et al. 2000). In Bangalore, India, 5-year survival for Wilms tumor in 1982–1989 was only 27 % (Nandakumar et al. 1996). Treatment can have a high success rate in specialist centres in developing countries, but overall survival is adversely affected by abandonment of therapy. For example, in a paediatric oncology department in Morocco, the 5-year overall survival of evaluable patients with Wilms tumor was 79 % and the corresponding event-free survival was 77 %, but event-free survival fell to 56 % if abandonment was included as an event (Madani et al. 2006).

As a result of high, and increasing, survival rates throughout several decades, there are now substantial numbers of long-term survivors of childhood renal tumors, especially Wilms tumor, in the general population. At the end of 2005, there were estimated to be more than 2,000 5-year survivors of childhood renal tumors alive in Great Britain, of whom well over 1,000 were adults (Stiller 2007a). At the beginning of 2005, there were estimated to be about 12,450 people aged 20 years and over in the United States who had been diagnosed with renal cancer in the first 20 years of life, of whom about 6,950 had been diagnosed more than 30 years earlier (Mariotto et al. 2009). Despite this success, survivors are at increased risk of morbidity and mortality from a range of causes. Chap. 13 deals with long-term survival and late effects from a clinical viewpoint. Here we review the main epidemiological features.

Overall, 5-year survivors in the NWTS who were originally diagnosed with a renal tumor during 1969–1995 had an almost 13-fold higher risk of death between 5 and 10 years after diagnosis compared with the general population, and the excess risk was still three- to fourfold at 10–25 years after diagnosis (Cotton et al. 2009). Of the 153 deaths of known cause occurring more than 5 years after diagnosis, 42 % were due to the original disease, 41 % to late effects and 18 % to nontreatment-related causes (Cotton et al. 2009). The percentages of these three categories among 42 deaths of 5-year survivors of Wilms tumor diagnosed in Britain during 1940–1985 were broadly similar (Hawkins et al. 1990; Robertson et al. 1994), as were those among 30 deaths of 5-year survivors of childhood renal cancer diagnosed in the Nordic countries during 1960–1989 (Möller et al. 2001).

As with other childhood cancers, one of the most serious sequelae of Wilms tumor is development of a subsequent primary neoplasm. The largest study to date of subsequent malignancies after Wilms tumor was based on a combined cohort of 13,351 patients diagnosed between 1960 and 2004 from the NWTS and the Childhood Cancer Survivor Study (CCSS) in North America and the population-based national registries of Great Britain and the Nordic countries (Breslow et al. 2010). The standardised incidence ratio (SIR) for leukaemia was 5.0. The leukaemias were predominantly acute myeloid leukaemia and myelodysplasia, and the risk was highest in the first 5 years after diagnosis of Wilms tumor. The SIR for solid tumors other than skin carcinoma was 5.1, with a cumulative incidence of 6.7 % by age 40 in those patients who had survived free of second malignancy to age 15. The most common primary sites for solid tumors were digestive organs, breast, thyroid, bone and CNS. CNS tumors tended to develop in the first decade following diagnosis of Wilms tumor, thyroid and bone tumors in the second decade and cancers of digestive organs and breast in the second decade onwards. The SIR for solid tumors was fairly constant with time since Wilms tumor diagnosis, but absolute risk increased with length of follow-up and attained age. Occurrence of a subsequent malignancy had a severe effect on survival. Two thirds of patients who developed leukaemia have died, with median time to death of 10 months from diagnosis of leukaemia. Age-specific mortality was increased 15-fold for subjects who developed a solid second malignancy. Risk of leukaemia was highest in the most recently diagnosed patients, whereas the risk of solid tumor decreased for more recent decades of Wilms tumor diagnosis. These patterns were consistent with increased use of potentially leukaemogenic chemotherapy and decreased use of radiotherapy in more recent treatment protocols for Wilms tumor. Skin carcinomas were excluded from this study and from many other studies of second malignancies because of difficulties in ascertainment and in calculating expected numbers, and because these tumors usually have an excellent prognosis. In the British Childhood Cancer Survivor Study (BCCSS), the cumulative incidence of skin carcinomas, all of which were basal cell carcinomas, following Wilms tumor was 6 % by age 50.

In the NWTS, the principal late effects that were causes of death among 5-year survivors were subsequent malignancies, cardiac (cardiomyopathy and congestive heart disease) and end-stage renal disease (Cotton et al. 2009). In the CCSS, cause-specific standardised mortality ratios (SMR) for deaths among 5-year survivors of renal tumors were 16.4 for subsequent malignancy and 12.7 for cardiac causes (Mertens et al. 2008); the SMR for cardiac causes was the highest for survivors of any type of cancer.

As is the case with childhood cancer in general, survivors of childhood renal tumors are also liable to a range of other predominantly nonlethal late effects. These are reviewed in detail in Chap. 13.

References

Ajiki W, Tsukuma H, Oshima A (2004) Survival rates of childhood cancer patients in Osaka, Japan. Jpn J Clin Oncol 34:50–54

Au KS, Williams AT, Roach ES, Batchelor L, Sparagana SP, Delgado MR, Wheless JW, Baumgartner JE, Roa BB, Wilson CM, Smith-Knuppel TK, Cheung MY,

Whittemore VH, King TM, Northrup H (2007) Genotype/phenotype correlation in 325 individuals referred for a diagnosis of tuberous sclerosis complex in the United States. Genet Med 9:88–100

Bernstein L, Linet M, Smith MA, Olshan AF (1999) Renal tumors. In: Gloeckler Ries LA, Smith MA, Gurney JG, Linet M, Tamra T, Young JL, Bunin GR (eds) Cancer incidence and survival among children and adolescents: United States SEER program 1975–1995. NIH Pub No 99–4649, Bethesda, pp 79–90

Biegel JA (2006) Molecular genetics of atypical teratoid/rhabdoid tumors. Neurosurg Focus 20:E11

Biegel JA, Zhou J-Y, Rorke LB, Stenstrom C, Wainwright LM, Fogelgren B (1999) Germ-line and acquired mutations of *INI1* in atypical teratoid and rhabdoid tumors. Cancer Res 59:74–79

Birch JM, Alston RD, Quinn M, Kelsey AM (2003) Incidence of malignant disease by morphological type, in young persons aged 12–24 years in England, 1979–1997. Eur J Cancer 39:2622–2631

Bjørge T, Cnattingius S, Lie RT, Tretli S, Engeland A (2008) Cancer risk in children with birth defects and in their families: a population based cohort study of 5.2 million children from Norway and Sweden. Cancer Epidemiol Biomarkers Prev 17:500–506

Blakely ML, Shamberger RC, Norkool P, Beckwith JB, Green DM, Ritchey ML, from the National Wilms' Tumor Study Group (2003) Outcome of children with cystic partially differentiated nephroblastoma treated with or without chemotherapy. J Pediatr Surg 38:897–900

Boman F, Hill DA, Williams GM, Chauvenet A, Fournet J-C, Bouron-Dal Soglio D, Messinger Y, Priest JR (2006) Familial association of pleuropulmonary blastoma with cystic nephroma and other renal tumors: a report from the International Pleuropulmonary Blastoma Registry. J Pediatr 149:850–854

Boschmonar MG, Alvarez YG, García AM, Soto TN, Roger MC, Garrote LF (2000) Childhood cancer survival in Cuba. Eur J Epidemiol 16:763–767

Breslow N, Olshan A, Beckwith JB, Moksness J, Feigl P, Green D (1994) Ethnic variation in the incidence, diagnosis, prognosis, and follow-up of children with Wilms' tumor. J Natl Cancer Inst 86:49–51

Breslow NE, Takashima JR, Ritchey ML, Strong LC, Green DM (2000) Renal failure in the Denys-Drash and Wilms' tumor-aniridia syndromes. Cancer Res 60:4030–4032

Breslow NE, Norris R, Norkool PA, Kang T, Beckwith JB, Perlman EJ, Ritchey ML, Green DM, Nichols KE, National Wilms Tumor Study Group (2003) Characteristics and outcomes of children with the Wilms tumor-Aniridia syndrome: a report from the National Wilms Tumor Study Group. J Clin Oncol 21:4579–4585

Breslow NE, Beckwith JB, Perlman EJ, Reeve AE (2006) Age distributions, birth weights, nephrogenic rests, and heterogeneity in the pathogenesis of Wilms tumor. Pediatr Blood Cancer 47:260–267

Breslow NE, Lange JM, Friedman DL, Green DM, Hawkins MM, Murphy MFG, Neglia JP, Olsen JH, Peterson SM, Stiller CA, Robison LL (2010) Secondary malignant neoplasms following Wilms Tumor: an International Collaborative Study. Int J Cancer 127:657–666

Bunin GR, Kramer S, Marrero O, Meadows AT (1987) Gestational risk factors for Wilms' tumor: results of a case-control study. Cancer Res 47:2972–2977

Bunin GR, Nass CC, Kramer S, Meadows AT (1989) Parental occupation and Wilms' tumor: results of a case-control study. Cancer Res 49:725–729

Carozza SE, Li B, Wang Q, Horel S, Cooper S (2009) Agricultural pesticides and risk of childhood cancers. Int J Hyg Environ Health 212:186–195

Cooney MA, Daniels JL, Ross JA, Breslow NE, Pollock BH, Olshan AF (2007) Household pesticides and the risk of Wilms tumor. Environ Health Perspect 115:134–137

Coppes MJ, Haber DA, Grundy PE (1994) Genetic events in the development of Wilms' tumor. N Engl J Med 331:586–590

Cotton CA, Peterson S, Norkool PA, Takashima J, Grigoriev Y, Breslow NE (2009) Early and late mortality after diagnosis of wilms tumor. J Clin Oncol 27:1304–1309

Crino PB, Nathanson KL, Henske EP (2006) The tuberous sclerosis complex. N Engl J Med 355:1345–1356

Cummins C, Winter H, Maric R, Cheng KK, Silcocks P, Varghese C, Batlle G (2001) Childhood cancer in the south Asian population of England (1990–1992). Br J Cancer 84:1215–1218

Daniels JL, Pan I-J, Olshan AF, Breslow NE, Bunin GR, Ross JA (2008) Obstetric history and birth characteristics and Wilms tumor: a report from the Children's Oncology Group. Cancer Causes Control 19:1103–1110

Ducore JM, Parikh-Patel A, Gold EB (2004) Cancer occurrence in Southeast Asian children in California. J Pediatr Hematol Oncol 26:613–618

Fear NT, Roman E, Reeves G, Pannett B (1998) Childhood cancer and paternal employment in agriculture: the role of pesticides. Br J Cancer 77:825–829

Fear NT, Vincent TJ, King JC, MacCarthy A, Bunch KJ, Murphy MFG (2009) Wilms tumour and paternal occupation: an analysis of data from the national registry of childhood tumours. Pediatr Blood Cancer 53:28–32

Felgenhauer JL, Barce JM, Benson RL, Nan B, Olson JM, Breslow NE (2001) No excess of early onset cancer in family members of Wilms tumor patients. Cancer 92:1606–1612

Flower KB, Hoppin JA, Lynch CF, Blair A, Knott C, Shore DL, Sandler DP (2004) Cancer risk and parental pesticide application in children of Agricultural Health Study participants. Environ Health Perspect 112:631–635

Fukuzawa R, Breslow NE, Morison IM, Dwyer P, Kusafuka T, Kobayashi Y, Becroft DM, Beckwith JB, Perlman EJ, Reeve AE (2004) Epigenetic differences between Wilms' tumours in white and east-Asian children. Lancet 363:446–451

Furtwaengler R, Reinhard H, Leuschner I, Schenk JP, Goebel U, Claviez A, Kulozik A, Zoubek A, von Schweinitz D, Graf N, and the Gesellschaft fur Pädiatrische Onkologie und Hämatologie (GPOH) Nephroblastoma Study Group (2006) Mesoblastic nephroma–a report from the Gesellschaft fur Pädiatrische Onkologie und Hämatologie (GPOH). Cancer 106:2275–2283

Gatta G, Zigon G, Capocaccia R, Coebergh JW, Desandes E, Kaatsch P, Pastore G, Peris-Bonet R, Stiller CA, the Eurocare Working Group (2009) Survival of European children and young adults with cancer diagnosed 1995–2002. Eur J Cancer 45:992–1005

Goel R, Olshan AF, Ross JA, Breslow NE, Pollock BH (2009) Maternal exposure to medical radiation and Wilms tumor in the offspring: a report from the Children's Oncology Group. Cancer Causes Control 20:957–963

Goodman MT, Yoshizawa CN, Kolonel LN (1989) Ethnic patterns of childhood cancer in Hawaii between 1960 and 1984. Cancer 64:1758–1763

Grønskov K, Olsen JH, Sand A, Pedersen W, Carlsen N, Jylling AMB, Lyngbye T, Brøndum-Nielson K, Rosenberg T (2001) Population-based risk estimates of Wilms tumor in sporadic aniridia: a comprehensive mutation screening procedure of PAX6 identifies 80 % of mutations in aniridia. Hum Genet 109:11–19

Hardell L, Dreifaldt AC (2001) Breast-feeding duration and the risk of malignant diseases in childhood in Sweden. Eur J Clin Nutr 55:179–185

Hasle H, Olsen JH, Nielsen J, Hansen J, Friedrich U, Tommerup N (1996) Occurrence of cancer in women with Turner syndrome. Br J Cancer 73:1156–1159

Hawkins MM, Kingston JE, Kinnier Wilson LM (1990) Late deaths after treatment for childhood cancer. Arch Dis Child 65:1356–1363

Hemminki K, Mutanen P (2001) Parental cancer as a risk factor for nine common childhood malignancies. Br J Cancer 84:990–993

Hersh JH, Cole TR, Bloom AS, Bertolone SJ, Hughes HE (1992) Risk of malignancy in Sotos syndrome. J Pediatr 120:572–574

Horner MJ, Ries LAG, Krapcho M, Neyman N, Aminou R, Howlader N, Altekruse SF, Feuer EJ, Huang L, Mariotto A, Miller BA, Lewis DR, Eisner MP, Stinchcomb DG, Edwards BK (2009) SEER Cancer Statistics Review, 1975–2006. http://seer.cancer.gov/csr/1975_2006/. Based on November 2008 SEER data submission, posted to the SEER web site, 2009. 2009. National Cancer Institute, Bethesda

Howell CG, Othersen HB, Kiviat NE, Norkool P, Beckwith JB, D'Angio GJ (1982) Therapy and outcome in 51 children with mesoblastic nephroma: a report of the National Wilms' Tumor Study. J Pediatr Surg 17:826–831

Hoyme HE, Seaver LH, Jones KL, Procopio F, Crooks W, Feingold M (1998) Isolated hemihyperplasia (hemihypertrophy): report of a prospective multicenter study of the incidence of neoplasia and review. Am J Med Genet 79:274–278

Innis MD (1972) Nephroblastoma: possible index cancer of childhood. Med J Aust 1:18–20

Jepsen P, Olsen ML, Mellemkjaer L, Olsen JH, Sorensen HT (2004) A registry-based study of gender, fetal growth, and risk of Wilms tumor. Pediatr Hematol Oncol 21:435–439

Kantor AF, McCrea Curnen MG, Wister Meigs J, Flannery JT (1979) Occupations of fathers of patients with Wilms' tumour. J Epidemiol Community Health 33:253–256

Kristensen P, Andersen A, Irgens LM, Bye AS, Sundheim L (1996) Cancer in offspring of parents engaged in agricultural activities in Norway: incidence and risk factors in the farm environment. Int J Cancer 65:39–50

Laurvick CL, Milne E, Blair E, de Klerk N, Charles AK, Bower C (2008) Fetal growth and the risk of childhood non-CNS solid tumours in Western Australia. Br J Cancer 99:179–181

Linabery AM, Ross JA (2008) Trends in childhood cancer incidence in the U.S. (1992–2004). Cancer 112:416–432

Lindblad P, Zack M, Adami H-O, Ericson A (1992) Maternal and perinatal risk factors for Wilms' tumor: a nationwide nested case-control study in Sweden. Int J Cancer 51:38–41

Little SE, Hanks SP, King-Underwood L, Jones C, Rapley EA, Rahman N, Pritchard-Jones K (2004) Frequency and heritability of *WT1* mutations in nonsyndromic Wilms' tumor patients: a UK Children's Cancer Study Group Study. J Clin Oncol 22:4140–4146

Madani A, Zafad S, Harif M, Yaakoubi M, Zamiati S, Sahraoui S, Benjelloun A, Fehri M, Benchekroun S (2006) Treatment of Wilms tumor according to SIOP 9 protocol in Casablanca, Morocco. Pediatr Blood Cancer 46:472–475

Mariotto AB, Rowland JH, Yabroff KR, Scoppa S, Hachey M, Ries L, Feuer EJ (2009) Long-term survivors of childhood cancers in the United States. Cancer Epidemiol Biomarkers Prev 18:1033–1040

McKinney PA, Stiller CA (1986) Maternal smoking during pregnancy and the risk of childhood cancer. Lancet 2:519–520

Merks JHM, Smets AM, Van Rijn RR, Kobes J, Caron HN, Maas M, Hennekam RCM (2005) Prevalence of RIB anomalies in normal Caucasian children and childhood cancer patients. Eur J Med Genet 48:113–129

Mertens AC, Liu Q, Neglia JP, Wasilewski K, Leisenring W, Armstrong GT, Robison LL, Yasui Y (2008) Cause-specific late mortality among 5-year survivors of childhood cancer: the Childhood Cancer Survivor Study. J Natl Cancer Inst 100:1368–1379

Mishra K, Mathur M, Logani KB, Kakkar N, Krishna A (1998) Precursor lesions of Wilms' tumor in Indian children A multiinstitutional study. Cancer 83:2228–2232

Mogren I, Damber L, Tavelin B, Högberg U (1999) Characteristics of pregnancy and birth and malignancy in the offspring (Sweden). Cancer Causes Control 10:85–94

Möller TR, Garwicz S, Barlow L, Falck Winther J, Glattre E, Olafsdottir G, Olsen JH, Perfekt R, Ritvanen A,

Sankila R, Tulinius H (2001) Decreasing late mortality among five-year survivors of cancer in childhood and adolescence: a population-based study in the Nordic countries. J Clin Oncol 19:3173–3181

Moutou C, Hochez J, Chompret A, Tournade M-F, Le Bihan C, Zucker J-M, Lemerle J, Bonaïti-Pellié C (1994) The French Wilms' tumour study: no clear evidence for cancer prone families. J Med Genet 31:429–434

Muto R, Yamamori S, Ohashi H, Osawa M (2002) Prediction by FISH analysis of the occurrence of Wilms tumor in aniridia patients. Am J Med Genet 108:285–289

Nandakumar A, Anantha N, Appaji L, Swamy K, Mukherjee G, Venugopal T, Reddy S, Dhar M (1996) Descriptive epidemiology of childhood cancers in Bangalore, India. Cancer Causes Control 7:405–410

Narchi H (2005) Risk of Wilms' tumour with multicystic kidney disease: a systematic review. Arch Dis Child 90:147–149

Neville H, Ritchey ML, Shamberger RC, Haase G, Perlman S, Yoshioka T (2002) The occurrence of Wilms tumor in horseshoe kidneys: a report from the National Wilms Tumor Study Group (NWTSG). J Pediatr Surg 37:1134–1137

Ng A, Griffiths A, Cole T, Davison V, Griffiths M, Larkin S, Parkes SE, Mann JR, Grundy RG (2007) Congenital abnormalities and clinical features associated with Wilms' tumour: a comprehensive study from a centre serving a large population. Eur J Cancer 43:1422–1429

Olsen JH, Boice JD, Seersholm N, Bautz A, Fraumeni JF (1995) Cancer in the parents of children with cancer. N Engl J Med 333:1594–1599

Olshan AF (2007) Meeting report: the use of newborn blood spots in environmental research: opportunities and challenges. Environ Health Perspect 115:1767–1779

Olshan AF, Breslow NE, Daling JR, Falletta JM, Grufferman S, Robison LL, Waskerwitz M, Hammond GD (1990) Wilms' tumor and paternal occupation. Cancer Res 50:3212–3217

Olshan AF, Breslow NE, Falletta JM, Grufferman S, Pendergrass PHT, Robison LL, Waskerwitz M, Woods WG, Vietti TJ, Hammond GD (1993) Risk factors for Wilms tumor. Report from the National Wilms Tumor Study. Cancer 72:938–944

Olson JM, Breslow NE, Beckwith JB (1993) Wilms' tumour and parental age: a report from the National Wilms' Tumour Study. Br J Cancer 67:813–818

Olson JM, Hamilton A, Breslow NE (1995) Non-11p constitutional chromosome abnormalities in Wilms' tumor patients. Med Pediatr Oncol 24:305–309

Ong KR, Woodward ER, Killick P, Lim C, Macdonald F, Maher ER (2007) Genotype-phenotype correlations in von Hippel-Lindau disease. Hum Mutat 28:143–149

Oue T, Fukuzawa M, Okita H, Mugishima H, Horie H, Hata J, Saito M, Nozaki M, Chin M, Nakadate H, Hinotsu S, Koshinaga T, Kaneko Y, Kitano Y, Tanaka Y, Japan Wilms Tumor Study (JWiTS) Group (2009) Outcome of pediatric renal tumor treated using the Japan Wilms Tumor Study-1 (JWiTS-1) protocol: a report from the JWiTS group. Pediatr Surg Int 25:923–929

Pang D, McNally R, Birch JM, on behalf of the UK Childhood Cancer Study Investigators (2003) Parental smoking and childhood cancer: results from the United Kingdom Childhood Cancer Study. Br J Cancer 88:373–381

Parkin DM, Kramárová E, Draper GJ, Masuyer E, Michaelis J, Neglia J, Qureshi S, Stiller CA, Kramárová E, Draper GJ (1998) International incidence of childhood cancer, vol 2. IARC Scientific Publications, No 144. International Agency for Research on Cancer, Lyon

Parkin DM, Ferlay J, Hamdi-Chérif M, Sitas F, Thomas JO, Wabinga H, Whelan SL (2003) Cancer in Africa: epidemiology and prevention. IARC Press, Lyon

Pastore G, Znaor A, Spreafico F, Graf N, Pritchard-Jones K, Steliarova-Foucher E (2006) Malignant renal tumours incidence and survival in European children (1978–1997): report from the Automated Childhood Cancer Information System project. Eur J Cancer 42:2103–2114

Pearce MS, Parker L (2001) Childhood cancer registrations in the developing world: still more boys than girls. Int J Cancer 91:402–406

Porteus MH, Narkool P, Neuberg D, Guthrie K, Breslow N, Green DM, Diller L (2000) Characteristics and outcome of children with Beckwith-Wiedemann syndrome and Wilms' tumor: a report from the National Wilms Tumor Study Group. J Clin Oncol 18:2026–2031

Puumala SE, Soler JT, Johnson KJ, Spector LG (2008) Birth characteristics and Wilms tumor in Minnesota. Int J Cancer 122:1368–1373

Rapley EA, Barfoot R, Bonaïti-Pellié C, Chompret A, Foulkes W, Perusinghe N, Reeve A, Royer-Pokora B, Schumacher V, Shelling A, Skeen J, de Toureil S, Weirich A, Pritchard-Jones K, Stratton MR, Rahman N (2000) Evidence for susceptibility genes to familial Wilms tumour in addition to *WT1*, *FWT1* and *FWT2*. Br J Cancer 83:177–183

Robertson CM, Hawkins MM, Kingston JE (1994) Late deaths and survival after childhood cancer: implications for cure. BMJ 309:162–166

Rodriguez-Galindo C, Marina NM, Fletcher BD, Parham DM, Bodner SM, Meyer WH (1997) Is primitive neuroectodermal tumor of the kidney a distinct entity? Cancer 79:2243–2250

Saddlemire S, Olshan AF, Daniels JL, Breslow NE, Bunin GR, Ross JA (2006) Breast-feeding and Wilms tumor: a report from the Children's Oncology Group. Cancer Causes Control 17:687–693

Schüz J, Forman MR (2007) Birthweight by gestational age and childhood cancer. Cancer Causes Control 18:655–663

Schüz J, Kaletsch U, Meinert R, Kaatsch P, Michaelis J (2001) High-birth weight and other risk factors for Wilms' tumour: results of a population-based case-control study. Eur J Pediatr 160:333–338

Scott RH, Stiller CA, Walker L, Rahman N (2006) Syndromes and constitutional chromosomal abnormalities associated with Wilms tumour. J Med Genet 43:705–715

Scott RH, Douglas J, Baskcomb L, Huxter N, Barker K, Hanks S, Craft A, Gerrard M, Kohler JA, Levitt GA, Picton S, Pizer B, Ronghe MD, Williams D, Factors Associated with Childhood Tumours (FACT) Collaboration, Cook JA, Pujol P, Maher ER, Birch JM, Stiller CA, Pritchard-Jones K, Rahman N (2008) Constitutional 11p15 abnormalities, including heritable imprinting center mutations, cause nonsyndromic Wilms tumor. Nat Genet 40:1329–1334

Selle B, Furtwängler R, Graf N, Kaatsch P, Bruder E, Leuschner I (2007) Population-based study of renal cell carcinoma in children in Germany, 1980–2005. More frequently localized tumors and underlying disorders compared with adult counterparts. Cancer 107:2906–2914

Sharpe CR, Franco EL (1996) Use of Dipyrone during pregnancy and risk of Wilms' tumor. Epidemiology 7:533–535

Sharpe CR, Franco EL, De Camargo B, Lopes LF, Barreto JH, Johnsson RR, Mauad MA (1995) Parental exposure to pesticides and risk of Wilms' tumor in Brazil. Am J Epidemiol 141:210–217

Sharpe CR, Franco EL, De Camargo B, Lopes LF, Barreto J, Johnsson R, Mauad M (1999) The influence of parental age on the risk of Wilm's tumour. Paediatr Perinat Epidemiol 13:138–143

Smulevich VB, Solionova LG, Belyakova SV (1999) Parental occupation and other factors and cancer risk in children: II Occupational factors. Int J Cancer 83:718–722

Spector LG, Puumala SE, Carozza SE, Chow EJ, Fox EE, Horel S, Johnson KJ, McLaughlin CC, Reynolds P, Von Behren J, Mueller BA (2009) Cancer risk among children with very low birth weights. Pediatrics 124:96–104

Steliarova-Foucher E, Stiller C, Lacour B, Kaatsch P (2005) International classification of childhood cancer, third edition. Cancer 103:1457–1467

Stiller C (2007a) Childhood cancer in Britain: incidence, survival, mortality. Oxford University Press, Oxford

Stiller CA (2007b) International patterns of cancer incidence in adolescents. Cancer Treat Rev 33:631–645

Stiller CA (2008) Epidemiology of childhood tumours. In: Carachi R, Grosfeld JL, Azmy AF (eds) The surgery of childhood tumours. Springer, Heidelberg

Stiller CA, Parkin DM (1990) International variations in the incidence of childhood renal tumours. Br J Cancer 62:1026–1030

Stiller CA, McKinney PA, Bunch KJ, Bailey CC, Lewis IJ (1991) Childhood cancer and ethnic group in Britain: a United Kingdom Children's Cancer Study Group (UKCCSG) study. Br J Cancer 64:543–548

Stiller CA, Desandes E, Danon SE, Izarzugaza I, Ratiu A, Vassileva-Valerinova Z, Steliarova-Foucher E (2006) Cancer incidence and survival in European adolescents (1978–1997). Report from the Automated Childhood Cancer Information System project. Eur J Cancer 42:2006–2018

Stjernfeldt M, Berglund K, Lindsten J, Ludvigsson J (1986) Maternal smoking during pregnancy and risk of childhood cancer. Lancet 1:1350–1352

Swartz MA, Karth J, Schneider DT, Rodriguez R, Beckwith JB, Perlman EJ (2002) Renal medullary carcinoma: clinical, pathologic, immunohistochemical, and genetic analysis with pathogenetic implications. Urology 60:1083–1089

Swerdlow AJ, Hermon C, Jacobs PA, Alberman E, Beral V, Daker M, Fordyce A, Youings S (2001) Mortality and cancer incidence in persons with numerical sex chromosome abnormalities: a cohort study. Ann Hum Genet 65:177–188

Swerdlow AJ, Schoemaker MJ, Higgins CD, Wright AF, Jacobs PA, on behalf of the UK Clinical Cytogenetics Group (2008) Cancer risk in patients with constitutional chromosome deletions: a nationwide British cohort study. Br J Cancer 98:1929–1933

Tatton-Brown K, Douglas J, Coleman K, Baujat G, Cole TRP, Das S, Horn D, Hughes HE, Temple IK, Faravelli F, Waggoner D, Türkmen S, Cormier-Daire V, Irrthum A, Rahman N, for the Childhood Overgrowth Collaboration (2005) Genotype-phenotype associations in Sotos syndrome: an analysis of 266 individuals with *NSD1* aberrations. Am J Hum Genet 77:193–204

Tsai J, Kaye WE, Bove FJ (2006) Wilms' tumor and exposures to residential and occupational hazardous chemicals. Int J Hyg Environ Health 209:57–64

Wilcox AJ, Weinberg CR, Lie RT (1998) Distinguishing the effects of maternal and offspring genes through studies of "case-parent triads". Am J Epidemiol 148:893–901

Wilkins JR, Sinks TH (1984a) Occupational exposures among fathers of children with Wilms' tumor. J Occup Med 26:427–435

Wilkins JR, Sinks TH (1984b) Paternal occupation and Wilms' tumour in offspring. J Epidemiol Community Health 38:7–11

Yeazel MW, Ross JA, Buckley JD, Woods WG, Ruccione K, Robison LL (1997) High birth weight and risk of specific childhood cancers: a report from the Children's Cancer Group. J Pediatr 131:671–677

Yip BH, Pawitan Y, Czene K (2006) Parental age and risk of childhood cancers: a population-based cohort study from Sweden. Int J Epidemiol 35:1495–1503

2 Genetic Predisposition to Wilms Tumor

Richard H. Scott and Nazneen Rahman

Contents

R.H. Scott • N. Rahman (✉)
Section of Cancer Genetics, Institute of Cancer Research, 15 Cotswold Road, Sutton, Surrey SM2 5NG, UK
e-mail: ScottR3@gosh.nhs.uk; nazneen.rahman@icr.ac.uk

K. Pritchard-Jones, J.S. Dome (eds.), *Renal Tumors of Childhood: Biology and Therapy*, Pediatric Oncology, DOI 10.1007/978-3-662-44003-2_2, © Springer-Verlag Berlin Heidelberg 2014

Abstract

Wilms tumor is a primarily sporadic disease, with only 1–2 % of affected individuals having a relative with Wilms tumor. However, bilateral Wilms tumors occur in approximately 5 % of cases, and Wilms tumor has been reported in association with more than 50 different genetic disorders, pointing to an underlying predisposition in further individuals. There is conclusive evidence of an increased risk of Wilms tumor in only a small number of disorders, including familial Wilms tumor, the *WT1*-related syndromes, certain overgrowth disorders including Beckwith-Wiedemann syndrome and a small number of other cancer predisposition syndromes. The identification of the molecular defects that underlie these Wilms predisposition syndromes clarifies the risks of Wilms tumor risks and assists in the targeting of Wilms surveillance to those at increased risk. For example, in some disorders such as the 11p15-overgrowth disorders, it has emerged that only a subset of individuals are at increased risk of Wilms tumor. The discovery of further Wilms predisposition alleles is set to continue and will improve our ability to identify and manage those at increased risk of Wilms tumor.

2.1 Introduction

Wilms tumor is primarily a sporadic disease with only 1–2 % of individuals with the tumor having a relative with Wilms tumor (Breslow et al. 1996). However, a number of strands of evidence indicate that underlying constitutional predisposition accounts for a substantial proportion of cases.

Firstly, Wilms tumors are frequently multifocal. Disease is bilateral in 5 % of cases and unilateral-multicentric in 10 % (Dinkel et al. 1988; Breslow et al. 1993; Ritchey et al. 2005). Precursor lesions – nephrogenic rests – are present in surrounding renal tissue in 40 % of cases (25 % perilobar; 15 % intralobar) (Beckwith et al. 1990).

Secondly, a wide range of syndromes, congenital anomalies and constitutional chromosome abnormalities have been reported in association with Wilms tumor (Scott et al. 2006a). Data from the British National Registry of Childhood Tumors showed that ~9 % of individuals with Wilms tumor have a congenital malformation and one study of long-term survivors of childhood cancer found a syndrome diagnosis in 23 of 136 (17 %) of those with Wilms tumor (Narod et al. 1997; Merks et al. 2005). This is the highest proportion seen in any malignancy. Conclusive evidence exists of an increased risk of Wilms tumor for only a minority of conditions reported in association with Wilms tumor (Table 2.1). In many of the other conditions reported, the rare co-occurrence of Wilms tumor is likely due to chance.

Identification of the underlying molecular basis of Wilms predisposition has furthered understanding of Wilms tumor predisposition. In some syndromes, for example, those caused by 11p15 abnormalities, evidence has emerged that an increased risk of Wilms tumor occurs only in a subset of individuals (Scott et al. 2006a; Gaston et al. 2001). In addition, it has emerged that some genetic defects originally identified in individuals with syndromic Wilms tumor also account for a proportion of cases with apparently sporadic isolated ('non-syndromic') disease, for example, 11p15 abnormalities and *WT1* mutations (Little et al. 2004; Scott et al. 2008).

The underlying cause of the large majority of Wilms tumors, including bilateral and familial cases, remains unexplained, and it is likely that further strongly predisposing genetic defects remain to be identified. It is also likely

Table 2.1 Conditions in which there is strong evidence of an increased risk of Wilms tumor

High risk (≥20 %)
Familial Wilms tumor
WT1 deletions (including WAGR syndrome)[a]
WT1 truncating mutations and pathogenic missense mutations (including Denys-Drash syndrome)
Perlman syndrome
Fanconi anaemia subtype D1 (biallelic *BRCA2* mutations) and subtype N (biallelic *PALB2* mutations)
Mosaic variegated aneuploidy
Moderate risk (5–20 %)
WT1 intron 9 splice mutations (Frasier syndrome)
11p15-overgrowth caused by *H19* DMR hypermethylation or paternal UPD 11p15[b]
Beckwith-Wiedemann syndrome without an 11p15 defect
Simpson-Golabi-Behmel syndrome caused by *GPC3* deletions or mutations
Low risk (≤5 %)
Isolated hemihypertrophy without an 11p15 defect
Bloom syndrome
Li-Fraumeni syndrome and Li-Fraumeni-like syndrome
Mulibrey nanism
Hereditary hyperparathyroidism-jaw tumor syndrome
Trisomy 18
Trisomy 13
2q37 deletions

[a]WAGR syndrome, Wilms tumor-aniridia-genitourinary abnormalities-growth retardation syndrome

[b]11p15-overgrowth caused by *H19* DMR hypermethylation or paternal UPD 11p15 includes individuals with Beckwith-Wiedemann syndrome, isolated hemihypertrophy as well as other presentations such as non-syndromic Wilms tumor

that lower-penetrance predisposition alleles exist, such those that have been identified in neuroblastoma and a number of adult malignancies (Capasso et al. 2009).

2.2 Conditions with an Increased Risk of Wilms Tumor

2.2.1 Familial Wilms Tumor

At least 50 familial Wilms tumor pedigrees are known (N Rahman, unpublished observation). Most families manifest with non-syndromic disease, and the underlying cause of the majority remains unknown. A minority are caused by syndromes described in the subsequent sections: *WT1* mutations/deletions (four families), 11p15 defects (two families), mosaic variegated aneuploidy (two families) and biallelic *BRCA2* mutations (one family) (Scott et al. 2008; Yunis and Ramsay 1980; Pelletier et al. 1991; Kaplinsky et al. 1996; Zirn et al. 2005; Sparago et al. 2007; Hanks et al. 2004; Reid et al. 2007).

An autosomal dominant non-syndromic familial Wilms tumor gene, *FWT1*, has been mapped to 17q21 but has not yet been identified (Rahman et al. 1996, 1998). Wilms tumor in *FWT1*-linked families tends to be diagnosed at a later age and more advanced stage than sporadic Wilms tumor (median age at diagnosis 6 years). The penetrance of *FWT1* is only ~30 %, and the wild-type allele is not lost in tumors (Rahman et al. 1997). These features suggest that *FWT1* does not operate as a classical tumor suppressor gene.

A second autosomal dominant non-syndromic Wilms tumor predisposition gene, *FWT2*, has been proposed to lie at 19q13 (McDonald et al. 1998). The evidence favouring this locus is inconclusive as no single family with a LOD score >3 has been identified. Although combining the LOD score of five smaller families gave a score >3, families unlinked at 19q13 were excluded from the analysis.

Several families not linked to *FWT1*, *FWT2*, *WT1* or 11p15 exist, indicating that further genetic heterogeneity in familial Wilms tumor exists (Rapley et al. 2000). A small number of families have been reported which show predisposition to both Wilms tumor and neuroblastoma, another embryonal tumor (Abbaszadeh et al. 2010). The gene(s) causing this previously unrecognised cancer syndrome are currently unknown.

2.2.2 *WT1*-Associated Syndromes

Constitutional monoallelic (heterozygous) mutations or deletions in the *WT1* gene cause predisposition to Wilms tumor. The gene behaves as a classical tumor suppressor gene, and the wild-type allele is inactivated in tumors occurring in individuals with constitutional monoallelic mutations or deletions. The median age of Wilms tumor diagnosis in such individuals is younger than in unselected Wilms tumor case series (approximately 1 year in *WT1*-associated syndromes; 3–4 years in unselected Wilms cases). Tumors are more frequently bilateral (38 % in WT1-assiociated syndromes; 5 % in unselected Wilms cases), and intralobar nephrogenic rests (ILNRs) are more frequently present. The tumors often show stromal predominant histology (Royer-Pokora et al. 2004).

Constitutional *WT1* defects are associated with a range of overlapping phenotypes, manifesting various combinations of three features: Wilms tumor predisposition, genitourinary abnormalities and renal dysfunction. A number of genotype-phenotype correlations have emerged.

2.2.2.1 WAGR Syndrome

WAGR (Wilms tumor-aniridia-genitourinary abnormalities-mental retardation) syndrome is found in approximately 7–8 per 1,000 individuals with Wilms tumor (Breslow et al. 2003). It manifests with complete or partial aniridia, ambiguous external genitalia/cryptorchidism in males and intellectual impairment. Additionally, there is a high risk of renal failure, which affects ~40 % of individuals by the age of 20 years (Breslow et al. 2000). The condition is caused by monoallelic deletions at 11p13 encompassing the *WT1* and *PAX6* genes. Deletion of *WT1* results in Wilms tumor predisposition and deletion of *PAX6* results in aniridia (Muto et al. 2002). Approximately 30 % of individuals with aniridia harbour *WT1-PAX6* deletions. Many of the remainder harbour point mutations or intragenic deletions of *PAX6*. Individuals with isolated *PAX6* defects are not at increased risk of Wilms tumor. A number of individuals have been reported with deletions or chromosomal aberrations that delete *WT1* but not *PAX6* (Royer-Pokora et al. 1991; Baird et al. 1992). These manifest with Wilms tumor predisposition and genitourinary abnormalities but not aniridia.

2.2.2.2 Denys-Drash Syndrome

Denys-Drash syndrome classically describes the combination of Wilms tumor, nephropathy and genitourinary abnormalities in males that are severe enough to result in pseudohermaphroditism (Denys et al. 1967; Drash et al. 1970). The nephropathy is usually a characteristic mesangial sclerosis, presenting with hypertension and proteinuria and typically progressing to renal failure requiring renal replacement therapy prior to the age of 10 years (Eddy and Mauer 1985). Genitourinary abnormalities in XY individuals are very common but vary in severity from mild hypospadias to female genitalia with streak gonads. Some XX individuals have gonadal dysgenesis, but the majority have normal genitourinary development. Most individuals with classical Denys-Drash syndrome harbour de novo missense *WT1* mutations targeting critical residues in the zinc finger domains that are responsible for DNA binding of the WT1 protein. These mutations are thought to act in a dominant-negative manner to result in this more severe phenotype (Royer-Pokora et al. 2004).

2.2.2.3 Frasier Syndrome

Frasier syndrome is the association of nephropathy, gonadal dysgenesis and gonadoblastoma (Frasier et al. 1964). The nephropathy is typically a focal segmental glomerulosclerosis which progresses to renal failure by the second or third decade of life (Demmer et al. 1999). Genitourinary abnormalities in XY individuals are severe and sex reversal is common. The syndrome is caused by mutations in intron 9 of *WT1* that alter splicing and prevent formation of WT1 isoforms that normally include a linker of three amino acids (KTS) between the third and fourth zinc finger domains (Barbaux et al. 1997).

2.2.2.4 Non-syndromic Wilms Tumor and Other Presentations of *WT1* Mutations

WT1 mutations have also been reported in individuals with one or two of the three features of *WT1*-associated syndromes, for example, with Wilms tumor and cryptorchidism, with isolated ('non-syndromic') Wilms tumor or with isolated nephropathy (Kohler et al. 2001). These individuals are more likely to harbour intragenic truncating mutations than missense mutations in the zinc finger domains. Most germline *WT1* mutations are de novo, but rare families have been reported with *WT1* defects that have presented with familial Wilms tumor (Little et al. 2004; Yunis and Ramsay 1980; Pelletier et al. 1991; Kaplinsky et al. 1996; Zirn et al. 2005).

2.2.2.5 The Risk of Wilms Tumor with *WT1* Mutations

The risk of Wilms tumor in individuals with *WT1* deletions, truncating mutations or pathogenic missense mutations targeting the zinc finger domains is probably at least 50 % (Royer-Pokora et al. 2004; Muto et al. 2002). Missense variants outside the zinc finger domains may be rare non-pathogenic polymorphisms, and caution should be exercised in their interpretation, particularly if they are not de novo.

The risk of Wilms tumor in individuals with *WT1* intron 9 splice mutations (Frasier syndrome) is considerably lower than for other mutations. Only four of 66 individuals (6 %) reported with Frasier syndrome developed Wilms tumor (Coppes et al. 1993; Barbosa et al. 1999; Loirat et al. 2003). However, the risk of gonadoblastomas is high in Frasier syndrome, whereas these tumors are rare in individuals with other classes of *WT1* mutation.

2.2.3 Overgrowth Syndromes

Childhood overgrowth syndromes are a heterogeneous group of disorders characterised by pre- and/or postnatal overgrowth often in association with other abnormal phenotypic features. It has previously been assumed that a wide variety of overgrowth disorders predispose to cancer in childhood including Wilms tumor. In part, this may be because high birth weight has been identified as a possible risk factor for Wilms tumor in a number of mainly population-based studies (Leisenring et al. 1994; Heuch et al. 1996; Yeazel et al. 1997; Schuz et al. 2001; Jepsen et al. 2004). However, as understanding of specific overgrowth disorders has improved, it has emerged that only a small subset of overgrowth syndromes predispose to Wilms tumor. Wilms tumor risk of children with overgrowth should therefore be evaluated on the basis of the specific syndrome rather than a collective basis.

2.2.3.1 11p15-Overgrowth Including Beckwith-Wiedemann Syndrome and Hemihypertrophy

Growth-promoting constitutional epigenetic and genetic abnormalities at the imprinted 11p15 region cause a spectrum of overgrowth phenotypes (Scott et al. 2008; Weksberg et al. 2005). The classical 11p15-overgrowth phenotype is Beckwith-Wiedemann syndrome (Weksberg et al. 2005; Thorburn et al. 1970; Elliott and Maher 1994). It is characterised by pre- and postnatal overgrowth, macroglossia, anterior abdominal wall defects, ear lobe creases and posterior helical pits, neonatal hypoglycaemia and hemihypertrophy (growth asymmetry). Non-malignant renal tract abnormalities also occur, including nephromegaly, renal cysts, medullary sponge kidney, medullary dysplasia and hydronephrosis. The overall risk of childhood cancer associated with Beckwith-Wiedemann syndrome has been estimated to be 4–21 %. Wilms tumor is the most frequently occurring childhood tumor, reported in 1–8 % of individuals (Sotelo-Avila et al. 1980; Elliott et al. 1994; Wiedemann 1997; DeBaun and Tucker 1998; Goldman et al. 2002). Perilobar nephrogenic rests (60 %) and bilateral disease (17 %) are seen more frequently than in unselected Wilms series (15 and 5 % respectively) (Ritchey et al. 2005; Beckwith et al. 1990; Porteus et al. 2000). Approximately 75 % of individuals fulfilling diagnostic criteria for Beckwith-Wiedemann syndrome have an identifiable 11p15 defect (Weksberg et al. 2005).

A substantial proportion of individuals with 11p15 defects do not fulfil the diagnostic criteria of Beckwith-Wiedemann syndrome. These individuals typically manifest with more subtle physical phenotypes such as isolated hemihypertrophy (Merks et al. 2005; Martin et al. 2005; Shuman et al. 2006; Bliek et al. 2008). This is in keeping with the recognised association between isolated hemihypertrophy and Wilms tumor. A prospective study of 168 patients with isolated hemihypertrophy identified ten tumors in nine individuals including five with Wilms tumor (3 %) (Hoyme et al. 1998). It is notable that tumors occur at similar frequency in the larger and smaller kidney in asymmetric individuals. Approximately 20 % of individuals with hemihypertrophy have an identifiable 11p15 defect (Martin et al. 2005; Shuman et al. 2006; Bliek et al. 2008).

Constitutional 11p15 Defects Cause Non-syndromic Wilms Tumor

More recently, it has emerged that some individuals with constitutional 11p15 defects manifest with non-syndromic Wilms tumor. A study of 437 British children with non-syndromic Wilms tumor found 11p15 defects in 12 (3 %) (Scott et al. 2008). These individuals could not be reliably distinguished from unselected cases based on physical phenotypic or histological features. As with individuals with Beckwith-Wiedemann syndrome, bilateral disease was more frequent in this group.

The Risk of Wilms Tumor with Constitutional 11p15 Defects

The detailed exposition of the 11p15 region and these defects is beyond the scope of this chapter. Briefly, the 11p15 region contains a number growth-controlling genes that show imprinted (i.e. parent-of-origin-specific) expression at 11p15 (Weksberg et al. 2005; Rahman 2005). The genes are arranged in two independent domains (imprinted domain 1 and imprinted domain 2), each controlled by differential DNA methylation at an imprinting control region (the H19 DMR at domain 1 and KvDMR at domain 2).

A variety of epigenetic and genetic defects have been reported that disrupt the region to result in a net increase in the expression of growth-promoting genes. Isolated KvDMR hypomethylation is the commonest cause of Beckwith-Wiedemann syndrome, accounting for approximately 50 % of cases. Paternal uniparental disomy of 11p15, which results in KvDMR hypomethylation and *H19* DMR hypermethylation, is found in 20 % of cases. Isolated *H19* DMR hypermethylation is found in approximately 5 % of cases. Maternally inherited *CDKN1C* mutations are found in a further 5 % of Beckwith-Wiedemann syndrome cases. A small number of cases are caused by duplications 11p15. These include interstitial paternal duplications encompassing only the *IGF2*/*H19* locus, as well as larger duplications extending to the 11p telomere as part of an unbalanced reciprocal chromosome translocation (Weksberg et al. 2005; Russo et al. 2006; Algar et al. 2007).

A number of studies have revealed strong epigenotype-Wilms tumor risk correlations in 11p15-overgrowth disorders. Studies of large numbers of individuals with Beckwith-Wiedemann syndrome and individuals with hemihypertrophy have each found a strong association between defects that result in *H19* DMR hypermethylation and Wilms tumor risk (Merks et al. 2005; Gaston et al. 2001; Martin et al. 2005; Shuman et al. 2006; Bliek et al. 2008; Bliek et al. 2001, 2004; Weksberg et al. 2001; DeBaun et al. 2002; Cooper et al. 2005). These defects include isolated hypermethylation of the *H19* DMR and UPD 11p15 and result in biallelic expression of *IGF2*. It has been assumed that it is biallelic *IGF2* expression which drives Wilms predisposition in these individuals. No individual to date has been identified with Wilms tumor and isolated KvDMR hypomethylation, despite this accounting for approximately 50 % of cases of Beckwith-Wiedemann syndrome. This strong correlation is confirmed by study of Wilms tumor case series, which has identified only 11p15 defects resulting in *H19* DMR hypermethylation (Scott et al. 2008).

The risk of Wilms tumor in individuals with features of 11p15-overgrowth but with no detectable 11p15 defect is dependent on their clinical presentation. The risk of Wilms tumor in individuals fulfilling diagnostic criteria for Beckwith-Wiedemann syndrome is likely to be moderately increased (>5 %), while the risk for those with isolated hemihypertrophy is likely to be low (<5 %) (Scott et al. 2006a).

It should be noted that there is no evidence of an increased risk of Wilms tumor in individuals with 11p15-growth retardation disorders such as Silver-Russell syndrome. This is in keeping with the observation that the molecular defects at 11p15 observed in these individuals result in *H19* DMR hypomethylation/reduced *IGF2* expression and are therefore reciprocal to those seen in 11p15-overgrowth disorders (Gicquel et al. 2005).

Heritability of 11p15 Defects

The majority of 11p15 defects are apparently isolated epigenetic abnormalities. These are typically non-heritable and therefore manifest with sporadic rather than familial disease. A small number of individuals have been identified with heritable genetic defects, usually *H19* DMR microdeletions or microinsertions, that cause *H19* DMR hypermethylation (Scott et al. 2008; Sparago et al. 2004; Cerrato et al. 2008). To allow accurate counselling regarding familial recurrence risks, 11p15 testing should be targeted to detect these heritable defects, for example, by using MS-MLPA (spell out in full). The risk of Wilms tumor in relatives of those with 11p15 defects is low assuming this group of defects have been eliminated.

2.2.3.2 Perlman Syndrome

Perlman syndrome is a rare autosomal recessive overgrowth disorder with high mortality in infancy. It is characterised by prenatal overgrowth with polyhydramnios, visceromegaly, cryptorchidism, facial dysmorphism, developmental delay, renal dysplasia and Wilms tumor (Perlman et al. 1973). It is caused by biallelic mutations in DIS3L2 gene (Astuti et al. 2012). Nine of 29 (31 %) reported cases developed Wilms tumor (Perlman et al. 1975; Neri et al. 1984; Greenberg et al. 1986; Grundy et al. 1992; Henneveld et al. 1999; Fahmy et al. 1998; Chitty et al. 1998; Piccione et al. 2005; Alessandri et al. 2008). No other tumors have been reported. Of note, nephroblastomatosis or renal hamartomas have been reported in all but one of the infants born at term. Of the nine individuals that survived beyond 28 days, six developed Wilms tumor.

2.2.3.3 Simpson-Golabi-Behmel Syndrome

Simpson-Golabi-Behmel syndrome is an X-linked recessive overgrowth disorder characterised by coarse facial features, cardiac abnormalities, polydactyly, accessory nipples and, in some individuals, learning difficulties. Renal dysplasia or nephromegaly have been reported in approximately 30 % of cases, and other renal abnormalities described include hydroureter and hydronephrosis (Mariani et al. 2003). The condition is caused by loss of function mutations or deletions of *glypican-3* (*GPC3*) located at Xq26 (Pilia et al. 1996; Li et al. 2001). Such mutations are identifiable in about 70 % of affected individuals. The cause of the remainder is unknown. GPC3 is a cell surface proteoglycan that modulates the effects of several growth factors and interacts with the Wnt pathway (Grisaru et al. 2001; Song et al. 2005).

Of the 51 cases with *GPC3* mutations reported with the condition, three (6 %) developed Wilms tumor (Hughes-Benzie et al. 1996; Lindsay et al. 1997; Rodriguez-Criado et al. 2005; Young et al. 2006; Romanelli et al. 2007; Sakazume et al. 2007; Li and McDonald 2009). Other embryonal tumors have been reported in a small number of cases. There is no evidence of increased risk of Wilms tumor in females carrying *GPC3* mutations/deletions or in individuals affected with a clinical diagnosis of Simpson-Golabi-Behmel syndrome without a *GPC3* mutation/deletion.

2.2.4 Other Tumor Predisposition Syndromes

There is evidence to support an increased risk of Wilms tumor associated with a small number of additional tumor predisposition syndromes.

2.2.4.1 Fanconi Anaemia Types D1 and N

Fanconi anaemia refers to a group of recessive chromosome breakage disorders with overlapping clinical and cellular phenotypes. Clinically, it is characterised by short stature, microcephaly, radial ray defects, hyper- and hypopigmented skin lesions and bone marrow failure. Myelodysplasia and acute myeloid leukaemia are common in childhood, and there is an increased risk of solid tumors of the head and neck in adulthood (Tischkowitz and Hodgson 2003). Cells from individuals with Fanconi anaemia show increased chromosome breakage to DNA crosslinking agents. It is this feature which allows confirmation of the diagnosis of Fanconi anaemia through the analysis of the response of peripheral blood lymphocytes to agents such as diepoxybutane (DEB). At least 13 subtypes of Fanconi anaemia have been described and 13 causative genes identified (Reid et al. 2007; Tischkowitz and Hodgson 2003; Thompson 2005). Two subtypes of Fanconi anaemia, subtypes D1 and N, show a high risk of Wilms tumor and other childhood solid tumors.

Heterozygous monoallelic mutations in *BRCA2*, which is involved in double-strand break DNA repair, cause high-penetrance predisposition to breast cancer and ovarian cancer in adulthood, but not to childhood cancers. Biallelic (homozygous or compound heterozygous) mutations in *BRCA2* cause Fanconi anaemia type D1. Affected children are less likely to have skeletal abnormalities than most Fanconi anaemia subtypes, and their cells often show spontaneous chromosome breakage (Howlett et al. 2002; Reid et al. 2005; Meyer et al. 2005). The cancer spectrum is also distinctive, with a greatly increased risk of childhood solid tumors including Wilms tumor, as well brain tumors. Ten of 32 individuals (30 %) reported with biallelic *BRCA2* mutations developed Wilms tumors (Reid et al. 2005; Meyer et al. 2005; Reid 2008).

Biallelic mutations in *PALB2*, which encodes a BRCA2 interacting protein, cause Fanconi anaemia type N (Reid et al. 2007; Xia et al. 2006, 2007). Unlike *BRCA2*, heterozygous monoallelic mutations in *PALB2* cause only a modest (approximately twofold) increase in breast cancer risk, and increased risk of ovarian cancer has not been observed (Rahman et al. 2007). However, the phenotype seen with biallelic *PALB2* mutations is very similar to that caused by biallelic *BRCA2* mutations. The cancer spectrum is strikingly similar, with frequent occurrence of Wilms tumor and other childhood solid tumors. Three of eight individuals (38 %) reported with biallelic *PALB2* mutations developed Wilms tumor (Reid et al. 2007; Reid 2008).

There is no evidence to suggest that there is an increased risk of Wilms tumor in other subtypes of Fanconi anaemia.

2.2.4.2 Mosaic Variegated Aneuploidy

Mosaic variegated aneuploidy is a rare autosomal recessive disorder characterised by constitutional mosaicism for gains and losses of whole chromosomes. Biallelic mutations in *BUB1B* – which encodes BUBR1, a key component of the mitotic spindle checkpoint – cause approximately half of cases (Hanks et al. 2004). The clinical features of the condition are variable and include developmental delay, microcephaly, CNS malformations, cataracts, congenital heart defects and other malformations. Childhood cancers are frequently reported in the condition, including Wilms tumor, leukaemia and rhabdomyosarcoma. Wilms tumor has occurred in nine (19 %) of 47 cases (N Rahman, unpublished observation) (Hanks et al. 2004; Nakamura et al. 1985; Kajii et al. 1998, 2001; Kawame et al. 1999; Matsuura et al. 2000; Jacquemont et al. 2002; Furukawa et al. 2003).

2.2.4.3 Bloom Syndrome

Bloom syndrome is an autosomal recessive DNA repair disorder caused by biallelic mutations in the *BLM* gene, which encodes a DNA helicase important in the response to aberrant recombination between sister chromatids and homologous chromosomes (Ellis et al. 1995). Diagnosis of the condition can be made through the analysis of peripheral blood lymphocytes following exposure to bromodeoxyuridine (BrdU). Clinically, the condition is characterised by short stature, microcephaly, sun-sensitivity and characteristic telangiectatic skin lesions in sun-exposed areas. In some cases, learning difficulties are also a feature. An increased frequency of a number of cancers has been reported, principally in adulthood (German 1997). Wilms tumor has been reported in a number of individuals and is known to have occurred in eight of 267 individuals (3 %) in the Bloom syndrome registry (J German, personal communication) (German 1997; Cairney et al. 1987; Berger et al. 1996; Jain et al. 2001; The Bloom's Syndrome Registry 2010).

2.2.4.4 Li-Fraumeni Syndrome

Li-Fraumeni is an autosomal dominant tumor predisposition disorder which is characterised by a high incidence of a range of tumors including breast cancer, sarcomas, adrenocortical carcinoma and brain tumors (Li et al. 1988). Approximately 70 % of families with classical Li-Fraumeni syndrome harbour heterozygous, monoallelic mutations in *TP53* – a key regulator of cell cycle arrest, apoptosis and DNA repair (Birch et al. 1994; Evans et al. 2002). Wilms tumor is not one of the cardinal tumors seen in the condition and is not included in the diagnostic criteria of Li-Fraumeni syndrome. However, it has been reported in at least 7 families with *TP53* mutations and in several Li-Fraumeni or Li-Fraumeni-like families without *TP53* mutations (Li and Fraumeni 1982; Hartley et al. 1993; Bardeesy et al. 1994; Evans et al. 1998; Verselis et al. 2000; Chompret et al. 2000; Birch et al. 2001; Olivier et al. 2002). Of note, five of the seven *TP53* mutations were splice site mutations despite splice mutations accounting for only 4 % of all reported germline *TP53* mutations, and it is possible that Wilms tumor risk is influenced by the type of *TP53* mutation. However, overall, the risk of Wilms tumor appears to be low, both in families with *TP53* mutations and in mutation-negative families with classical Li-Fraumeni syndrome or a Li-Fraumeni-like phenotype.

2.2.4.5 Mulibrey Nanism

Mulibrey nanism (MUscle-LIver-BRain-EYe nanism) is an autosomal recessive disorder characterised by short stature, facial dysmorphism, muscle wasting, hepatogmegaly, J-shaped sella turcica radiographically and distinctive yellow spots on the retina (Karlberg et al. 2004a, b). Hepatic hamartomas and ovarian fibrothecomas are also seen. The condition is caused by biallelic mutations in the *TRIM37* gene, which has ubiquitin E3 ligase activity (Avela et al. 2000). At least 130 individuals with mulibrey nanism have been reported, of whom six (4–5 %) have developed Wilms tumor (Karlberg et al. 2004a; Simila et al. 1980; Seemanova and Bartsch 1999; Karlberg et al. 2009).

2.2.4.6 Hyperparathyroidism-Jaw Tumor Syndrome

Hyperparathyroidism-jaw tumor syndrome is an autosomal dominant disorder caused by heterozygous, monoallelic mutations in the *HRPT2* gene, which is thought to be involved in RNA elongation (Carpten et al. 2002). It is characterised by parathyroid tumors and fibro-osseous lesions of the maxilla and mandible (Jackson et al. 1990). More than 150 individuals from more than 50 families have been reported (Kakinuma et al. 1994; Teh et al. 1996; Wassif et al. 1999; Tan and Teh 2004; Mizusawa et al. 2006; Masi et al. 2008; Iacobone et al. 2009). A variety of renal abnormalities and tumors occur including renal cysts, renal cortical adenomas, benign mixed epithelial-stromal renal tumors and papillary renal cell carcinomas. Wilms tumor has been reported in three individuals (<2 %), including one individual who apparently developed bilateral Wilms tumor at the age of 53 years.

2.2.5 Constitutional Chromosome Abnormalities

Abnormalities at 11p13 (*WT1*) and 11p15 are the most frequent constitutional chromosome abnormalities associated with Wilms tumor. There is evidence of Wilms tumor predisposition in a small number of other chromosome disorders.

2.2.5.1 Trisomy 18

Trisomy 18 (Edwards syndrome) occurs in approximately 1 in 13,000 live births (Nielsen and Wohlert 1991). It is associated with multiple congenital malformations and has high infant mortality, with 90 % of individuals dying before the age of 1 year. Renal malformations including horseshoe kidney are present in the majority of cases (Kinoshita et al. 1989). There have been at least 12 cases of Wilms tumor in individuals with trisomy 18 (Geiser and Schindler 1969;

Shanklin and Sotelo-Avila 1969; Miller 1971; Karayalcin et al. 1981; Sheng et al. 1990; Faucette and Carey 1991; Olson et al. 1995; Kullendorff and Wiebe 1997; Anderson et al. 2003). In addition, perilobar nephrogenic rests and/or nephroblastomatosis have been reported in a number of cases without Wilms tumor (Bove et al. 1969). The median age of diagnosis of Wilms tumor in trisomy 18 (5 years) is higher than in sporadic disease. Given the high early mortality of trisomy 18, the risk of Wilms tumor to long-term survivors is clearly increased.

2.2.5.2 Trisomy 13

Trisomy 13 (Patau syndrome) occurs in approximately 1 in 10,000 live births. Like trisomy 18, it is associated with multiple congenital malformations including renal abnormalities (Nielsen and Wohlert 1991). It has a high early mortality, with a median survival of 1 week. Two cases of Wilms tumor have been reported in trisomy 13, one of which arose in a horseshoe kidney (Olson et al. 1995; Sweeney and Pelegano 2000). Nephroblastomatosis was also identified in one foetus following termination at 24 weeks of gestation [cite 1] ADD REF. Given the very high mortality of trisomy 13, it is likely that there is an increased risk to those that survive the early neonatal period.

2.2.5.3 2q37 Deletion

Three individuals with constitutional terminal deletions of chromosome 2q37 have been reported with Wilms tumor. Two had isolated deletions of 2q37 with a centromeric breakpoint at 2q37.1 (Conrad et al. 1995; Viot-Szoboszlai et al. 1998). A further child had a paternally inherited unbalanced translocation resulting in monosomy 2q37-qter and trisomy 15q22-qter (Olson et al. 1995). The location of the breakpoint within 2q37 was not reported. Almost 100 individuals have been reported with 2q37 deletions (Casas et al. 2004; Falk and Casas 2007). The most frequent centromeric breakpoint is 2q37.3. In approximately a quarter of cases, the deletion extends to 2q37.1. The overall risk of Wilms tumor may be as high as 3 % (two of 66). However, it is possible that the risk is primarily in those in which the deletion extends to 2q37.1 and who may be at higher risk.

2.3 Conditions in Which Wilms Tumor Predisposition Is Unclear or Uncertain

In addition to the conditions described above in previous sections of this chapter, Wilms tumor has been reported in association with a substantial number of other genetic disorders (Scott et al. 2006a). For some, relatively common, disorders in which few cases of Wilms have been reported, it is likely that the occurrence(s) of Wilms tumor is coincidental and not because of a predisposition. For example, fragile-X syndrome, Marfan syndrome and tuberous sclerosis are all relatively common and readily diagnosed genetic disorders in which only a single case of Wilms has been reported (Newbold et al. 1982; Grether et al. 1987; Drouin et al. 1992). Only six cases of trisomy 21 (Down) syndrome have been reported with Wilms tumor despite the condition affecting approximately 1 in 800 live births (Fabia and Drolette 1970; Kusumakumary et al. 1995; Spreafico et al. 2007). Seven individuals with neurofibromatosis type 1 have been reported (Ito et al. 1997). However, neurofibromatosis type 1 occurs in approximately 1 in 3,000 individuals and a number of population-based, cohort and cancer registry studies have failed to detect an association with Wilms tumor (Sorensen et al. 1986; Huson et al. 1988; Friedman and Birch 1997; Walker et al. 2006).

For other disorders, the possibility of a small increased risk of Wilms tumor cannot be excluded. For example, four individuals with Turner syndrome (45,XO) were reported in one American Wilms tumor case series (Olson et al. 1995). However, no case was found in a British series of 400 cases and only one case was found in a Danish series of 597 individuals (Hasle et al. 1996; Swerdlow et al. 2001). It is likely therefore that the absolute Wilms tumor risk in Turner syndrome is close to that of the general population.

In the case of Sotos syndrome, an overgrowth disorder caused by heterozygous monoallelic mutations in *NSD1*, molecular testing has clarified the risk of Wilms tumor. The syndrome can be difficult for those without experience of the condition to diagnose on clinical grounds alone. A number of individuals with a clinical diagnosis of Sotos syndrome were reported with Wilms tumor, and it had been thought that the risk was appreciable in the condition. Following the introduction of molecular testing for the condition, it has emerged that the risk of Wilms tumor is very low (Tatton-Brown et al. 2005).

In the case of the rarer disorders reported on one or only a small number of occasions with Wilms tumor and the many reported individuals with Wilms tumor with a presentation that is not readily classifiable, it is hard to be certain whether the occurrence of Wilms tumor represents a predisposition or a coincidental finding. These conditions are not set out individually here, but the interested reader is referred to Table 2 in Scott et al. (2006a).

Similarly, a number of discrete chromosomal abnormalities have been reported on one occasion in association with Wilms tumor (Table 2.2). It is likely that in some of these, the chromosomal defect targets a Wilms predisposition gene. For example, two individuals have been reported with overlapping abnormalities that result in copy number gain at chromosome 15q (Hu et al. 2002; Schluth et al. 2005). This region contains the *IGF1R* gene, which may underlie predisposition to Wilms tumor in these individuals. One child with bilateral Wilms tumor was reported with a de novo apparently balanced reciprocal chromosome translocation with breakpoints at 5q21 and 6q21 (Table 2.2) (Hoban et al. 1997; Slade et al. 2010). The 6q21 breakpoint transects the *HACE1* gene and would be predicted to truncate the gene product. This, and the subsequent identification of a further child with unilateral Wilms tumor harbouring a truncating point mutation in *HACE1*, identified *HACE1* as a likely Wilms predisposition gene (Slade et al. 2010). This study found that *HACE1* mutations are rare in Wilms tumor and are likely to make only a small contribution to Wilms tumor predisposition.

2.4 Wilms Tumor Surveillance in Predisposed Individuals

Surveillance for Wilms tumor is recommended in children at substantially increased risk, and Wilms tumor surveillance has become widespread. However, there is limited evidence regarding its efficacy and the balance of risks and benefits of Wilms tumor surveillance (Scott et al. 2006b). This has resulted in the use of different surveillance strategies in different countries and even different units within the same country as well as the inclusion of children at different levels of risk. In some cases, children close to population risk have been enrolled in surveillance.

Because of the high survival rate in Wilms tumor, it is unlikely that surveillance will lead to a substantial decrease in mortality. However, surveillance may identify tumors at a more favourable stage. This could be important because the resultant reduced intensity of chemotherapy and radiotherapy is likely to result in reduced long-term treatment-related morbidity. There have been three small retrospective evaluations of Wilms tumor surveillance published, only one of which reported a significant difference in stage distribution between screened and unscreened individuals (Green et al. 1993; Craft et al. 1995; Choyke et al. 1999). It is notable that three of 15 screened individuals in this study had false-positive scans that resulted in further imaging and major surgery, indicating that significant negative sequelae of surveillance can occur. In addition, the anxiety and practical difficulties associated with regular surveillance can be appreciable.

Although there is no clear evidence that surveillance results in a significant decrease in mortality or tumor stage, tumors detected by Wilms tumor surveillance would be anticipated to be on average smaller than tumors that present clinically. In Germany, where abdominal ultrasound in children is common and 10 % of Wilms tumors are diagnosed prior to symptoms, there are some data to suggest that asymptomatic tumors are of lower stage than those that present due to clinical symptoms (N Graf, personal communication). On this basis, it is felt reasonable to offer surveillance

Table 2.2 Constitutional chromosome abnormalities reported in association with Wilms tumor

Karyotype	Comment	Clinical features	Reference
t(1;16)(p22;p13.2)	Apparently balanced	Unilateral Wilms	Olson et al. (1995)
del(1)(p36pter)		Unilateral Wilms	Scott et al. (2006a)
del(1)(p36pter) dup(1)(q24qter)	De novo unbalanced translocation with breakpoints at 1p36 and 1q24. Mosaic in amniocytes and normal renal tissue. Present in all tumor cells examined	Bilateral Wilms, agenesis corpus callosum, cardiac malformations, facial dysmorphism, developmental delay	Mark et al. (2005)
dup(1)(q2?2;q2?3)			Bache et al. (2006)
t(1;7)(q42;p15)	Apparently balanced, de novo	Unilateral Wilms, nephrogenic rest contralateral kidney, bilateral radial aplasia, short tibiae and fibulae; transient thrombocytopenia	Hewitt et al. (1991)
del (2)(p11.2p12)	Maternally inherited	Speech delay, mildly dysmorphic	Barber et al. (2005)
t(5;6)(q21;q21)	Apparently balanced, de novo, *HACE1* interrupted at 6q21; see text	Bilateral Wilms	Hoban et al. (1997), Slade et al. (2010)
t(7;19)(q11.2;q13.3)	Apparently balanced, de novo	Bilateral Wilms, thick corpus callosum, large cisterna magna, facial dysmorphism	Cavicchioni et al. (2005)
t(7;13)(q36;q13)	Apparently balanced, de novo	Unilateral Wilms, facial dysmorphism, developmental delay, umbilical hernia, testicular ectopia	Bernard et al. (1984)
8p+	Additional material of unknown origin at 8p	Wilms in a single kidney	Olson et al. (1995)
del(9)(q22q32)	De novo, encompasses *PTCH*	Synchronous rhabdomyosarcoma, features of Gorlin syndrome	Alvarez-Franco et al. (2000)
t(9;12)(q22.3;q15)	Apparently balanced, de novo		Betts et al. (2001)
del(11)(q14.1q21)	De novo	Horseshoe kidney, nephrogenic rests	Stratton et al. (1994)
del(12)(q11q13.1)	De novo, LOH 12q in tumor	Unilateral Wilms, growth retardation, developmental delay, facial dysmorphism	Rapley et al. (2001)
dup(12)(q24.3qter) del(22)(q13.3qter)	Inherited from mother with balanced t(12;22)(q24.3;q13.3)	Unilateral Wilms, overgrowth, developmental delay	Turner et al. (2001)
Tetrasomy 15q24.3-qter	Mosaic in lymphocytes	Unilateral Wilms, developmental delay, arachnodactyly, facial dysmorphism	Schluth et al. (2005)
Tetrasomy 15q25.3-qter	Mosaic constitutionally, present in all tumor cells	Bilateral, arachnodactyly, overgrowth, craniosynostosis	Hu et al. (2002)
Ring chromosome of unknown origin	Mother and two children with ring chromosome	Both children developed Wilms, one unilaterally, one bilaterally	Kakati et al. (1991)

to children at substantially increased risk of Wilms tumor (Scott et al. 2006b).

In the United Kingdom, surveillance is performed by renal ultrasound scanning, and, given the rapid tumor doubling time, this is recommended to be performed at 3–4-month intervals (Scott et al. 2006b). Alternative methods of surveillance have been proposed and used, including regular parental examination for abdominal masses and CT or MRI scanning. However, renal ultrasound scan is the preferred modality because it is sensitive to relatively small tumors and does not require sedation to perform (Schmidt et al. 2003).

In the United Kingdom, it is recommended that children at >5 % risk of Wilms tumor are offered this surveillance (Table 2.1) (Scott et al. 2006b). Screening begins at syndrome diagnosis and continues to cover the age range of diagnosis of at least 90–95 % of tumors for the predisposing syndrome. For the *WT1*-associated syndromes, Fanconi anaemia types D1 and N, mosaic variegated aneuploidy and Perlman syndrome virtually all tumors occur before 5 years and thus surveillance is not recommended beyond this age. Surveillance is recommended to continue to 7 years for individuals with constitutional 11p15 defects, Simpson-Golabi-Behmel syndrome and those from familial Wilms tumor pedigrees in which Wilms tumor has occurred above the age of 5 years.

2.5 Future Directions

2.5.1 Identification of Further High-Penetrance Predisposition Alleles

Despite the successes in the clinical and molecular delineation of Wilms tumor predisposition syndromes, further high-penetrance Wilms tumor predisposition alleles remain to be identified. The cause of the majority of familial Wilms tumor pedigrees remains unknown. The causative gene(s) are likely to be identifiable using linkage-based approaches and/or next-generation sequencing techniques. The genes underlying some recognised syndromic Wilms tumor predisposition syndromes also remain to be identified, for example, *BUB1B* mutation-negative mosaic variegated aneuploidy cases. In addition, it is likely that there are other Wilms tumor predisposition syndromes that are as yet unrecognised as illustrated by the recent emergence of Fanconi anaemia type add types as a new, highly penetrant Wilms predisposition syndrome. Next-generation sequencing approaches may be particularly applicable to gene identification in these rare syndromes, which may not be amenable to linkage analysis.

Some cases of bilateral Wilms tumor are accounted for by known Wilms predisposition genes, most notably *WT1* and 11p15. However, the majority remain unexplained and the underlying predisposition alleles remain to be identified (Little et al. 2004; Scott et al. 2008). In some cases, the underlying allele will be identifiable using the approaches above. However, recent evidence suggests that in some cases the underlying predisposition may be caused by a mosaic, tissue-specific defect at 11p15 which has arisen early during development such that it is present in the precursors of both kidneys (N Rahman, unpublished observation). Further investigation of this possibility is warranted.

2.5.2 Clarification of Wilms Tumor Risks and Identification of Further Genotype-Tumor Risk Correlations

The study of larger number of individuals with known Wilms tumor predisposition syndromes or syndromes where predisposition remains uncertain will improve estimates of the risk of Wilms tumor in these conditions. Accurate estimation of risk is difficult in the absence of large, prospective trials. These are rarely possible in the disorders in question, which are rare and in some cases difficult to diagnose before the occurrence of Wilms tumor. This is particularly problematic in conditions where Wilms tumor is a diagnostic criterion. It is likely that for many syndromes, cases with tumors are more likely to be reported than those without. This reporting bias is likely to have led to an overestimate of Wilms tumor risk. The availability of cheaper molecular testing and its application in a wider range of clinical presentations may assist by improving diagnosis of cases without Wilms tumor (or prior to its diagnosis), as it has in the *WT1*- and 11p15-related disorders (Little et al. 2004; Scott et al. 2008; Kohler et al. 2001; Martin et al. 2005).

Molecular analysis of larger number of cases also has the potential to detect further genotype-tumor risk correlations. The success in this regard in 11p15-overgrowth disorders points to the importance of these findings in targeting Wilms surveillance to those at highest risk and allowing the release of individuals at low risk from unnecessary surveillance (Scott et al. 2008).

2.5.3 Identification of Further Common, Low-Penetrance Predisposition Alleles

Following the advent of high-density SNP array technology and the development of the required statistical expertise, genome-wide association studies have been performed in a wide range of disorders (Donnelly 2008). These large case-control experiments have identified common low-penetrance predisposition alleles for a wide range of disorders including a number of cancers. Typically, odds ratios for disease seen with alleles identified by such studies are between 1.2 and 2.0. Of particular relevance is the genome-wide association study led by John Maris at the Children's Hospital of Philadelphia which has identified low-penetrance predisposition alleles for the childhood embryonal tumor neuroblastoma (Maris et al. 2008; Capasso et al. 2009; Diskin et al. 2009). In 2012, a genome-wide association study of British and American Wilms tumor cases identified loci at chromosome 2p24.3 and chromosome 11p14.1 at which common variants are associated with increased risk of Wilms tumor (Turnbull et al. 2012). The risk variants at these loci had odds ratios for disease of approximately 1.2 and 1.4 respectively. The mechanism by which the risk association of these loci is conferred remains unclear. At 2p24, the most likely candidate genes for the effect include *DDX1* and *MYCN*. At 11p14.1, the most likely candidate is *DLG2*. Further sequencing studies and functional analyses may assist in determining mechanism of these effects. Further genome-wide association studies may identify further such common, low-penetrance predisposition alleles.

References

Abbaszadeh F, Barker KT, McConville C, Scott RH, Rahman N (2010) A new familial cancer syndrome including predisposition to Wilms tumor and neuroblastoma. Fam Cancer 9(3):425–430

Alessandri JL, Cuillier F, Ramful D et al (2008) Perlman syndrome: report, prenatal findings and review. Am J Med Genet A 146A(19):2532–2537

Algar EM, St Heaps L, Darmanian A et al (2007) Paternally inherited submicroscopic duplication at 11p15.5 implicates insulin-like growth factor II in overgrowth and Wilms' tumorigenesis. Cancer Res 67(5):2360–2365

Alvarez-Franco M, Bale AE, Reyes-Mugica M (2000) Expanding the spectrum of Gorlin Syndrome: Wilms tumor in a patient with 9q22.3 deletion. Pediatr Dev Pathol 3:306–311

Anderson CE, Punnett HH, Huff V, de Chadarevian JP (2003) Characterization of a Wilms tumor in a 9-year-old girl with trisomy 18. Am J Med Genet 121A(1):52–55

Astuti D, Morris MR, Cooper WN et al (2012) Germline mutations in DIS3L2 cause the Perlman syndrome of overgrowth and Wilms tumor susceptibility. Nature Genet. 44:277–284

Avela K, Lipsanen-Nyman M, Idanheimo N et al (2000) Gene encoding a new RING-B-box-Coiled-coil protein is mutated in mulibrey nanism. Nat Genet 25(3):298–301

Bache I, Hasle H, Tommerup N, Olsen JH (2006) Population-based study of cancer among carriers of a constitutional structural chromosomal rearrangement. Genes Chromosomes Cancer 45(3):231–246

Baird PN, Groves N, Haber DA, Housman DE, Cowell JK (1992) Identification of mutations in the WT1 gene in tumours from patients with the WAGR syndrome. Oncogene 7(11):2141–2149

Barbaux S, Niaudet P, Gubler MC et al (1997) Donor splice-site mutations in WT1 are responsible for Frasier syndrome. Nat Genet 17(4):467–470

Barber JC, Thomas NS, Collinson MN et al (2005) Segmental haplosufficiency: transmitted deletions of 2p12 include a pancreatic regeneration gene cluster and have no apparent phenotypic consequences. Eur J Hum Genet 13(3):283–291

Barbosa AS, Hadjiathanasiou CG, Theodoridis C et al (1999) The same mutation affecting the splicing of WT1 gene is present on Frasier syndrome patients with or without Wilms' tumor. Hum Mutat 13(2):146–153

Bardeesy N, Falkoff D, Petruzzi MJ et al (1994) Anaplastic Wilms' tumour, a subtype displaying poor prognosis, harbours p53 gene mutations. Nat Genet 7(1):91–97

Beckwith JB, Kiviat NB, Bonadio JF (1990) Nephrogenic rests, nephroblastomatosis, and the pathogenesis of Wilms' tumor. Pediatr Pathol 10(1–2):1–36

Berger C, Frappaz D, Leroux D et al (1996) Wilms tumor and Bloom syndrome. Arch Pediatr 3(8):802–805

Bernard JL, Baeteman MA, Mattei JF, Raybaud C, Giraud F (1984) Wilms' tumor, malformative syndrome, mental retardation and de novo constitutional translocation, t(7;13)(q36;q13). Eur J Pediatr 141(3):175–177

Betts DR, Greiner J, Feldges A, Caflisch U, Niggli FK (2001) Constitutional balanced chromosomal rearrangements and neoplasm in children. J Pediatr Hematol Oncol 23(9):582–584

Birch JM, Hartley AL, Tricker KJ et al (1994) Prevalence and diversity of constitutional mutations in the p53 gene among 21 Li-Fraumeni families. Cancer Res 54(5):1298–1304

Birch JM, Alston RD, McNally RJ et al (2001) Relative frequency and morphology of cancers in carriers of germline TP53 mutations. Oncogene 20(34): 4621–4628

Bliek J, Maas SM, Ruijter JM et al (2001) Increased tumour risk for BWS patients correlates with aberrant H19 and not KCNQ1OT1 methylation: occurrence of KCNQ1OT1 hypomethylation in familial cases of BWS. Hum Mol Genet 10(5):467–476

Bliek J, Gicquel C, Maas S, Gaston V, Le Bouc Y, Mannens M (2004) Epigenotyping as a tool for the prediction of tumor risk and tumor type in patients with Beckwith-Wiedemann syndrome (BWS). J Pediatr 145(6):796–799

Bliek J, Maas S, Alders M, Merks JH, Mannens M (2008) Epigenotype, phenotype, and tumors in patients with isolated hemihyperplasia. J Pediatr 153(1):95–100

Bove KE, Koffler H, McAdams AJ (1969) Nodular renal blastema. Definition and possible significance. Cancer 24(2):323–332

Breslow N, Olshan A, Beckwith JB, Green DM (1993) Epidemiology of Wilms tumor. Med Pediatr Oncol 21(3):172–181

Breslow NE, Olson J, Moksness J, Beckwith JB, Grundy P (1996) Familial Wilms' tumor: a descriptive study. Med Pediatr Oncol 27(5):398–403

Breslow NE, Takashima JR, Ritchey ML, Strong LC, Green DM (2000) Renal failure in the Denys-Drash and Wilms' tumor-aniridia syndromes. Cancer Res 60(15):4030–4032

Breslow NE, Norris R, Norkool PA et al (2003) Characteristics and outcomes of children with the Wilms tumor-Aniridia syndrome: a report from the National Wilms Tumor Study Group. J Clin Oncol 21(24):4579–4585

Cairney AE, Andrews M, Greenberg M, Smith D, Weksberg R (1987) Wilms tumor in three patients with Bloom syndrome. J Pediatr 111(3):414–416

Capasso M, Devoto M, Hou C et al (2009) Common variations in BARD1 influence susceptibility to high-risk neuroblastoma. Nat Genet 41(6):718–723

Carpten JD, Robbins CM, Villablanca A et al (2002) HRPT2, encoding parafibromin, is mutated in hyperparathyroidism-jaw tumor syndrome. Nat Genet 32(4):676–680

Casas KA, Mononen TK, Mikail CN et al (2004) Chromosome 2q terminal deletion: report of 6 new patients and review of phenotype-breakpoint correlations in 66 individuals. Am J Med Genet 130A(4): 331–339

Cavicchioni O, Gomes DM, Leroy B et al (2005) Prenatal diagnosis of de novo (7;19)(q11.2;q13.3) translocation associated with a thick corpus callosum and Wilms tumor of the kidneys. Prenat Diagn 25(10):876–878

Cerrato F, Sparago A, Verde G et al (2008) Different Mechanisms Cause Imprinting defects at the IGF2/H19 locus in Beckwith-Wiedemann Syndrome and Wilms' Tumour. Hum Mol Genet 17(10):1427–1435

Chitty LS, Clark T, Maxwell D (1998) Perlman syndrome–a cause of enlarged, hyperechogenic kidneys. Prenat Diagn 18(11):1163–1168

Chompret A, Brugieres L, Ronsin M et al (2000) P53 germline mutations in childhood cancers and cancer risk for carrier individuals. Br J Cancer 82(12): 1932–1937

Choyke PL, Siegel MJ, Craft AW, Green DM, DeBaun MR (1999) Screening for Wilms tumor in children with Beckwith-Wiedemann syndrome or idiopathic hemihypertrophy. Med Pediatr Oncol 32(3):196–200

Conrad B, Dewald G, Christensen E, Lopez M, Higgins J, Pierpont ME (1995) Clinical phenotype associated with terminal 2q37 deletion. Clin Genet 48(3):134–139

Cooper WN, Luharia A, Evans GA et al (2005) Molecular subtypes and phenotypic expression of Beckwith-Wiedemann syndrome. Eur J Hum Genet 13(9): 1025–1032

Coppes MJ, Campbell CE, Williams BR (1993) The role of WT1 in Wilms tumorigenesis. FASEB J 7(10):886–895

Craft AW, Parker L, Stiller C, Cole M (1995) Screening for Wilms' tumour in patients with aniridia, Beckwith syndrome, or hemihypertrophy. Med Pediatr Oncol 24(4):231–234

DeBaun MR, Tucker MA (1998) Risk of cancer during the first four years of life in children from The Beckwith-Wiedemann Syndrome Registry. J Pediatr 132(3 Pt 1):398–400

DeBaun MR, Niemitz EL, McNeil DE, Brandenburg SA, Lee MP, Feinberg AP (2002) Epigenetic alterations of H19 and LIT1 distinguish patients with Beckwith-Wiedemann syndrome with cancer and birth defects. Am J Hum Genet 70(3):604–611

Demmer L, Primack W, Loik V, Brown R, Therville N, McElreavey K (1999) Frasier syndrome: a cause of focal segmental glomerulosclerosis in a 46, XX female. J Am Soc Nephrol 10(10):2215–2218

Denys P, Malvaux P, Van den BH, Tanghe W, Proesmans W (1967) Association of an anatomo-pathological syndrome of male pseudohermaphroditism, Wilms' tumor, parenchymatous nephropathy and XX/XY mosaicism. Arch Fr Pediatr 24(7): 729–739

Dinkel E, Britscho J, Dittrich M, Schulte-Wissermann H, Ertel M (1988) Renal growth in patients nephrectomized for Wilms tumour as compared to renal agenesis. Eur J Pediatr 147(1):54–58

Diskin SJ, Hou C, Glessner JT et al (2009) Copy number variation at 1q21.1 associated with neuroblastoma. Nature 459(7249):987–991

Donnelly P (2008) Progress and challenges in genome-wide association studies in humans. Nature 456(7223): 728–731

Drash A, Sherman F, Hartmann WH, Blizzard RM (1970) A syndrome of pseudohermaphroditism, Wilms' tumor, hypertension, and degenerative renal disease. J Pediatr 76(4):585–593

Drouin V, Vannier JP, Moirot H, Mitrofanoff P, Tron P (1992) Nephroblastoma and fragile X syndrome. Arch Fr Pediatr 49(5):477

Eddy AA, Mauer SM (1985) Pseudohermaphroditism, glomerulopathy, and Wilms tumor (Drash syndrome): frequency in end-stage renal failure. J Pediatr 106(4): 584–587

Elliott M, Maher ER (1994) Beckwith-Wiedemann syndrome. J Med Genet 31(7):560–564

Elliott M, Bayly R, Cole T, Temple IK, Maher ER (1994) Clinical features and natural history of Beckwith-Wiedemann syndrome: presentation of 74 new cases. Clin Genet 46(2):168–174

Ellis NA, Groden J, Ye TZ et al (1995) The Bloom's syndrome gene product is homologous to RecQ helicases. Cell 83(4):655–666

Evans SC, Mims B, McMasters KM et al (1998) Exclusion of a p53 germline mutation in a classic Li-Fraumeni syndrome family. Hum Genet 102(6):681–686

Evans DG, Birch JM, Thorneycroft M, McGown G, Lalloo F, Varley JM (2002) Low rate of TP53 germline mutations in breast cancer/sarcoma families not fulfilling classical criteria for Li-Fraumeni syndrome. J Med Genet 39(12):941–944

Fabia J, Drolette M (1970) Malformations and leukemia in children with Down's syndrome. Pediatrics 45(1): 60–70

Fahmy J, Kaminsky CK, Parisi MT (1998) Perlman syndrome: a case report emphasizing its similarity to and distinction from Beckwith-Wiedemann and prune-belly syndromes. Pediatr Radiol 28(3):179–182

Falk RE, Casas KA (2007) Chromosome 2q37 deletion: clinical and molecular aspects. Am J Med Genet C Semin Med Genet 145(4):357–371

Faucette KJ, Carey JC (1991) Trisomy 18 and Wilms' tumor-is there an association? Clin Res 39:96

Frasier S, Bashore R, Mosier H (1964) Gonadoblastoma associated with pure gonadal dysgenesis in monozygous twins. J Pediatr 64:740–745

Friedman JM, Birch PH (1997) Type 1 neurofibromatosis: a descriptive analysis of the disorder in 1,728 patients. Am J Med Genet 70(2):138–143

Furukawa T, Azakami S, Kurosawa H, Ono Y, Ueda Y, Konno Y (2003) Cystic partially differentiated nephroblastoma, embryonal rhabdomyosarcoma, and multiple congenital anomalies associated with variegated mosaic aneuploidy and premature centromere division: a case report. J Pediatr Hematol Oncol 25(11):896–899

Gaston V, Le Bouc Y, Soupre V et al (2001) Analysis of the methylation status of the KCNQ1OT and H19 genes in leukocyte DNA for the diagnosis and prognosis of Beckwith-Wiedemann syndrome. Eur J Hum Genet 9(6):409–418

Geiser CF, Schindler AM (1969) Long survival in a male with 18-trisomy syndrome and Wilms' tumor. Pediatrics 44(1):111–116

German J (1997) Bloom's syndrome. XX. The first 100 cancers. Cancer Genet Cytogenet 93(1):100–106

Gicquel C, Rossignol S, Cabrol S et al (2005) Epimutation of the telomeric imprinting center region on chromosome 11p15 in Silver-Russell syndrome. Nat Genet 37(9):1003–1007

Goldman M, Smith A, Shuman C et al (2002) Renal abnormalities in beckwith-wiedemann syndrome are associated with 11p15.5 uniparental disomy. J Am Soc Nephrol 13(8):2077–2084

Green DM, Breslow NE, Beckwith JB, Norkool P (1993) Screening of children with hemihypertrophy, aniridia, and Beckwith-Wiedemann syndrome in patients with Wilms tumor: a report from the National Wilms Tumor Study. Med Pediatr Oncol 21(3):188–192

Greenberg F, Stein F, Gresik MV et al (1986) The Perlman familial nephroblastomatosis syndrome. Am J Med Genet 24(1):101–110

Grether P, Carnevale A, Pasquel P (1987) Wilms' tumor in an infant with tuberous sclerosis. Ann Genet 30(3): 183–185

Grisaru S, Cano-Gauci D, Tee J, Filmus J, Rosenblum ND (2001) Glypican-3 modulates BMP- and FGF-mediated effects during renal branching morphogenesis. Dev Biol 231(1):31–46

Grundy RG, Pritchard J, Baraitser M, Risdon A, Robards M (1992) Perlman and Wiedemann-Beckwith syndromes: two distinct conditions associated with Wilms' tumour. Eur J Pediatr 151(12):895–898

Hanks S, Coleman K, Reid S et al (2004) Constitutional aneuploidy and cancer predisposition caused by biallelic mutations in BUB1B. Nat Genet 36(11):1159–1161

Hartley AL, Birch JM, Tricker K et al (1993) Wilms' tumor in the Li-Fraumeni cancer family syndrome. Cancer Genet Cytogenet 67(2):133–135

Hasle H, Olsen JH, Nielsen J, Hansen J, Friedrich U, Tommerup N (1996) Occurrence of cancer in women with Turner syndrome. Br J Cancer 73(9):1156–1159

Henneveld HT, van Lingen RA, Hamel BC, Stolte-Dijkstra I, van Essen AJ (1999) Perlman syndrome: four additional cases and review. Am J Med Genet 86(5):439–446

Heuch JM, Heuch I, Kvale G (1996) Birth characteristics and risk of Wilms' tumour: a nationwide prospective study in Norway. Br J Cancer 74(7):1148–1151

Hewitt M, Lunt PW, Oakhill A (1991) Wilms' tumour and a de novo (1;7) translocation in a child with bilateral radial aplasia. J Med Genet 28(6):411–412

Hoban PR, Cowen RL, Mitchell EL et al (1997) Physical localisation of the breakpoints of a constitutional translocation t(5;6)(q21;q21) in a child with bilateral Wilms' tumour. J Med Genet 34(4):343–345

Howlett NG, Taniguchi T, Olson S et al (2002) Biallelic inactivation of BRCA2 in Fanconi anemia. Science 297(5581):606–609

Hoyme HE, Seaver LH, Jones KL, Procopio F, Crooks W, Feingold M (1998) Isolated hemihyperplasia (hemihypertrophy): report of a prospective multicenter study of the incidence of neoplasia and review. Am J Med Genet 79(4):274–278

Hu J, McPherson E, Surti U, Hasegawa SL, Gunawardena S, Gollin SM (2002) Tetrasomy 15q25.3 → qter resulting from an analphoid supernumerary marker chromosome in a patient with multiple anomalies and bilateral Wilms tumors. Am J Med Genet 113(1):82–88

Hughes-Benzie RM, Pilia G, Xuan JY et al (1996) Simpson-Golabi-Behmel syndrome: genotype/phenotype analysis of 18 affected males from 7 unrelated families. Am J Med Genet 66(2):227–234

Huson SM, Harper PS, Compston DA (1988) Von Recklinghausen neurofibromatosis. A clinical and population study in South-East Wales. Brain 111(Pt 6):1355–1381

Iacobone M, Masi G, Barzon L et al (2009) Hyperparathyroidism-jaw tumor syndrome: a report of three large kindred. Langenbecks Arch Surg 394(5): 817–825

Ito F, Watanabe Y, Ito T (1997) Synchronous occurrence of Wilms tumor and ganglioneuroblastoma in a child with neurofibromatosis. Eur J Pediatr Surg 7(5): 308–310

Jackson CE, Norum RA, Boyd SB et al (1990) Hereditary hyperparathyroidism and multiple ossifying jaw fibromas: a clinically and genetically distinct syndrome. Surgery 108(6):1006–1012

Jacquemont S, Boceno M, Rival JM, Mechinaud F, David A (2002) High risk of malignancy in mosaic variegated aneuploidy syndrome. Am J Med Genet 109(1):17–21

Jain D, Hui P, McNamara J, Schwartz D, German J, Reyes-Mugica M (2001) Bloom syndrome in sibs: first reports of hepatocellular carcinoma and Wilms tumor with documented anaplasia and nephrogenic rests. Pediatr Dev Pathol 4(6):585–589

Jepsen P, Olsen ML, Mellemkjaer L, Olsen JH, Sorensen HT (2004) A registry-based study of gender, fetal growth, and risk of Wilms tumor. Pediatr Hematol Oncol 21(5):435–439

Kajii T, Kawai T, Takumi T et al (1998) Mosaic variegated aneuploidy with multiple congenital abnormalities: homozygosity for total premature chromatid separation trait. Am J Med Genet 78(3):245–249

Kajii T, Ikeuchi T, Yang ZQ et al (2001) Cancer-prone syndrome of mosaic variegated aneuploidy and total premature chromatid separation: report of five infants. Am J Med Genet 104(1):57–64

Kakati S, Xiao H, Siddiqui SY et al (1991) Constitutional extra chromosomal element in a family with Wilms' tumor. Hum Genet 87(2):183–188

Kakinuma A, Morimoto I, Nakano Y et al (1994) Familial primary hyperparathyroidism complicated with Wilms' tumor. Intern Med 33(2):123–126

Kaplinsky C, Ghahremani M, Frishberg Y, Rechavi G, Pelletier J (1996) Familial Wilms' tumor associated with a WT1 zinc finger mutation. Genomics 38(3):451–453

Karayalcin G, Shanske A, Honigman R (1981) Wilms' tumor in a 13-year old girl with trisomy 18. Am J Dis Child 135(7):665–666

Karlberg N, Jalanko H, Perheentupa J, Lipsanen-Nyman M (2004a) Mulibrey nanism: clinical features and diagnostic criteria. J Med Genet 41(2):92–98

Karlberg S, Tiitinen A, Lipsanen-Nyman M (2004b) Failure of sexual maturation in Mulibrey nanism. N Engl J Med 351(24):2559–2560

Karlberg N, Karlberg S, Karikoski R, Mikkola S, Lipsanen-Nyman M, Jalanko H (2009) High frequency of tumours in Mulibrey nanism. J Pathol 218(2):163–171

Kawame H, Sugio Y, Fuyama Y et al (1999) Syndrome of microcephaly, Dandy-Walker malformation, and Wilms tumor caused by mosaic variegated aneuploidy with premature centromere division (PCD): report of a new case and review of the literature. J Hum Genet 44(4):219–224

Kinoshita M, Nakamura Y, Nakano R et al (1989) Thirty-one autopsy cases of trisomy 18: clinical features and pathological findings. Pediatr Pathol 9(4):445–457

Kohler B, Schumacher V, l'Allemand D, Royer-Pokora B, Gruters A (2001) Germline Wilms tumor suppressor gene (WT1) mutation leading to isolated genital malformation without Wilms tumor or nephropathy. J Pediatr 138(3):421–424

Kullendorff CM, Wiebe T (1997) Chromosomal aberrations in Wilms' tumour. Eur J Pediatr Surg 7(5):286–287

Kusumakumary P, Ninan M, Chellam VG, Jacob R, Nair MK (1995) Wilms tumor in a child with Down syndrome. J Pediatr Hematol Oncol 17(3):276

Leisenring WM, Breslow NE, Evans IE, Beckwith JB, Coppes MJ, Grundy P (1994) Increased birth weights of National Wilms' Tumor Study patients suggest a growth factor excess. Cancer Res 54(17):4680–4683

Li FP, Fraumeni JF Jr (1982) Prospective study of a family cancer syndrome. JAMA 247(19):2692–2694

Li CC, McDonald SD (2009) Increased nuchal translucency and other ultrasound findings in a case of simpson-golabi-behmel syndrome. Fetal Diagn Ther 25(2):211–215

Li FP, Fraumeni JF Jr, Mulvihill JJ et al (1988) A cancer family syndrome in twenty-four kindreds. Cancer Res 48(18):5358–5362

Li M, Shuman C, Fei YL et al (2001) GPC3 mutation analysis in a spectrum of patients with overgrowth expands the phenotype of Simpson-Golabi-Behmel syndrome. Am J Med Genet 102(2):161–168

Lindsay S, Ireland M, O'Brien O et al (1997) Large scale deletions in the GPC3 gene may account for a minority of cases of Simpson-Golabi-Behmel syndrome. J Med Genet 34(6):480–483

Little SE, Hanks SP, King-Underwood L et al (2004) Frequency and heritability of WT1 mutations in nonsyndromic Wilms' tumor patients: a UK Children's Cancer Study Group Study. J Clin Oncol 22(20):4140–4146

Loirat C, Andre JL, Champigneulle J et al (2003) WT1 splice site mutation in a 46, XX female with minimal-change nephrotic syndrome and Wilms' tumour. Nephrol Dial Transplant 18(4):823–825

Mariani S, Iughetti L, Bertorelli R et al (2003) Genotype/phenotype correlations of males affected by Simpson-Golabi-Behmel syndrome with GPC3 gene mutations: patient report and review of the literature. J Pediatr Endocrinol Metab 16(2):225–232

Maris JM, Mosse YP, Bradfield JP et al (2008) Chromosome 6p22 locus associated with clinically aggressive neuroblastoma. N Engl J Med 358(24):2585–2593

Mark HF, Wyandt H, Pan A, Milunsky JM (2005) Constitutional partial 1q trisomy mosaicism and Wilms tumor. Cancer Genet Cytogenet 162(2):166–171

Martin RA, Grange DK, Zehnbauer B, DeBaun MR (2005) LIT1 and H19 methylation defects in isolated hemihyperplasia. Am J Med Genet A 134A(2):129–131

Masi G, Barzon L, Iacobone M et al (2008) Clinical, genetic, and histopathologic investigation of CDC73-related familial hyperparathyroidism. Endocr Relat Cancer 15(4):1115–1126

Matsuura S, Ito E, Tauchi H, Komatsu K, Ikeuchi T, Kajii T (2000) Chromosomal instability syndrome of total premature chromatid separation with mosaic variegated aneuploidy is defective in mitotic-spindle checkpoint. Am J Hum Genet 67(2):483–486

McDonald JM, Douglass EC, Fisher R et al (1998) Linkage of familial Wilms' tumor predisposition to chromosome 19 and a two-locus model for the etiology of familial tumors. Cancer Res 58(7): 1387–1390

Merks JH, Caron HN, Hennekam RC (2005) High incidence of malformation syndromes in a series of 1,073 children with cancer. Am J Med Genet A 134(2):132–143

Meyer S, Fergusson WD, Oostra AB et al (2005) A cross-linker-sensitive myeloid leukemia cell line from a 2-year-old boy with severe Fanconi anemia and biallelic FANCD1/BRCA2 mutations. Genes Chromosomes Cancer 42(4):404–415

Miller RW (1971) Relation between cancer and congenital malformations. The value of small series, with a note on pineal tumors in native and migrant Japanese. Isr J Med Sci 7(12):1461–1464

Mizusawa N, Uchino S, Iwata T et al (2006) Genetic analyses in patients with familial isolated hyperparathyroidism and hyperparathyroidism-jaw tumour syndrome. Clin Endocrinol (Oxf) 65(1):9–16

Muto R, Yamamori S, Ohashi H, Osawa M (2002) Prediction by FISH analysis of the occurrence of Wilms tumor in aniridia patients. Am J Med Genet 108(4):285–289

Nakamura Y, Nakashima H, Fukuda S, Hashimoto T, Maruyama M (1985) Bilateral cystic nephroblastomas and multiple malformations with trisomy 8 mosaicism. Hum Pathol 16(7):754–756

Narod SA, Hawkins MM, Robertson CM, Stiller CA (1997) Congenital anomalies and childhood cancer in Great Britain. Am J Hum Genet 60(3):474–485

Neri G, Martini-Neri ME, Katz BE, Opitz JM (1984) The Perlman syndrome: familial renal dysplasia with Wilms tumor, fetal gigantism and multiple congenital anomalies. Am J Med Genet 19(1):195–207

Newbold SG, Shafer AD, Goodwin CD, Nanagas VN, Dimlich SH (1982) Stage III Wilms' tumor of a solitary kidney in a patient with Marfan's syndrome: a 5-yr survival. J Pediatr Surg 17(6):841–842

Nielsen J, Wohlert M (1991) Chromosome abnormalities found among 34,910 newborn children: results from a 13-year incidence study in Arhus. Denmark Hum Genet 87(1):81–83

Olivier M, Eeles R, Hollstein M, Khan MA, Harris CC, Hainaut P (2002) The IARC TP53 database: new online mutation analysis and recommendations to users. Hum Mutat 19(6):607–614

Olson JM, Hamilton A, Breslow NE (1995) Non-11p constitutional chromosome abnormalities in Wilms' tumor patients. Med Pediatr Oncol 24(5):305–309

Pelletier J, Bruening W, Li FP, Haber DA, Glaser T, Housman DE (1991) WT1 mutations contribute to abnormal genital system development and hereditary Wilms' tumour. Nature 353(6343):431–434

Perlman M, Goldberg GM, Bar-Ziv J, Danovitch G (1973) Renal hamartomas and nephroblastomatosis with fetal gigantism: a familial syndrome. J Pediatr 83(3):414–418

Perlman M, Levin M, Wittels B (1975) Syndrome of fetal gigantism, renal hamartomas, and nephroblastomatosis with Wilms' tumor. Cancer 35(4):1212–1217

Piccione M, Cecconi M, Giuffre M et al (2005) Perlman syndrome: clinical report and nine-year follow-up. Am J Med Genet A 139A(2):131–135

Pilia G, Hughes-Benzie RM, MacKenzie A et al (1996) Mutations in GPC3, a glypican gene, cause the Simpson-Golabi-Behmel overgrowth syndrome. Nat Genet 12(3):241–247

Porteus MH, Narkool P, Neuberg D et al (2000) Characteristics and outcome of children with Beckwith-Wiedemann syndrome and Wilms' tumor: a report from the National Wilms Tumor Study Group. J Clin Oncol 18(10):2026–2031

Rahman N (2005) Mechanisms predisposing to childhood overgrowth and cancer. Curr Opin Genet Dev 15(3): 227–233

Rahman N, Arbour L, Tonin P et al (1996) Evidence for a familial Wilms' tumour gene (FWT1) on chromosome 17q12-q21. Nat Genet 13(4):461–463

Rahman N, Arbour L, Tonin P et al (1997) The familial Wilms' tumour susceptibility gene, FWT1, may not be a tumour suppressor gene. Oncogene 14(25): 3099–3102

Rahman N, Abidi F, Ford D et al (1998) Confirmation of FWT1 as a Wilms' tumour susceptibility gene and phenotypic characteristics of Wilms' tumour attributable to FWT1. Hum Genet 103(5):547–556

Rahman N, Seal S, Thompson D et al (2007) PALB2, which encodes a BRCA2-interacting protein, is a breast cancer susceptibility gene. Nat Genet 39(2):165–167

Rapley EA, Barfoot R, Bonaiti-Pellie C et al (2000) Evidence for susceptibility genes to familial Wilms tumour in addition to WT1, FWT1 and FWT2. Br J Cancer 83(2):177–183

Rapley EA, Hargrave D, Persinguhe N et al (2001) Case of interstitial 12q deletion in association with Wilms tumor. Am J Med Genet 104(3):246–249

Reid SL (2008) Identification and characterisation of genes predisposing to Wilms tumour. Institute of Cancer Research, University of London, London

Reid S, Renwick A, Seal S et al (2005) Biallelic BRCA2 mutations are associated with multiple malignancies in childhood including familial Wilms tumour. J Med Genet 42(2):147–151

Reid S, Schindler D, Hanenberg H et al (2007) Biallelic mutations in PALB2 cause Fanconi anemia subtype FA-N and predispose to childhood cancer. Nat Genet 39(2):162–164

Ritchey ML, Shamberger RC, Hamilton T, Haase G, Argani P, Peterson S (2005) Fate of bilateral renal lesions missed on preoperative imaging: a report from the National Wilms Tumor Study Group. J Urol 174(4 Pt 2):1519–1521

Rodriguez-Criado G, Magano L, Segovia M et al (2005) Clinical and molecular studies on two further families

with Simpson-Golabi-Behmel syndrome. Am J Med Genet A 138(3):272–277
Romanelli V, Arroyo I, Rodriguez JI et al (2007) Germinal mosaicism in Simpson-Golabi-Behmel syndrome. Clin Genet 72(4):384–386
Royer-Pokora B, Ragg S, Heckl-Ostreicher B et al (1991) Direct pulsed field gel electrophoresis of Wilms' tumors shows that DNA deletions in 11p13 are rare. Genes Chromosomes Cancer 3(2):89–100
Royer-Pokora B, Beier M, Henzler M et al (2004) Twenty-four new cases of WT1 germline mutations and review of the literature: genotype/phenotype correlations for Wilms tumor development. Am J Med Genet A 127A(3):249–257
Russo S, Finelli P, Recalcati MP et al (2006) Molecular and genomic characterisation of cryptic chromosomal alterations leading to paternal duplication of the 11p15.5 Beckwith-Wiedemann region. J Med Genet 43(8):e39
Sakazume S, Okamoto N, Yamamoto T et al (2007) GPC3 mutations in seven patients with Simpson-Golabi-Behmel syndrome. Am J Med Genet A 143A(15): 1703–1707
Schluth C, Mattei MG, Mignon-Ravix C et al (2005) Intrachromosomal triplication for the distal part of chromosome 15q. Am J Med Genet A 136(2):179–184
Schmidt T, Hohl C, Haage P et al (2003) Diagnostic accuracy of phase-inversion tissue harmonic imaging versus fundamental B-mode sonography in the evaluation of focal lesions of the kidney. AJR Am J Roentgenol 180(6):1639–1647
Schuz J, Kaletsch U, Meinert R, Kaatsch P, Michaelis J (2001) High-birth weight and other risk factors for Wilms tumour: results of a population-based case-control study. Eur J Pediatr 160(6):333–338
Scott RH, Stiller CA, Walker L, Rahman N (2006a) Syndromes and constitutional chromosomal abnormalities associated with Wilms tumour. J Med Genet 43(9):705–715
Scott RH, Walker L, Olsen OE et al (2006b) Surveillance for Wilms tumour in at-risk children: pragmatic recommendations for best practice. Arch Dis Child 91(12):995–999
Scott RH, Douglas J, Baskcomb L et al (2008) Constitutional 11p15 abnormalities, including heritable imprinting center mutations, cause nonsyndromic Wilms tumor. Nat Genet 40(11):1329–1334
Seemanova E, Bartsch O (1999) Mulibrey nanism and Wilms tumor. Am J Med Genet 85(1):76–78
Shanklin DR, Sotelo-Avila C (1969) In situ tumors in fetuses, newborns and young infants. Biol Neonat 14(5):286–316
Sheng WW, Soukup S, Bove K, Gotwals B, Lampkin B (1990) Chromosome analysis of 31 Wilms' tumors. Cancer Res 50(9):2786–2793
Shuman C, Smith AC, Steele L et al (2006) Constitutional UPD for chromosome 11p15 in individuals with isolated hemihyperplasia is associated with high tumor risk and occurs following assisted reproductive technologies. Am J Med Genet A 140(14):1497–1503
Simila S, Timonen M, Heikkinen E (1980) A case of Mulibrey nanism with associated Wilms' tumor. Clin Genet 17(1):29–30
Slade I, Stephens P, Douglas J et al (2010) Constitutional translocation breakpoint mapping by genome-wide paired-end sequencing identifies HACE1 as a putative Wilms tumour susceptibility gene. J Med Genet 47(5): 342–347
Song HH, Shi W, Xiang YY, Filmus J (2005) The loss of glypican-3 induces alterations in Wnt signaling. J Biol Chem 280(3):2116–2125
Sorensen SA, Mulvihill JJ, Nielsen A (1986) Long-term follow-up of von Recklinghausen neurofibromatosis. Survival and malignant neoplasms. N Engl J Med 314(16):1010–1015
Sotelo-Avila C, Gonzalez-Crussi F, Fowler JW (1980) Complete and incomplete forms of Beckwith-Wiedemann syndrome: their oncogenic potential. J Pediatr 96(1):47–50
Sparago A, Cerrato F, Vernucci M, Ferrero GB, Silengo MC, Riccio A (2004) Microdeletions in the human H19 DMR result in loss of IGF2 imprinting and Beckwith-Wiedemann syndrome. Nat Genet 36(9):958–960
Sparago A, Russo S, Cerrato F et al (2007) Mechanisms causing imprinting defects in familial Beckwith-Wiedemann syndrome with Wilms' tumour. Hum Mol Genet 16(3):254–264
Spreafico F, Terenziani M, Lualdi E et al (2007) Non-chromosome 11-p syndromes in Wilms tumor patients: Clinical and cytogenetic report of two Down syndrome cases and one Turner syndrome case. Am J Med Genet A 143(1):85–88
Stratton RF, Lazarus KH, Ritchie EJ, Bell AM (1994) Deletion (11)(q14.1q21). Am J Med Genet 49(3): 294–298
Sweeney H, Pelegano J (2000) Wilms tumor in a child with trisomy 13. J Pediatr Hematol Oncol 22(2): 171–172
Swerdlow AJ, Hermon C, Jacobs PA et al (2001) Mortality and cancer incidence in persons with numerical sex chromosome abnormalities: a cohort study. Ann Hum Genet 65(Pt 2):177–188
Tan MH, Teh BT (2004) Renal neoplasia in the hyperparathyroidism-jaw tumor syndrome. Curr Mol Med 4(8):895–897
Tatton-Brown K, Douglas J, Coleman K et al (2005) Genotype-phenotype associations in Sotos syndrome: an analysis of 266 individuals with NSD1 aberrations. Am J Hum Genet 77(2):193–204
Teh BT, Farnebo F, Kristoffersson U et al (1996) Autosomal dominant primary hyperparathyroidism and jaw tumor syndrome associated with renal hamartomas and cystic kidney disease: linkage to 1q21-q32 and loss of the wild type allele in renal hamartomas. J Clin Endocrinol Metab 81(12): 4204–4211
The Bloom's Syndrome Registry (2010) http://www.med.cornell.edu/bsr/. Ref Type: Generic
Thompson LH (2005) Unraveling the Fanconi anemia-DNA repair connection. Nat Genet 37(9):921–922

Thorburn MJ, Wright ES, Miller CG, Smith-Read EH (1970) Exomphalos-macroglossia-gigantism syndrome in Jamaican infants. Am J Dis Child 119(4): 316–321

Tischkowitz MD, Hodgson SV (2003) Fanconi anaemia. J Med Genet 40(1):1–10

Turnbull C, Perdeaux ER, Pernet D et al (2012) A genome-wide association study identifies susceptibility loci for Wilms tumor. Nat Genet 44(6):681–684

Turner AM, Rosier M, Cohn R, Turner G, Battese K, Yip M (2001) "Weaver Syndrome" and Wilms Tumour in a child with an Unbalanced Cryptic Translocation. 7 Individuals with Mental Retardation in the One Family due to Translocation – t(12;22)(q24.33;q13.31). International Congress of Human Genetics P0430

Verselis SJ, Rheinwald JG, Fraumeni JF Jr, Li FP (2000) Novel p53 splice site mutations in three families with Li-Fraumeni syndrome. Oncogene 19(37):4230–4235

Viot-Szoboszlai G, Amiel J, Doz F et al (1998) Wilms' tumor and gonadal dysgenesis in a child with the 2q37.1 deletion syndrome. Clin Genet 53(4):278–280

Walker L, Thompson D, Easton D et al (2006) A prospective study of neurofibromatosis type 1 cancer incidence in the UK. Br J Cancer 95(2):233–238

Wassif WS, Farnebo F, Teh BT et al (1999) Genetic studies of a family with hereditary hyperparathyroidism-jaw tumour syndrome. Clin Endocrinol (Oxf) 50(2):191–196

Weksberg R, Nishikawa J, Caluseriu O et al (2001) Tumor development in the Beckwith-Wiedemann syndrome is associated with a variety of constitutional molecular 11p15 alterations including imprinting defects of KCNQ1OT1. Hum Mol Genet 10(26):2989–3000

Weksberg R, Shuman C, Smith AC (2005) Beckwith-Wiedemann syndrome. Am J Med Genet C Semin Med Genet 137(1):12–23

Wiedemann HR (1997) Frequency of Wiedemann-Beckwith syndrome in Germany; rate of hemihyperplasia and of tumours in affected children. Eur J Pediatr 156(3):251

Xia B, Sheng Q, Nakanishi K et al (2006) Control of BRCA2 cellular and clinical functions by a nuclear partner, PALB2. Mol Cell 22(6):719–729

Xia B, Dorsman JC, Ameziane N et al (2007) Fanconi anemia is associated with a defect in the BRCA2 partner PALB2. Nat Genet 39(2):159–161

Yeazel MW, Ross JA, Buckley JD, Woods WG, Ruccione K, Robison LL (1997) High birth weight and risk of specific childhood cancers: a report from the Children's Cancer Group. J Pediatr 131(5): 671–677

Young EL, Wishnow R, Nigro MA (2006) Expanding the clinical picture of Simpson-Golabi-Behmel syndrome. Pediatr Neurol 34(2):139–142

Yunis JJ, Ramsay NK (1980) Familial occurrence of the aniridia-Wilms tumor syndrome with deletion 11p13-14.1. J Pediatr 96(6):1027–1030

Zirn B, Wittmann S, Gessler M (2005) Novel familial WT1 read-through mutation associated with Wilms tumor and slow progressive nephropathy. Am J Kidney Dis 45(6):1100–1104

Clinical Presentation

3

Elizabeth Mullen and Norbert Graf

Contents

E. Mullen (✉)
Harvard Medical School, Dana Farber Cancer Institute, 450 Brookline Avenue, Boston, MA 02115, USA
e-mail: elizabeth_mullen@dfci.harvard.edu

N. Graf
Department of Pediatric Oncology and Hematology, Saarland University, Campus Homburg, Building 9, 66421, Homburg, Germany
e-mail: norbert.graf@uniklinikum-saarland.de

Abstract

The classic clinical presentation of children with Wilms tumor (WT) overlaps with many aspects of the general presentation of abdominal mass in children. However, specific details of the history, physical exam and laboratory evaluation can raise the suspicion of WT even prior to imaging or surgical procedures. Other renal tumors, such as rhabdoid tumor of the kidney (RTK), congenital mesoblastic nephroma (CMN), clear cell sarcoma of the kidney (CCSK), and renal cell carcinoma (RCC), also have particular presenting characteristics that can steer the clinician towards the consideration of those diagnoses.

This chapter will largely address the presentation of children with WT, as the leading renal tumor in children, but will also give brief attention to these less common renal tumors of childhood. We will review both common and uncommon presentations of Wilms tumor through discussion of an evaluation for a child suspected to have either an abdominal mass or a renal tumor. We will review the basic elements of evaluation which should be performed, including history, thorough physical exam, and initial laboratory and radiologic evaluation.

3.1 Introduction

Renal tumors account for approximately 7 % of childhood cancer in both North America and Europe. Within renal tumors, Wilms tumor (WT)

K. Pritchard-Jones, J.S. Dome (eds.), *Renal Tumors of Childhood: Biology and Therapy*, Pediatric Oncology, DOI 10.1007/978-3-662-44003-2_3, © Springer-Verlag Berlin Heidelberg 2014

is by far the most commonly occurring tumor, accounting for approximately 95 % of renal tumors (Pastore et al. 2006).

In the majority of children diagnosed with Wilms tumor, clinical presentation overlaps with the general presentation of abdominal mass in children. Specific details of the history, physical exam, and laboratory evaluation, however, can raise the suspicion of Wilms tumor even prior to imaging or surgical procedures. Other renal tumors, such as rhabdoid tumor of the kidney (RTK), congenital mesoblastic nephroma (CMN), clear cell sarcoma of the kidney (CCSK), and renal cell carcinoma (RCC) each also have particular presenting characteristics that can steer the clinician towards the consideration of those diagnosis.

This chapter will largely address the presentation of children with WT, as the leading renal tumor in children, but will also give brief attention to the less common renal tumors of childhood. We will review both common and uncommon presentations of Wilms tumor through discussion of an evaluation for a child suspected to have either an abdominal mass or a renal tumor. We will review the basic elements of evaluation which should be performed, including history, thorough physical exam, and initial laboratory and radiologic evaluation.

As there is overlap of topics in the discussion of the clinical presentation of children with renal tumors that are discussed in much greater depth in other chapters of this book, specifically chapters on WT Genetics, Imaging, Surgery, Pathology, and Non-Wilms Tumors, the reader is also referred to those chapters for additional detail.

3.2 Presentation

The classic presentation of a child with a Wilms tumor (WT) is of an asymptomatic palpable mass in the abdomen (Fig. 3.1). In most cases, this mass is found by parents who are convinced that it was not there a day before. Asymptomatic children also frequently present to their primary care doctor in a well child visit, where an incidental abdominal mass is appreciated. Complaints or symptoms are found in only about 20 % or less of children with new Wilms tumor (Gutjahr et al. 1990; Graf et al. 2003) (Table 3.1). Abdominal pain, abdominal distension, and symptoms of constipation are the most common complaints associated with the presentation of WT. Microscopic or gross hematuria, a typical presenting symptom on adult renal tumors, is uncommon in children, occurring in less than 20 %. It is seen most frequently in patients who have ureteral extension of Wilms tumor (Ritchey et al. 2008) Fever, flank pain, and weight gain or weight loss, are among symptoms that are seen at presentation in less than 10 % of patients. Signs and symptoms of anemia can be present in patients with internal blood loss due to tumor hemorrhage.

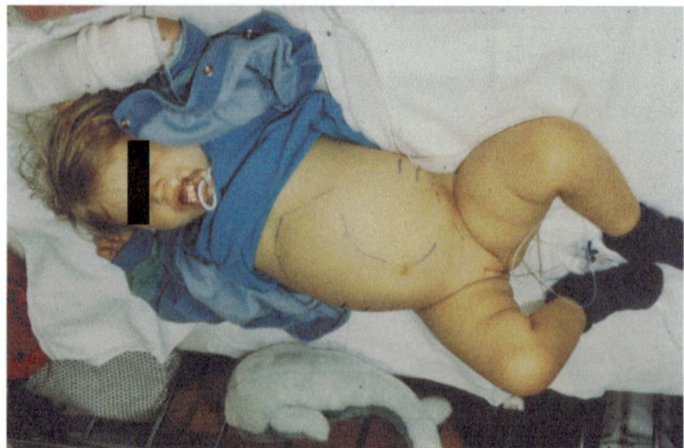

Fig. 3.1 Clinical presentation of a child with nephroblastoma with marked abdominal distension

Table 3.1 Initial symptoms in children with nephroblastoma at the time of diagnosis (Gutjahr et al. 1990; Graf et al. 2003)

Symptom	Frequency
Asymptomatic, incidental finding during regular examination	10
Incidental finding during consultation for other reasons	15
Asymptomatic mass	56
Pain	25
Hematuria	18
Fever	10
Urinary tract infection	6
Weight loss	5
Constipation	6
Enteritis	4
Vomiting	6
Others	19

3.3 History

After establishing an initial presenting complaint, a further detailed history should be obtained. History should include any family history of childhood cancer, specifics of the patient's birth, birth weight, hypoglycemia at birth, growth and development, and known physical or developmental abnormalities.

Wilms tumor has been reported in association with more than 50 different syndromes (Scott et al. 2006a). Conclusive evidence of an increased risk exists in only a minority of these conditions (Scott et al. 2006b). About 12 % of patients with a WT have an underlying syndrome (Fig. 3.2). These syndromes can be divided in overgrowth syndromes and others. One third of the syndromes affect the urogenital system and in 15 % a hemihypertrophy can be diagnosed. All other syndromes or malformations are rare including aniridia, Denys–Drash syndrome, and Beckwith–Wiedemann syndrome (Coppes et al. 1994; Graf et al. 2003). A summary of the different malformations and syndromes is given in Table 3.2. Familial WTs do occur in about 2 % of patients (Ruteshouser and Huff 2004).

History should also include any known preexisting medical conditions that might increase the child's risk of treatment morbidity. History of cardiac defect, past pulmonary issues, and history of bleeding disorders in patient or family should be identified.

3.4 Physical Exam

Physical exam should take into consideration the general appearance of the child, as well close attention to vital signs.

Increased respiratory rate, increased work of breathing, and decreased oxygen saturation can indicate pulmonary or pleural spread of disease. Increased work of breathing can also occur from elevation of the diaphragm from the underlying abdominal mass. Occasionally, accompanying peritoneal fluid can also add to abdominal distension. The degree of abdominal distension can be extreme on occasion to the extent of precipitating respiratory failure (Fig. 3.3). A small percentage of patients (4.3 % in a small series of patients at St Jude's Hospital) present with pleural effusion (Corey et al. 2004). Pleural effusions can be sympathetic or malignant and should be tapped when feasible if results will change therapy. Presence of pleural effusion at diagnosis has not been correlated with worse prognosis.

Patients that have spontaneous tumor rupture with contained loss of blood can present with signs and symptoms consistent with acute anemia (Ramsay et al. 1977). Usually this is accompanied

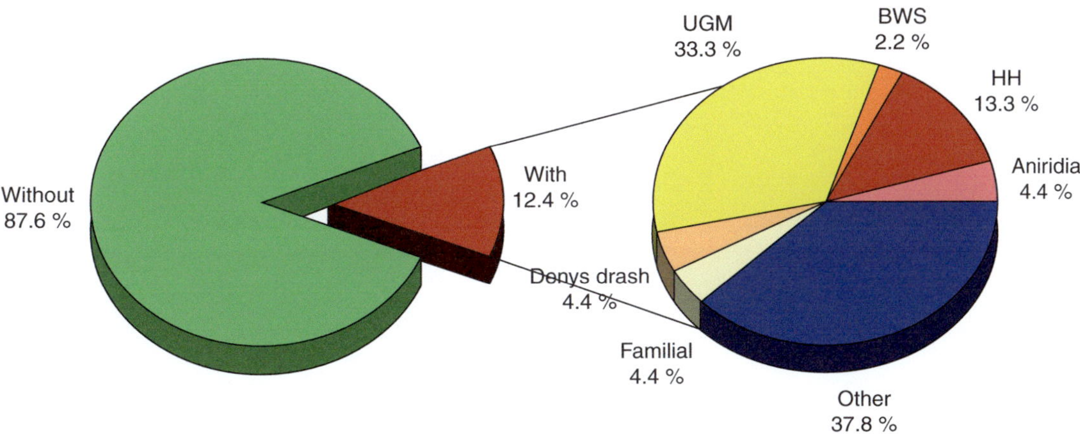

Fig. 3.2 Proportion of children with Wilms Tumor and malformations or syndromes treated in Germany in the prospective study and trials SIOP 9 and SIOP 93-01. (*UGM* urogenital malformations, *BWS* Beckwith–Wiedemann syndrome, *HH* Hemihypertrophy, *Denys–Drash* Denys–Drash syndrome)

Table 3.2 Malformations and syndromes in children with Wilms tumor (Bürger et al. 1986; Cowell et al. 1989; Gronskov et al. 2001; Rump et al. 2005; Scott et al. 2006a, b)

Syndrome Link to OMIM[a]	Characteristics	Gene	Risk [%]	Incidence [%]	
				SIOP	NWTSG/COG
Overgrowth syndromes					
Hemihypertrophy http://www.ncbi.nlm.nih.gov/entrez/dispomim.cgi?id=235000	Hemihypertrophy	11p15 WT2	3–5	3.13	2.47
Beckwith–Wiedemann **EMG** syndrome http://www.ncbi.nlm.nih.gov/entrez/dispomim.cgi?id=130650	**E**xomphalos **M**acroglossia **G**igantismus	11p15.5 WT2, IGF2, H19	10–20 %	<1	
Sotos syndrome http://www.ncbi.nlm.nih.gov/entrez/dispomim.cgi?id=117550	Rapid growth, acromegalic features; nonprogressive cerebral disorder with mental retardation	5q35 *NSD1*		<1	
Simpson–Golabi–Behmel syndrome http://www.ncbi.nlm.nih.gov/entrez/dispomim.cgi?id=312870	Postnatal overgrowth Coarse facies Congenital heart defects other congenital abnormalities	Xq26 *GPC3*		<1	
Klippel–Trenaunay syndrome http://www.ncbi.nlm.nih.gov/entrez/dispomim.cgi?id=149000	Cutaneous hemangiomata Hypertrophy of the related bones and soft tissues	5q13.3 VG5Q		<1	
Perlman syndrome http://www.ncbi.nlm.nih.gov/entrez/dispomim.cgi?id=267000	Renal hamartomas Nephroblastomatosis Fetal gigantismus	?		<1	
Other syndromes					
Aniridia http://www.ncbi.nlm.nih.gov/entrez/dispomim.cgi?id=106210	Aniridia	11p13 PAX6	30 %	<1	0.84
WAGR http://www.ncbi.nlm.nih.gov/entrez/dispomim.cgi?id=194072	**W**ilms tumor **A**niridia **G**enitourinary anomalies Mental **R**etardation	11p13 WT1		<1	
Denys–Drash http://www.ncbi.nlm.nih.gov/entrez/dispomim.cgi?id=194080	Nephropathy Wilms tumor Genital anomalies	11p13 WT1	30 %	<1	

GUM http://www.ncbi.nlm.nih.gov/entrez/dispomim.cgi?id=137357	Genitourinary malformations	11p13 GUD		4.41	4.61
Mosaic variegated aneuploidy syndrome http://www.ncbi.nlm.nih.gov/entrez/dispomim.cgi?id=257300	Constitutional losses or gains of whole chromosomes	15q15 BUB1B	>20 %	?	
Li–Fraumeni syndrome http://www.ncbi.nlm.nih.gov/entrez/dispomim.cgi?id=151623	Inherited cancer syndrome	17p13 p53		<1	
Neurofibromatosis I Morbus Recklinghausen http://www.ncbi.nlm.nih.gov/entrez/dispomim.cgi?id=162200	Cafe-au-lait spots fibromatous tumors of the skin	17q11.2 NF1		<1	

[a]Online Mendelian Inheritance in Man: http://www.ncbi.nlm.nih.gov/entrez/query.fcgi?db=OMIM

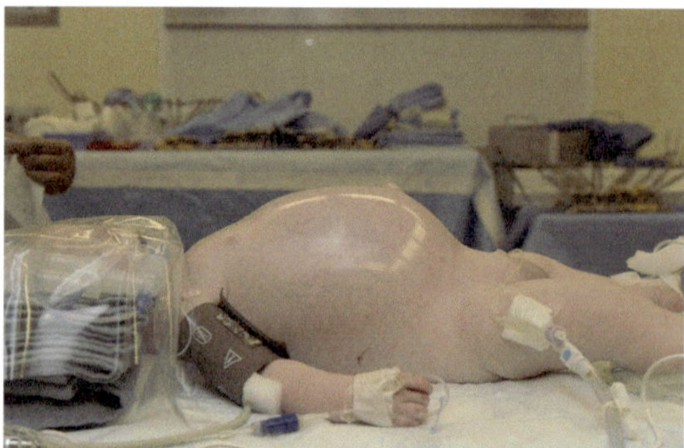

Fig. 3.3 Child with a renal mass, presenting with massive abdominal distension, leading to respiratory failure

by marked abdominal pain and distension, as well as pallor and tachycardia. Volume and blood product resuscitation should be initiated rapidly in this situation.

Hypertension can be a presenting sign, and may be asymptomatic, or accompanied by complaint of headache or pain. Consideration of a renal cause, including possibility of renal tumor should be included on the differential diagnosis of any young child with noted hypertension. Hypertension associated with renal tumors has been shown to be caused by an increase in renin activity (Maas et al. 2007). Sometimes blood pressure is difficult to control especially in children receiving preoperative chemotherapy. In the retrospective study of Maas et al., in at least a subset of patients, ACE inhibitors may be a good therapeutic option. After tumor nephrectomy, the blood pressure returns to normal values without any medication in nearly all of these children.

There are many specific physical exam findings that can heighten the suspicion of a diagnosis of a Wilms tumor in a child with abdominal mass. After initial vital signs, the examination of the abdomen should include the size and location of mass, presence of contralateral mass, clinical ascites, and observation of whether the mass moves with respiration. Tenderness to palpation raises the concern for the possibility of tumor rupture and hemorrhage with subsequent peritoneal irritation. There is a historic teaching to avoid deep palpation in patients with WT because of the concern of causing tumor rupture.

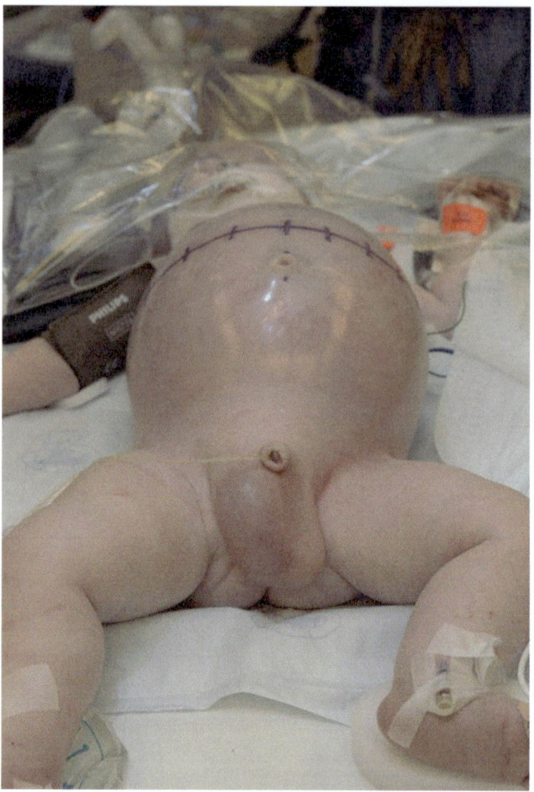

Fig. 3.4 Physical exam can also reveal presence of hydroceles or varicoceles, related to compression of the mass

On exam, mass associated with WT usually does not cross the midline, or move with respiration, which can help differentiate from a mass associated with neuroblastoma. Increased respiratory rate, observation of increased work of breathing, and/or absence of breath sounds as indicators of pulmonary spread of disease are important factors in deciding the risk of anesthesia for the patient, both for imaging or any surgical procedure.

Genital urinary abnormalities can be seen in several of the syndromes associated with increased risk of WT and should be carefully documented. The presence of hernias, hydroceles, or varicoceles (Fig. 3.4) may be related to compression of vascular and vital structures affected by the mass. Ureteral prolapse of WT observed on physical exam has also been reported in a small number of patients (Ritchey et al. 2008).

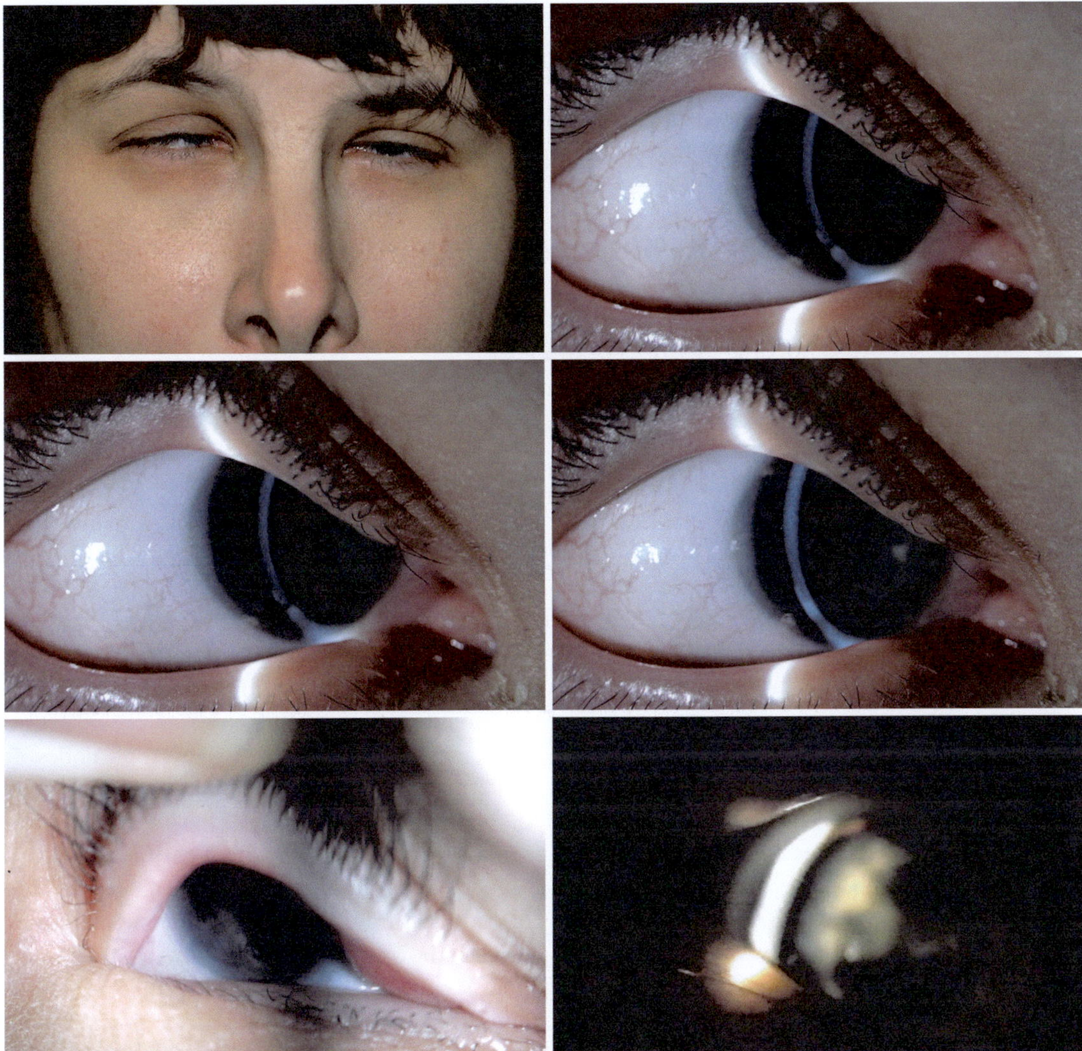

Fig. 3.5 Aniridia on exam of adolescent

An extremity exam, including extremity measurements, should be done, to investigate the possibility of subtle hemihypertrophy. An ophthalmologic finding of aniridia in a patient would markedly increase the chance of a finding of Wilms tumor (Fig. 3.5).

3.5 Laboratory Evaluation

Initial assessment of patient with suspected renal mass should include a complete blood count with differential, with special attention to the hematocrit. Renal function should be assessed through a full panel of electrolytes, including magnesium, phosphorous, and calcium, as well as blood urea nitrogen (BUN) and creatinine (Cr.). It is rare for a patient with a renal tumor to present with renal failure, but compression from mass effect can lead to ureteral compression, more often in patients with bilateral disease. These patients often have expected severe hypertension. Ca has been observed to be markedly elevated in some infants with renal tumors (Bayindir et al. 2009; Amar et al. 2001; Glick 2004). Most commonly, these patients are found to have congenital mesoblastic nephroma or rhabdoid tumor. The hypercalcemia associated with these tumors can be clinically significant and require careful medical management. The underlying cause though is most likely to be from increased secretion of parathyroid hormone. The calcium levels usually improve after surgical resection of the tumor, but can persist for some time and can require medical and pharmaceutical management.

A clotting screen should be performed in every child with a nephroblastoma, including a PT and PTT. Very rarely, a coagulopathy caused by an acquired von Willebrand syndrome (AVWS) is diagnosed during routine laboratory tests (Coppes et al. 1992; Leung et al. 2004). These children do need vWF concentrate or fresh frozen plasma prior to and after surgical procedures (Hickman line insertion, tumor nephrectomy or biopsy). After tumor nephrectomy, the AVWS is always resolved.

A complete urinalysis should be performed. Although uncommon in children with renal tumors relative to adults presenting with renal tumors, hematuria can be the only presenting sign of a renal tumor. This suggests invasion of the tumor into the renal pelvis or less commonly ureter (Senthilnathan et al. 2004) Depending on the location of the tumor in relation to the renal sinus, even a very small tumor unable to be palpated on exam can produce hematuria.

In children presenting with fever, coincident urinary tract infection (UTI) should be ruled out with urine culture, as obstruction can contribute to increased incidence of UTI at diagnosis.

Urinary b-fibroblastic growth factor (b-FGF) has been shown to be elevated in some children with WT, but is currently not a clinically useful test, as it is not a specific or constant finding (Sköldenberg et al. 2001).

Intra-tumoral hemorrhage may occur, resulting sometimes in an emergency situation with a rapid abdominal enlargement and profound and symptomatic anemia. In such a situation, emergent surgery is required. In most of these children, presurgical tumor rupture occurs. This can be a rupture into the abdominal cavity but also to the retroperitoneal space. Sometimes the bleeding into the tumor is compressed by the tumor capsule without a rupture. Only then preoperative chemotherapy might be possible to apply, but one should be aware that shrinkage of the tumor releases the pressure of the intratumoral vessels resulting in a second bleeding. Such children need to stay in the hospital to handle a possible emergency situation. Surgeons should always be involved in such a decision process.

3.6 Imaging Evaluation

If a renal tumor is suspected, either by finding of a mass or unexplained hematuria, hypertension, or other concerning findings, diagnostic imaging should be obtained promptly. Initial radiologic evaluation should be aimed at identifying the presence and origin of the tumor. Once a tumor is confirmed, imaging should be aimed at assessing important staging factors, such as possible rupture, metastatic spread to local lymph nodes or other organs, (primarily liver and lung,) presence of bilateral kidney lesions, and involvement of renal veins as well as the inferior vena cava (IVC). Abdominal and chest radiographs can often identify presence of primary and metastatic disease; however, a thorough diagnostic evaluation should include additional imaging techniques. Although some patients present with massive pulmonary metastasis (Fig. 3.6), computed tomography (CT) scan of the chest is more sensitive for the detection of small, but clinically

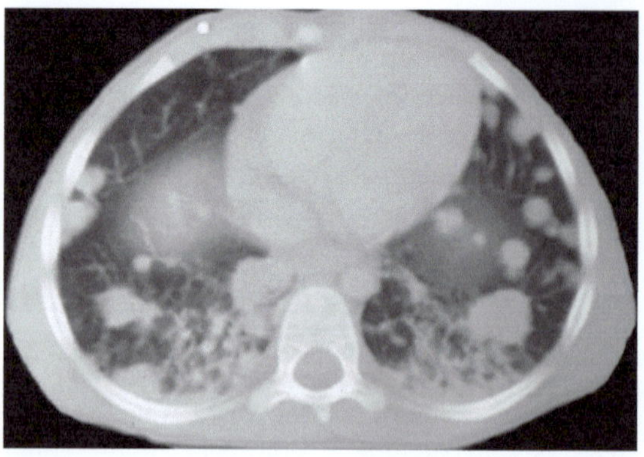

Fig. 3.6 Lung metastasis in a child with Wilms tumor

important pulmonary metastatic lesions (Cohen 2008). Detection of CXR negative but CT positive lesions has been shown to be important to the staging and appropriate therapeutic assignment of patients (Owens 2002).

Abdominal ultrasound provides much valuable information about origin of mass, presence of bilateral lesions, and vascular involvement. It is important to identify patients that present with involvement of tumor thrombus in the renal veins and IVC (Fig. 3.7). This can complicate the risk of upfront surgery, particularly if the tumor thrombus extends through the hepatic portion of the IVC. It can also increase the risk of mortality for the patient. An extension of the tumor and a related thrombus may involve the inferior vena cava and can grow into the right atrium. This is a potential cause of death due to massive cardiac insufficiency. Pulmonary emboli can occur, mandating hospitalization during initial diagnostic and therapeutic period. Immediate surgery is not routinely recommended; as such thrombi can often be successfully managed with initial chemotherapy. In many situations, with good chemotherapy response, the thrombus will shrink and facilitate further surgical procedures. In other cases, surgery has to be done under cardiopulmonary bypass.

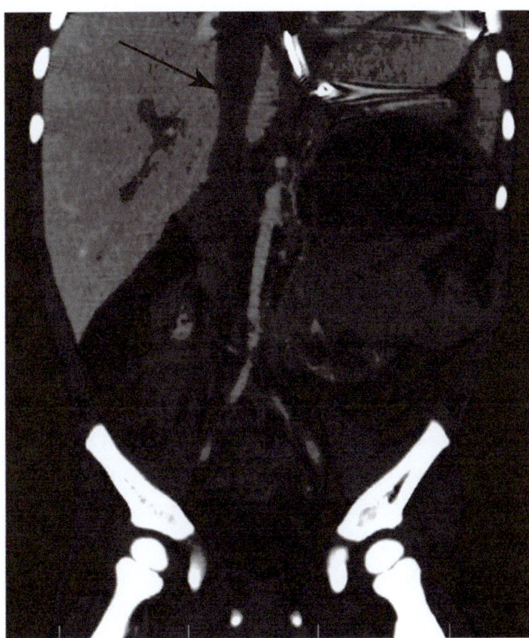

Fig. 3.7 V. cava thrombus in a child with Wilms tumor. The *arrow* indicates the V. cava thrombus

Magnetic resonance imaging (MRI) has been increasingly employed in the initial diagnostic evaluation of renal tumors, but its use is still being studied. It may be useful for more detailed characterization of vessel involvement and for establishing the presence of nephrogenic rests versus tumor.

3.7 Histologic Diagnosis

The use of preoperative chemotherapy versus upfront nephrectomy and the discussion of the merits and flaws of various biopsy techniques are covered in depth in other chapters in this text and will not be discussed here.

3.7.1 Characteristics of Patients as Regards to Stage and Histology at Diagnosis

NWTS V registered 2,596 patients with WT (Dome et al. 2006). Patients were staged according to NWTS staging system (Table 3.3). Although there was central review of pathology and imaging, it was not real time, and assignment of histological type and stage was entered by the local institution.

The overwhelming majority of patients (2,315 of 2,596) had favorable histology WT. Slightly less than one third were under 2 years of age, 1/3 were between ages 2 and 3, and 38 % were over age 4. 82 % of these patients had localized disease (stages 1–III), 13.1 % had metastatic (stage IV) disease, and 5.6 % had bilateral disease.

The incidence of focal anaplasia (FA) and diffuse anaplasia (DA) was much lower and demonstrated different clinical characteristics than the group of FH WT patients. There was a marked increase incidence in female over male patients (FA 74.6 % female, DA 64.9 %). Patients tended to present at older ages, less than 10 % were under age 2, in FA the majority (52.5 %) were between ages 2 and 3, and in DA almost 60 %

Table 3.3 NWTS staging

Stage I
(a) Tumor limited to the kidney and completely excised (b) The tumor was not ruptured before or during removal (c) The vessels of the renal sinus are not involved beyond 2 mm (d) No residual tumor apparent beyond the margins of excision
Stage II (a) Tumor extends beyond the kidney but is completely excised (b) No residual tumor is apparent at or beyond the margins of excision (c) Tumor thrombus in vessels outside the kidney is stage II if the thrombus is removed en bloc with the tumor
Stage III Residual tumor confined to the abdomen: (a) Regional lymph nodes in the renal hilum, the periaortic chains, or beyond shown to contain tumor (b) Diffuse peritoneal contamination by the tumor (c) Peritoneal tumor implants (d) Tumor extends beyond the surgical margins either microscopically or grossly (e) Tumor is not completely resectable because of local infiltration into vital structures
Stage IV Presence of hematogenous metastases or metastases to distant lymph nodes
Stage V Bilateral renal involvement at the time of initial diagnosis

were greater than 4. There was also a higher percentage of metastatic and bilateral disease in both FA and DA groups (FA 25.4 % stage IV, 18.6 % stage V, DA 18.9 % stage IV, 10.8 % stage V).

The NWTS patients are grouped through different staging systems in SIOP and UK protocols (Table 3.4); however, it is still possible to compare the number of patients that present with metastatic and bilateral disease.

European data on overall characteristics of children with WT supports similar rates of metastatic disease found at presentation.

Thirteen percent of patients will be diagnosed with metastatic disease at presentation (Pastore et al. 2006). These children are older with a median age of 5.2 years compared to 3.4 years in localized tumors and they present with larger tumors of more than 600 ml as median tumor volume compared to 400 ml in localized tumors.

Table 3.4 Revised SIOP (after chemotherapy) staging

I	(a) Tumor is limited to kidney or surrounded with fibrous pseudocapsule if outside of the normal contours of the kidney, and the renal capsule or pseudocapsule may be infiltrated with the tumor, but it does not reach the outer surface and is completely resected (resection margins "clear") (b) The tumor may be protruding into the pelvic system and "dipping" into the ureter (but it is not infiltrating their walls) (c) The vessels of the renal sinus are not involved (d) Intrarenal vessel involvement may be present
II	(a) The tumor extends beyond kidney or penetrates through the renal capsule and/or fibrous pseudocapsule into perirenal fat but is completely resected (resection margins "clear") (b) The tumor infiltrates the renal sinus and/or invades blood and lymphatic vessels outside the renal parenchyma but is completely resected (c) The tumor infiltrates adjacent organs or vena cava but is completely resected
III	(a) Incomplete excision of the tumor, which extends beyond resection margins (gross or microscopical tumor remains postoperatively) (b) Any abdominal lymph nodes are involved (c) Tumor rupture before or intraoperatively (irrespective of other criteria for staging) (d) The tumor has penetrated through the peritoneal surface (e) Tumor thrombi present at resection margins of vessels or ureter, transected or removed piecemeal by surgeon (f) The tumor has been surgically biopsied (wedge biopsy) prior to preoperative chemotherapy or surgery
IV	Hematogenous metastases (lung, liver, bone, brain, etc.) or lymph node metastases outside the abdominopelvic region
V	Bilateral renal tumors at diagnosis

More than 60 % of these patients have isolated metastases to the lung and more than 10 % to the liver. Extra-regional lymph node involvement occurs in less than 10 % of patients with metastatic disease. Metastases to bone and brain are uncommon. In case of bone metastasis, diagnosis of clear cell sarcoma of the kidney (CCSK) is more likely. If metastatic disease occurs in infants with a renal tumor, a rhabdoid tumor of the kidney should be considered, for metastases are very unlikely in WTs in this age group.

3.8 Prenatal Diagnosis

Prenatal diagnoses of nephroblastoma are described (Siemer et al. 2004). Such tumors are found during regular ultrasound screens in pregnancy. Interdisciplinary workout between gynecologists, pediatric surgeons, neonatologists, and pediatric oncologist is needed to provide the best treatment for such a child in terms of prolonging pregnancy, way of delivery, and optimal time for surgical removal of the tumor. A sectio Caesarea is always recommended. In most cases, histology shows a mesoblastic nephroma.

3.9 Diagnosis in Patients with Associated Syndromes and Malformations

Patients with syndromes known to have an associated increased risk of developing WT usually undergo routine interval surveillance screening, most often by ultrasound. Therefore, patients with syndromes may present asymptomatically and with lower stage disease. A higher incidence of synchronous and metachronous bilateral WT is associated with many of these syndromes.

3.10 Early Diagnosis: Children Diagnosed on Routine Surveillance

In Germany in about 10 % of patients, an early diagnosis of WT is made during routine scheduled pediatric well-child care, by exam on an asymptomatic child (Gutjahr et al. 1990). Another 15 % of patients are diagnosed during a consultation for other reasons without tumor-related symptoms (Graf et al. 2003). This results in 25 % of children being asymptomatic at the time of diagnosis in Germany.

A comparison between the group of children with and without symptoms was done for children treated according SIOP 93-01 in Germany (Graf et al. 2003). During the time period between April 1994 and December 2001, 947 patients with a Wilms tumor were analyzed. 687 (72.5 %) of them did show tumor-related symptoms at the time of diagnosis (group A), whereas 260 patients (27.5 %) were diagnosed without having such symptoms (group B). Ninety seven patients of group B had no symptoms at all and were diagnosed by casual ultrasound. In 163 patients other symptoms – but not related to the tumor – did lead to the diagnosis. Twenty percent of patients in group B compared to 11.9 % in group A had an underlying syndrome. Age and tumor volume were significantly lower in group B than in group A (median age: 1.73 years versus 3.10 years, $p<0.001$; tumor volume: 222 ml versus 344 ml, $p<0.001$). Stage distribution and histology were in favor of group B. There were less patients with metastatic disease in group B (17 (6.5 %) versus 130 (18.9 %), $p<0.001$). The 5-year relapse-free survival was insignificant better for group B compared to group A (90 % versus 84 %, $p=0.0502$), whereas the overall survival was not different between both groups (91 % versus 90 %). For more detailed information, see Table 3.5. In summary, an earlier diagnosis of WT results in less treatment because of lower stages and a favorable distribution of histological subtypes (Graf et al. 2003). As a regular screening by abdominal ultrasound may contribute to an earlier diagnosis, the question of screening for Wilms tumor has to be answered.

3.10.1 Surveillance in Children with Increased Risk of Wilms Tumor

Regular surveillance in children thought to be at increased risk of Wilms tumor has become widespread in parts of Europe and North America. In the UK, a working group of clinical geneticists, pediatricians, pediatric oncologists, and radiologists was formed to formulate recommendations for Wilms tumor surveillance. These recommendations are based on available evidence from literature, current practice, and expert opinion (Scott et al. 2006a). In their summary, they state the following:

1. Surveillance should be offered to children at 5 % risk of Wilms tumor.
2. Surveillance should be offered only after review by a clinical geneticist.

Table 3.5 Patients treated in Germany according to SIOP 93-01

	all patients		patients with tumor related symptoms or unknown symptoms		patients without symptoms or with symptoms not related to the tumor	
	n	%	n	%	n	%
registered	**947**	**100**	**687**	**72.5**	**260**	**27.5**
Syndromes						
unknown	**74**	**7.8**	**66**	**9.6**	**8**	**3.1**
no	**739**	**78.0**	**539**	**78.5**	**200**	**76.9**
				p <0.05		
yes	**134**	**14.1**	**82**	**11.9**	**52**	**20.0**
Aniridia	7		2		5	
Hemihypertrophy	14		8		6	
Beckwith-Wiedemann	9		2		7	
Denys Drash	3		2		1	
Urogenital malform	41		24		17	
other	83		53		30	

Table 3.6 Molecular genetic investigations to define the risk of Wilms tumor development and indication for screening by ultrasound every 3 months (Scott et al. 2006a, b)

Phenotype	Method	Result	Screening
Aniridia	FISH for PAX6/WT1	Del(WT1)	Yes
WAGR		WT1 normal	No
Denys–Drash syndrome	WT1-Mutation	Yes	Yes
		No	No
Fanconi anemia	BRCA2	Biallelic	Yes
		Monoallelic	No
Mosaic variegated aneuploidy	Karyotype	All	Yes
	BUB1B mutation screen		
Beckwith–Wiedemann syndrome	LOI, UPD 11p15	LOI KvDMR1	No
		LOI CDKN1C	No
		All others	Yes
Simpson–Golabi–Behmel syndrome	GPC3-mutation/deletion	Male	Yes
		Female	No
Perlman syndrome	Unknown	All	Yes
Hemihypertrophy	UPD 11p15	Yes	Yes
		No	No

WAGR Wilms–aniridia–genitourinary–mental retardation, *FISH* fluorescence in situ hybridization, *LOI* loss of imprinting, *UPD* uniparental disomia

3. Surveillance should be carried out by renal ultrasonography every 3 month.
4. Surveillance should continue until 5 years in all conditions except Beckwith–Wiedemann syndrome, Simpson–Golabi–Behmel syndrome and some familial Wilms' tumor pedigrees, where it should continue until 7 years.
5. Surveillance can be undertaken at a local center, but should be carried out by someone with experience of pediatric ultrasonography.
6. Screen-detected lesions should be managed at a specialist center.

The reason to offer surveillance only after review by a clinical geneticist is obvious as there are some malformations and syndromes in which the risk of developing a Wilms tumor can be better excluded after molecular genetic testing. Table 3.6 lists the molecular genetic investigations to define the risk of Wilms tumor development and indication for screening by ultrasound

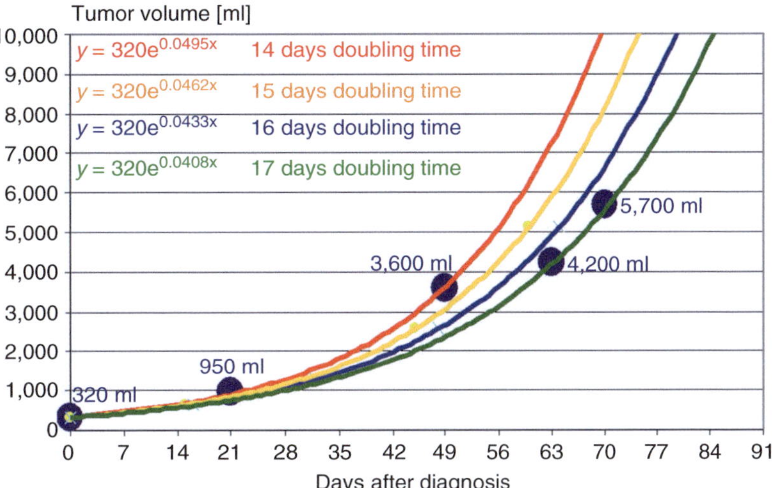

Fig. 3.8 Natural course of a Wilms tumor (Zoubek et al. 1999)

every 3 months (Scott et al. 2006a). In cases where surveillance is indicated, abdominal ultrasound should be done in 3-month intervals. Longer time intervals are not recommended as the doubling time of Wilms tumors is between 2 and 3 weeks (Zoubek et al. 1999) (Fig. 3.8).

References

Amar AM, Tomlinson G, Green DM et al (2001) Clinical presentation of rhabdoid tumors of the kidney. J Pediatr Hematol Oncol 23:105–108

Bayindir P, Guillerman RP, Hicks MJ et al (2009) Cellular mesoblastic nephroma (infantile renal fibrosarcoma): institutional review of the clinical, diagnostic imaging, and pathologic features of a distinctive neoplasm of infancy. Pediatr Radiol 39:1066–1074

Bürger D, Feickert HJ, Mildenberger H (1986) Current status of nephroblastoma treatment. Monogr Paediatr 18:224–242

Cohen M (2008) Wilms tumor: a new method for quantification of lung metastatic tumor burden. Pediatr Radiol 38:817–818

Coppes MJ, Zandvoort SWH, Sparling CR et al (1992) Acquired von Willebrand disease in Wilms' tumor patients. J Clin Oncol 10:422–427

Coppes MJ, Haber DA, Grundy PE (1994) Genetic events in the development of Wilms' tumor. N Engl J Med 331:586–590

Corey B, Yang CH, Wilimas J, Davidoff A, Dome J (2004) Significance of pleural effusion at diagnosis of Wilms tumor. Pediatr Blood Cancer 42:145–148

Cowell JK, Wadey RB, Buckle BB, Pritchard J (1989) The aniridia Wilms' tumor association: molecular and genetic analysis of chromosome deletions on the short arm of chromosome 11. Hum Genet 82:123–126

Dome JS, Cotton CA, Perlman E et al (2006) Treatment of anaplastic Wilms' tumor: results from the fifth National Wilms Tumor Study. J Clin Oncol 24(15): 2352–2358

Glick RD, Hicks MJ, Nuchtern JG et al (2004) Renal tumors in infants less than 6 months of age. J Pediatr Surg 39:522–525

Graf N, Reinhard H, Aliani S et al (2003) Wilms tumour with or without tumour related symptoms at diagnosis. Med Pediatr Oncol 41:266 O036 (abstract)

Gronskov K, Olsen JH, Sand A, Pedersen W, Carlsen N, Bak Jylling AM, Lyngbye T, Brondum-Nielsen K, Rosenberg T (2001) Population-based risk estimates of Wilms tumor in sporadic aniridia. A comprehensive mutation screening procedure of PAX6 identifies 80% of mutations in aniridia. Hum Genet 109: 11–18

Gutjahr P, Kaatsch P, Spaar HJ et al (1990) Klinik, Therapie und Prognose bei 373 Kindern mit Wilms-Tumoren – Ergebnisse der bundesweiten Studie 1980–1988. Akt Urol 121:132–141

Leung RS, Liesner R, Brock P et al (2004) Coagulopathy as a presenting feature of Wilms tumour. Eur J Pediatr 163:369–373

Maas MH, Cransberg K, van Grotel M et al (2007) Renin-induced hypertension in Wilms tumor patients. Pediatr Blood Cancer 48:500–503

Owens CM, Veys PA, Pritchard J et al (2002) Role of chest computed tomography at diagnosis in the management of Wilms' tumor: a study by the United Kingdom Children's Cancer Study Group. J Clin Oncol 20:2768–2773

Pastore G, Znaor A, Spreafico F, Graf N et al (2006) Malignant renal tumours incidence and survival in European children (1978–1997): report from the

Automated Childhood Cancer Information System project. Eur J Cancer 42:2103–2114
Ramsay NK, Dehner LP, Coccia PF et al (1977) Acute hemorrhage into Wilms tumor: a cause of rapidly developing abdominal mass with hypertension, anemia, and fever. J Pediatr 91:763–765
Ritchey M, Daleya S, Shamberg R, Ehrlich P, Hamilton T, Haased G, Sawine R (2008) Ureteral extension in Wilms' tumor: a report from the National Wilms' Tumor Study Group. J Pediatr Surg 43(9):1625–1629
Rump P, Zeegers MP, van Essen AJ (2005) Tumor risk in Beckwith-Wiedemann syndrome: a review and meta-analysis. Am J Med Genet A 136:95–104
Ruteshouser EC, Huff V (2004) Familial Wilms tumor. Am J Med Genet C Semin Med Genet 129C:29–34
Sköldenberg EG, Christiansson J, Sandstedt B et al (2001) Angiogenesis and angiogenic growth factors in Wilms tumor. J Urol 165:2274–2279
Scott RH, Walker L, Olsen ØE et al (2006a) Surveillance for Wilms Tumour in at-risk children: pragmatic recommendations for best practice. Arch Dis Child 91:995–999
Scott RH, Stiller CA, Walker L et al (2006b) Syndromes and constitutional chromosomal abnormalities associated with Wilms tumour. J Med Genet 43: 705–715
Senthilnathan R, Bagdi RK, Senthilganesh K, Senthilbarathi (2004) Interesting presentations of Wilms' tumor. J Indian Assoc Pediatr Surg 9: 193–197
Siemer S, Lehmann J, Reinhard H et al (2004) Prenatal diagnosis of congenital mesoblastic nephroma associated with renal hypertension in a premature child. Int J Urol 11:50–51
Zoubek A, Slavc I, Mann G et al (1999) Natural course of a Wilms' tumour. Lancet 354:344

Pathology of Renal Tumors of Childhood

4

Gordan M. Vujanic

Contents

Abstract

Postoperative treatment of renal tumors of childhood is based on their histological diagnosis and subtyping and their stage (for localised tumors), which are determined by pathological examination of the nephrectomy specimen. In order to ensure that the child is treated appropriately, it is vital that pathological examination provides an accurate diagnosis and stage. In the COG (Children's Oncology Group, former National Wilms Tumor Study Group) trials, postoperative treatment is also influenced by molecular markers (loss of heterozygosity for chromosomes 1p and 16q), age of the patient and size of the tumor (Perlman, Pediatr Dev Pathol 8:320–338, 2005).

G.M. Vujanic, MD, PhD, FRCPath
Department of Cellular Pathology,
Cardiff University School of Medicine, Heath Park,
Cardiff CF14 4XN, UK
e-mail: vujanic@cf.ac.uk

K. Pritchard-Jones, J.S. Dome (eds.), *Renal Tumors of Childhood: Biology and Therapy*, Pediatric Oncology,
DOI 10.1007/978-3-662-44003-2_4,

4.1 Classification/Subtypes

Presently, there are two principal histological classifications of renal tumors of childhood: the COG and SIOP (International Society of Paediatric Oncology) classifications (Perlman 2005; Vujanic et al. 2002). They differ only in the subclassification of Wilms' tumor, whereas other renal tumors of childhood are classified in the same way (Table 4.1).

It is worth emphasising that there are differences in terminology between the SIOP and COG classifications as different criteria are used for subclassifying tumors, making a direct comparison problematic. The key differences are that in the SIOP, chemotherapy-induced changes are taken into account for subclassifying tumors (and they do not exist in primarily operated tumors) and that the amount of blastema in defining the stromal and epithelial types is critical (*see below*).

Table 4.1 Comparison of the SIOP and COG classifications

SIOP	COG
Low-risk tumor	
CPDN	CPDN
Mesoblastic nephroma	Mesoblastic nephroma
WT – completely necrotic	
Intermediate risk	*Favourable histology*
	Favourable histology (non-anaplastic) WTs
WT – mixed type	Mixed
WT – regressive type	Blastemal predominant
WT – epithelial type	Epithelial predominant
WT – stromal type	Stromal predominant
WT – focal anaplasia	
High risk	*Unfavourable histology*
WT – blastemal type	
WT – diffuse anaplasia	WT – anaplastic (focal and diffuse anaplasia)
Clear cell sarcoma of the kidney	Clear cell sarcoma of the kidney
Rhabdoid tumor of the kidney	Rhabdoid tumor of the kidney

SIOP International Society of Paediatric Oncology, *COG* Children's Oncology Group, *CPDN* cystic partially differentiated nephroblastoma, *WT* Wilms' tumor

In both classifications, there are two main groups: non-anaplastic and anaplastic tumors. Subtyping of non-anaplastic Wilms' tumor is based on the percentages of tumor's components. If all three components are present and none of them is predominant (occupying more than 2/3 of the tumor), tumor is regarded as mixed (also called triphasic of classical) type. Similarly, if only two components are present and none of them is predominant, tumor is still regarded as mixed. When only one component is present (monophasic tumors), tumors are assigned according to that component.

In the COG classification, which is used for primarily operated Wilms' tumors, if one component comprises more than 2/3 of tumor mass, tumor is labelled accordingly (blastemal or epithelial or stromal predominant), irrespectively of what the remaining component is (Murphy et al. 2004).

The SIOP classification is used when Wilms' tumors are treated with preoperative chemotherapy followed by surgery, and it contains more types which are separated into three risk groups: low, intermediate and high risk (Table 4.1). The criteria for subclassification include the assessment of percentage of chemotherapy-induced changes and the amount of blastema in the viable tumor (Table 4.2) (Vujanic et al. 2002). Stromal- and epithelial-type tumors may contain only up to 10 % of blastema, irrespectively on the percentage of the predominant component (which may be even up to 90 %) – if more than 10 % of blastema is present, tumor is subclassified as mixed (Vujanic et al. 2002). The reason for introducing these criteria in the SIOP subtyping was to investigate whether the stromal and epithelial subtypes with <10 % of blastemal could be treated with less therapy and even moved to low-risk tumors.

For these reasons, it is important to bear in mind that although the terms used in the COG and SIOP subtyping of Wilms' tumor are similar, they do not necessarily describe the same histology and make a direct comparison of the prognosis more complicated.

Table 4.2 SIOP histological criteria for subtyping of Wilms' tumors

WT – completely necrotic type
No viable tumor persists
WT – mixed type
Three or two components present, none of which occupies more than 2/3 of the viable tumor
WT – epithelial type
Epithelial component comprises more than 2/3 of the viable tumor
The remaining viable tumor comprises stromal (up to 1/3) and blastemal (up to 10 %) components
WT – stromal type
Stromal component comprises more than 2/3 of the viable tumor
The remaining viable tumor comprises epithelial (up to 1/3) and blastemal (up to 10 %) components
WT – regressive type
Chemotherapy-induced changes comprise more than 2/3 of the tumor
The remaining tumor comprise one, two or three WT components in any proportion
WT – focal anaplasia type
Localised anaplasia in any of WT types
WT – blastemal type
Blastemal component comprises more than 2/3 of the viable tumor
The remaining viable tumor comprises epithelial and/or stromal components in any proportion
WT – diffuse anaplasia type
Non-localised anaplasia in any of WT types

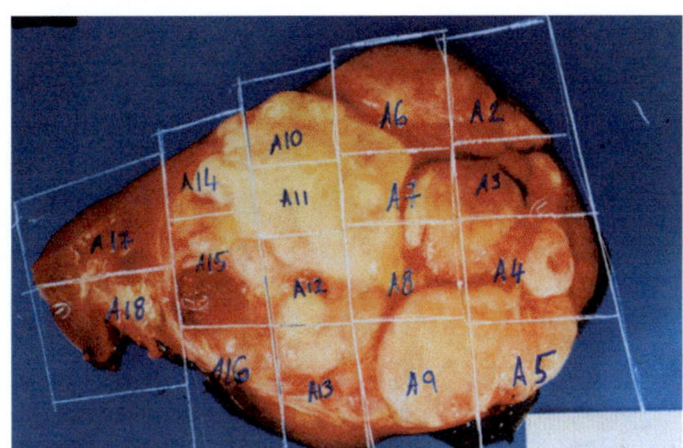

Fig. 4.1 Tumor sampling should include at least one whole slice of the tumor with a block guide

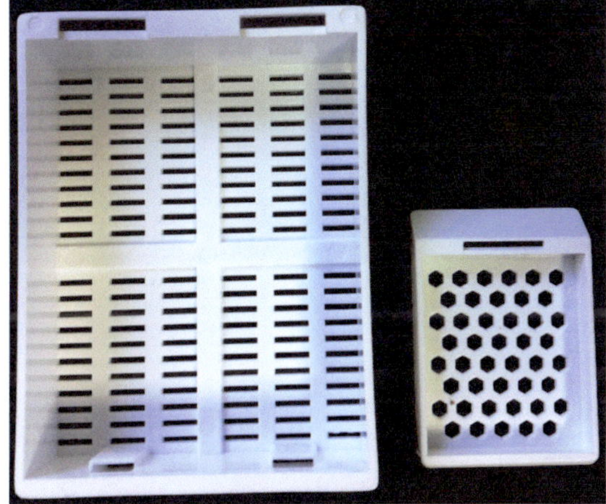

Fig. 4.2 Mega-cassettes vs. normal-sized cassettes which make sampling and microscopic assessment of tumor components easier

Since the accurate assessment of different tumor's component is critical for SIOP subclassification, it is important to sample the tumor according to the established protocol (Vujanic and Sandstedt 2010) which requires that *at least* one whole slice of tumor surface is blocked (Fig. 4.1). The first step in assessing a pretreated tumor is to determine the percentage of chemotherapy-induced changes. After that, the percentages of viable tumor's components are assessed and tumors subclassified accordingly (Table 4.2).

The accurate assessment of the percentages of different tumor components is not simple. There is no objective way of doing that, as it is a semi-quantitative exercise based on review of many slides and on pathologist's experience, so it is not surprising that there are significant discrepancies between institutional pathologists' and central pathology review's results (Vujanic et al. 2009). A way forward might be a replacement of normal-sized blocks with mega blocks (Fig. 4.2) which make the whole exercise easier.

Another problem is that preoperative chemotherapy alters histological features, and, not infrequently, it is challenging to distinguish genuine histological features from chemotherapy-induced changes. Occasionally, it may be even difficult to evaluate whether the tumor is viable or not, and, again, there are no perfect criteria on the basis on

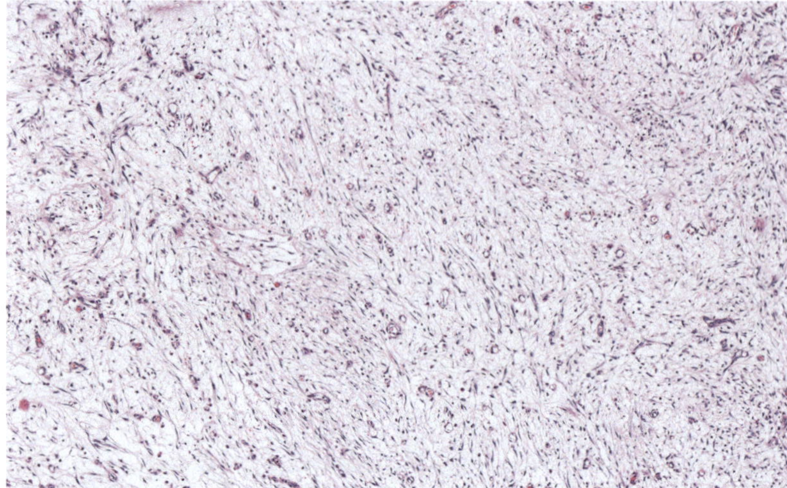

Fig. 4.3 Hypocellular tumor stroma which may be difficult to distinguish from stroma with chemotherapy-induced changes

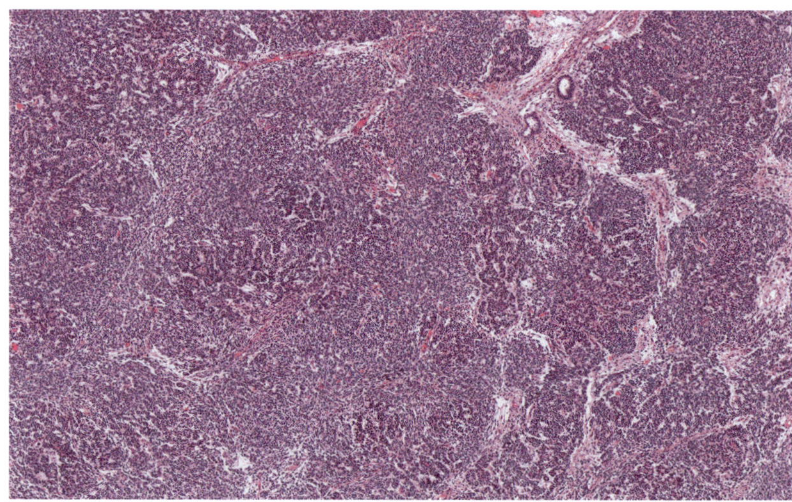

Fig. 4.4 A blastemal tumor component with areas of epithelial differentiation

which one could be absolutely certain about it. Further, distinguishing between a genuine hypocellular tumor stroma and chemotherapy-induced changes resulting in a stroma-like appearance may be difficult (Fig. 4.3). The finding of foamy macrophages would favour the latter.

Even more difficult is how to distinguish between blastema and early epithelial differentiation (Fig. 4.4) as no firm histological or immunohistochemical criteria are of any help.

Still, the vast majority of tumors can be subclassified relatively confidently and treated appropriately. But it may be a real challenge in a small number of so-called borderline cases where the amount of regressive or blastemal component is close to 2/3 of the tumor, where a particular tumor may be subclassified in either intermediate- or high-risk group with very serious and important therapeutic consequences. For example, if the tumor shows widespread chemotherapy-induced changes and a viable part is predominantly or all blastemal and if a pathologist estimates that chemotherapy-induced changes occupy just over 2/3 of tumor mass, tumor will be labelled as regressive type, intermediate risk. If, however, the estimate of chemotherapy-induced changes is that they occupy just under 2/3 of tumor, then it will be labelled as blastemal type, high-risk tumor. Similarly, if blastemal component in the tumor is close to 2/3 of the viable tumor, judging it as over 2/3 would mean blastemal type, high-risk tumor, and less than 2/3 would mean mixed type, intermediate risk.

As discussed elsewhere, the results of the latest SIOP 2001 Trial indicate that the volume rather than percentage of blastema is the most critical prognostic factor in non-anaplastic case (Graf et al. 2011), but the formula used to calculate the volume is based on the percentages of tumor components, so the problem will remain until some biological markers of 'bad' blastema are found and replace this semi-quantitative method.

4.2 Staging

Together with a histological subtype, stage is the second determining factor for postoperative treatment of Wilms' tumor in the SIOP protocol. Again, the COG and SIOP staging criteria differ in some details (Tables 4.3 and 4.4) and should be applied depending on pre-nephrectomy treatment. However, in both primarily operated and pretreated Wilms' tumors, staging is difficult

Table 4.3 SIOP WT 2001 staging criteria for renal tumors of childhood

Stage I
(a) The tumor is limited to the kidney or surrounded with a fibrous (pseudo)capsule if outside of the normal contours of the kidney. The renal capsule or pseudocapsule may be infiltrated by the tumor but it does not reach the outer surface
(b) The tumor may be protruding ('bulging') into the pelvic system and 'dipping' into the ureter, but it is not infiltrating their walls
(c) The renal sinus (its vessels and soft tissues) is not involved
(d) Intrarenal vessels may be involved
Notes: Fine needle aspiration or percutaneous core needle ('tru-cut') biopsy does not upstage the tumor, but the size of the needle gauge should be mentioned to the pathologist
The presence of necrotic tumor or chemotherapy-induced change in the renal sinus and/or within the perirenal fat should not be regarded as a reason for upstaging a tumor provided it is completely excised and does not reach the resection margins
Stage II
(a) Viable tumor penetrates through the renal capsule and/or fibrous pseudocapsule into perirenal fat but is completely resected (resection margins 'clear')
(b) Viable tumor infiltrates the soft tissues and/or blood and/or lymphatic vessels of the renal sinus
(c) Viable tumor infiltrates the perirenal tissue but it is completely resected
(d) Viable tumor infiltrates the renal pelvic or ureter's wall
(e) Viable tumor infiltrates adjacent organs or vena cava but is completely resected
Notes: Infiltration of the adrenal gland is not regarded as stage II if there is a (pseudo)capsule. Equally, tumor adherence to the liver is not regarded as stage II for which there should be a genuine infiltration of the liver parenchyma
Stage III
(a) Viable or non-viable tumor present at resection margins
(b) Any abdominal lymph nodes are involved
(c) Tumor rupture before or intraoperatively (irrespective of other criteria for staging)
(d) Tumor penetration through the peritoneal surface
(e) Tumor implants are found on the peritoneal surface
(f) Tumor thrombi present at resection margins of extra-renal vessels, transsected or removed piecemeal by surgeon
(g) The tumor has been surgically biopsied (wedge biopsy) prior to preoperative chemotherapy or surgery
Note: The presence of necrotic tumor or chemotherapy-induced changes in a lymph node or at the resection margins is regarded as proof of previous tumor with microscopic residue, and therefore the tumor is assigned stage III (because of the possibility that some viable tumor is left behind in the adjacent lymph node or beyond the resection margins)
Stage IV
Haematogenous metastases (lung, liver, bone, brain, etc.) or lymph node metastases outside the abdominopelvic region
Stage V
Bilateral renal tumors at diagnosis. Each side should be substaged according to the above criteria

Table 4.4 COG staging criteria for renal tumors (Perlman 2005)

Stage I
Tumor limited to the kidney and completely resected
Intact renal capsule
No previous rupture or biopsy
Renal sinus vessels not involved
No evidence of tumor at or beyond the margins of resection
Stage II
Tumor completely resected
No evidence of tumor at or beyond the margins of resection
Tumor extends beyond the kidney, as evidenced by one of the following:
Penetration through the renal capsule
Extensive invasion of the soft tissue of the renal sinus
Blood vessels within the nephrectomy specimen outside the renal parenchyma, including those of the renal sinus, contain tumor
Stage III
Residual non-haematogenous tumor confined to the abdomen is present after surgery as evidenced by any one of the following:
Involvement of lymph nodes with the abdomen or pelvis
Penetration through the peritoneal surface
Tumor implants on the peritoneal surface
Tumor present at the margin of surgical resection
Tumor not resectable because of local infiltration into vital structures
Biopsy of tumor prior to removal of kidney
Tumor spillage of any degree or localisation occurring before or during surgery
Tumor removed in greater than one piece
Stage IV
Haematogenous metastases (lung, liver, bone, brain, etc.)
Lymph node metastases outside the abdominopelvic region
Stage V
Bilateral renal involvement at diagnosis
Each side should be separately staged according to the above criteria

because tumors are often very large and distort normal anatomical structures (renal sinus, renal capsule, etc.).

With the aim of achieving the correct stage of the tumor, tumor sampling has to be done following the recommended approach/protocol (Tables 4.5 and 4.6) (Vujanic and Sandstedt 2010).

Table 4.5 Handling of the nephrectomy specimen

1. The specimen must be weighed, measured (in all three dimensions) and photographed. Areas with suspected ruptures and/or invasion should be inked in different colours from the rest of the specimen. A tumor capsule must not be stripped as it would make determination of growth beyond the capsule impossible
2. Perirenal and perihilar lymph nodes should be searched for and sampled separately
3. The renal vein, artery and ureter should be identified and sampled near the resection margin
4. The surface of the whole specimen should be inked and let it dry before opening the specimen. This is a crucial step and should always be done or else it might not be possible to stage the tumor
5. The specimen should be opened by a longitudinal incision to reveal the tumor and its relation to the kidney, capsule and renal sinus
6. The cut surface should be photographed and its macroscopic appearance recorded. The tumor dimensions should be measured and the percentage of necrosis assessed
7. Samples of fresh tumor and normal renal tissue should be taken for tumor banking and molecular studies
8. The specimen should be fixed in 4 % buffered formalin for 24–48 h, according to the usual procedure of the laboratory. Several additional cuts can be made parallel to the initial cut to divide the specimen into 'slabs' for better fixation
9. After fixation, blocks should be taken according to the recommended protocol (see Table 4.6)

It is critical to ink the surface and all suspicious areas on the nephrectomy specimen and to have a photo block guide showing clearly where the blocks have been taken from. Since histological features within one tumor vary from field to field, one whole slice (including necrotic areas) is regarded as a minimum acceptable sample, but further blocks (including another whole slice or two) should be taken whenever possible. With introduction of mega-cassettes, it has become much easier and more convenient, and often one slice can be blocked in 4–6 mega-cassettes.

It is important to emphasise that in the SIOP, staging is done on the basis of the findings *at the time of nephrectomy*, so, for example, even the finding of a viable tumor in the perirenal fat but covered by a pseudocapsule (its formation in this site is usually chemotherapy-induced) is regarded as stage I. The presence of

Table 4.6 Required sampling of renal tumors

1. *At least* one slice of the tumor should be sampled and carefully recorded
2. Areas of doubtful resection, as marked by the surgeon or pathologist
3. Sinus lymph nodes when present
4. Other lymph nodes
5. Renal sinus, ureter and sinus vessels. The renal vein should be scrutinised for evidence of tumor thrombus; if present, it is critical to assess whether it is completely resected
6. Each nodule away from the main mass (in multifocal tumors)
7. Tumor–kidney interface
8. Tumor–kidney capsule
9. Areas of the capsule that are suspected of being invaded by the tumor
10. Areas of perirenal fat suspected for tumor infiltration (important for assessment whether the tumor is completely resected)
11. Areas of adhesions of the tumor to surrounding tissues
12. At least 2 blocks of the normal kidney and blocks from abnormal-looking areas in the remaining renal tissue

chemotherapy-induced changes in the renal sinus (soft tissues and its vessels) and perirenal fat, even with no pseudocapsule, is disregarded for staging purposes. Only if a clearly non-viable tumor and/or chemotherapy-induced changes (foamy macrophages) are present at the resection margins, it is taken into account and regarded as evidence of stage III. Similarly, the finding of both viable and non-viable tumor in a lymph node is regarded as a positive finding (Vujanic and Sandstedt 2010).

4.3 Wilms' Tumor (Nephroblastoma)

4.3.1 Gross Features

Wilms' tumor usually presents as a unilateral, solitary, spherical mass sharply demarcated from the renal parenchyma, rising anywhere in the kidney and distorting its counters. In ~7 % of cases, it may be bilateral and in ~10 % of cases multicentric (Birch and Breslow 1995; Breslow et al. 1993; Murphy et al. 2004). They are usually large with a median weight of 550 g, but their weight varies from 60 to 6,000 g (Murphy et al. 2004). The appearances on the cut surface depend on the preoperative treatment. In primarily operated tumor, areas of necrosis and haemorrhage are usually not extensive. Tumor tissue is clearly demarcated from the renal parenchyma and there is usually a well-formed capsule. Tumor is grey-white or pink-grey in colour, lobulated, soft and friable. Some tumors may have a prominent cystic appearance, but there are usually solid areas too, making a differential diagnosis from cystic nephroma/cystic partially differentiated nephroblastoma easier. Rarely, tumor may show a botryoid growth pattern in the renal pelvis. In pretreated case, areas of necrosis and haemorrhage are usually more prominent and widespread, and viable tumor may be difficult to find. However, for SIOP subclassification purpose, it is important to sample not only areas of an apparently viable tumor but also what on gross examination appears non-viable and confirm that on microscopic examination. In very rare cases, tumor may grow into the inferior vena cava and reach the right atrium.

4.3.2 Microscopic Features

Wilms' tumor comprises three components: blastemal, epithelial and stromal, which may be present in any proportion, resulting in triphasic, biphasic or monophasic tumors (Murphy et al. 2004). Furthermore, the blastemal component may show different patterns, and the epithelial and stromal components may show different lines and degrees of differentiation, resulting in innumerable patterns with no two Wilms' tumors looking the same. Some Wilms' tumors may display prominent teratoid features which are of no prognostic significance, and such tumors are subclassified on the basis of their other components. Preoperative chemotherapy destroys some tumor's components, most commonly the blastemal, or results in maturation of others, particularly the stromal component (Weirich et al. 2001).

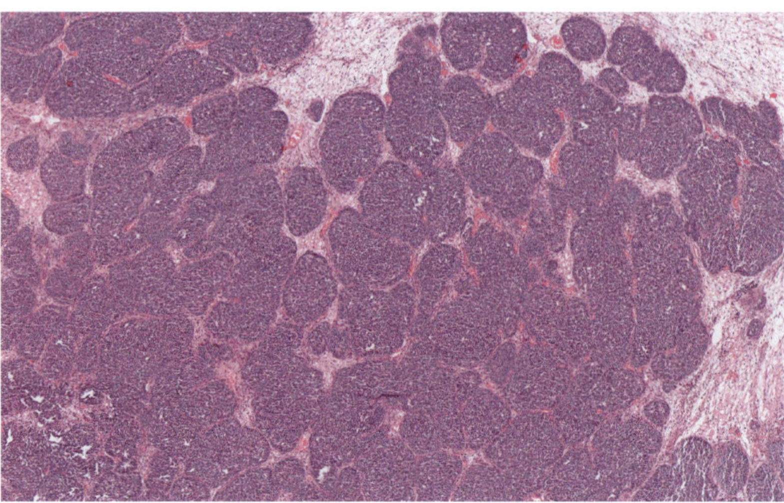

Fig. 4.5 Nodular blastemal pattern

Blastema is the least differentiated component consisting of small- to medium-sized blastemal cells with relatively small, regular nuclei and small nucleoli. The blastema may show different patterns including diffuse, serpentine, nodular and basaloid patterns which may be found in the same tumor and are of no prognostic significance (Fig. 4.5). A characteristic feature of blastemal cells is finely dispersed chromatin and overlapping nuclei (Murphy et al. 2004). A mitotic activity is usually very high. Being the most primitive, undifferentiated component, blastema is also the most aggressive component. However, it is very chemotherapy sensitive and usually disappears under preoperative chemotherapy, except for a small number of cases in which it resists this therapy. The recent SIOP Trial 2001 results indicate that the volume of blastema after preoperative chemotherapy is a significant prognostic factor which may be used in a new SIOP treatment stratification scheme (Graf et al. 2011).

An *epithelial component* is present in most WT. It may show nephrogenic epithelial elements which can be poorly differentiated, such as rosette-like structures, moderately differentiated, such as tubules and papillary structures, and well differentiated, such as glomerular-like structures and mature tubules (Fig. 4.6a–d). Heterologous epithelial elements such as squamous epithelium, respiratory type and gastrointestinal epithelium are more frequently found in tumor treated with preoperative chemotherapy. Epithelial-type Wilms' tumor occurs in much younger children than other types (median age is 15 months vs. 40 months for all other Wilms' tumors), and in over 80 % of cases, it is stage I (Verschuur et al. 2010).

A *stromal component* may also show nephrogenic and heterologous elements. Nephrogenic elements may vary from undifferentiated myxoid and spindle cell or hypocellular areas well-differentiated stroma with rhabdomyoblastic differentiation (Fig. 4.7a). Heterologous elements include adipose tissue, cartilage (Fig. 4.7b), osteoid and even neuroglial tissue (Murphy et al. 2004). In some cases stromal component may be predominantly or entirely composed of mature rhabdomyoblasts prompting the name fetal rhabdomyomatous Wilms' tumor. However, apart from being an interesting observation, this feature has no influence on prognosis, and these tumors should not be separated from other stromal Wilms' tumors. Stromal-type Wilms' tumor also tends to occur in younger children (median age is 28 months); they have a tendency for intra-pelvic, botryoid growth pattern and are bilateral in ~30 % of cases (Murphy et al. 2004; Verschuur et al. 2010).

Anaplasia is a histological feature which occurs in 5–8 % of WT and is associated with adverse prognosis (Dome et al. 2006). Anaplasia may occur in any of the tumor's components but it is rare in the stroma. Histological criteria for anaplasia include the presence of enlarged, atypical, tri- or multipolar mitotic figures, marked nuclear enlargement and hyperchromasia (Fig. 4.8). All three features have to be present, although in tumors with low mitotic activity, it may be more difficult to find more than one or two atypical mitoses. In atypical mitotic figures, each arm should be larger than the one of a normal mitosis. Marked nuclear enlargement means that these nuclei are at least three times larger than normal adjacent nuclei (Faria et al. 1996).

Anaplasia is subclassified as focal and diffuse. Focal anaplasia (or localised anaplasia) is now defined as the presence of anaplastic changes in one or few sharply defined foci within the tumor (Fig. 4.9), with no evidence of marked nuclear atypia elsewhere in the tumor. The diagnosis of diffuse anaplasia should be made in the following cases: the finding of a non-localised (multifocal) anaplasia, anaplasia which is not sharply demarcated from non-anaplastic tumor, focal anaplasia with marked 'nuclear unrest' elsewhere in the tumor, anaplasia beyond the original tumor capsule (such as in intrarenal vessels) and/or in metastases and anaplasia in a random biopsy sample (Faria et al. 1996). Focal anaplasia is less common than diffuse anaplasia (21 % vs. 79 %,

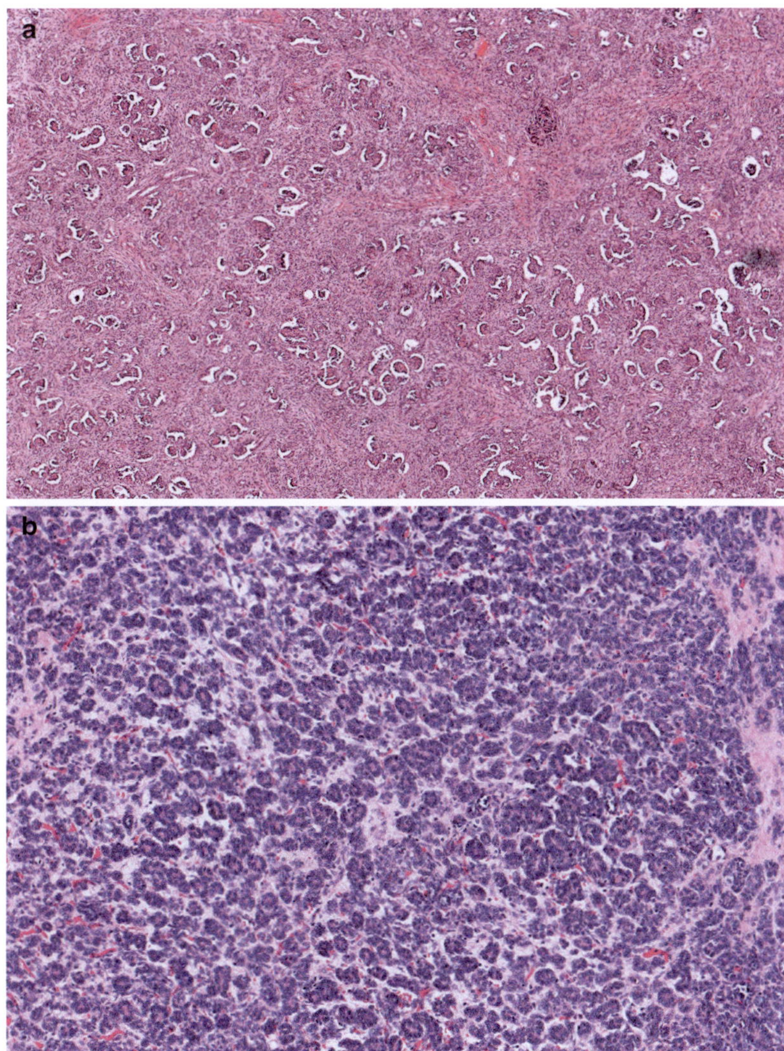

Fig. 4.6 Different epithelial elements including (**a**) glomeruli, (**b**) well-differentiated tubules, (**c**) moderately differentiated tubules and (**d**) squamous epithelium

Fig. 4.6 (continued)

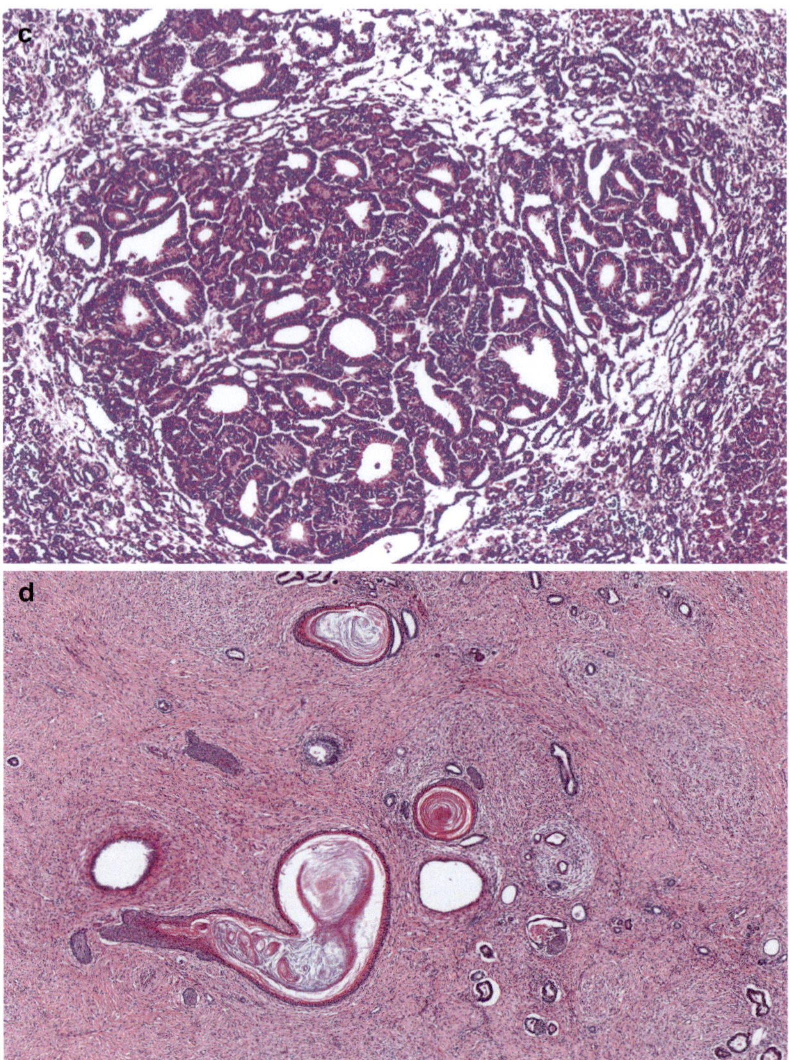

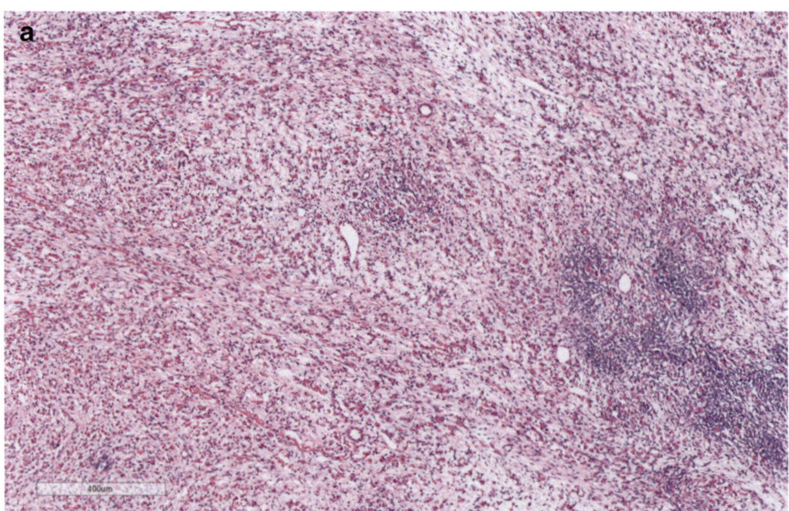

Fig. 4.7 A stromal component with (**a**) skeletal muscle and (**b**) cartilaginous differentiation

Fig. 4.7 (continued)

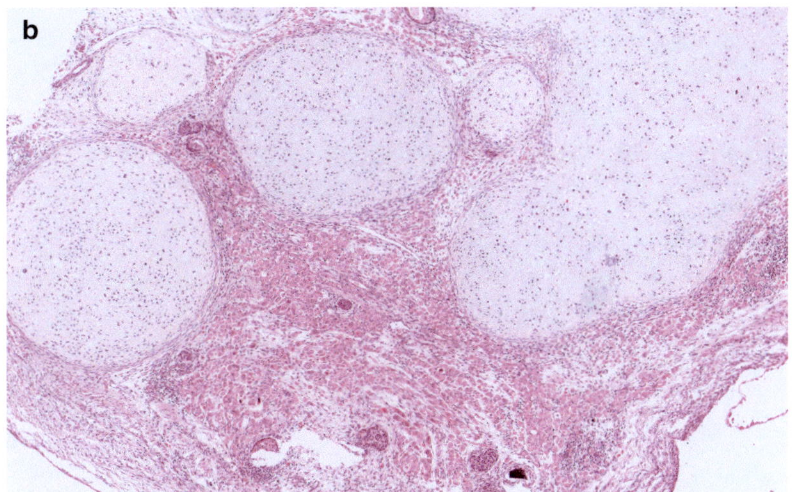

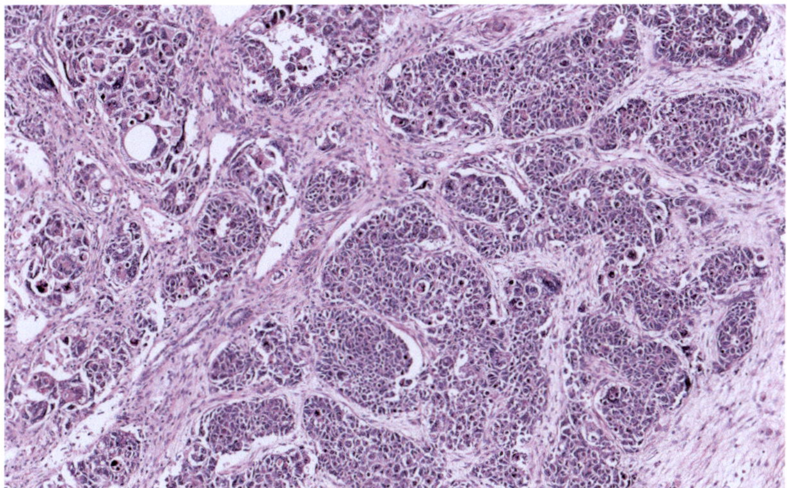

Fig. 4.8 Wilms' tumor showing anaplastic features including atypical mitoses, nuclear enlargement and hyperchromasia

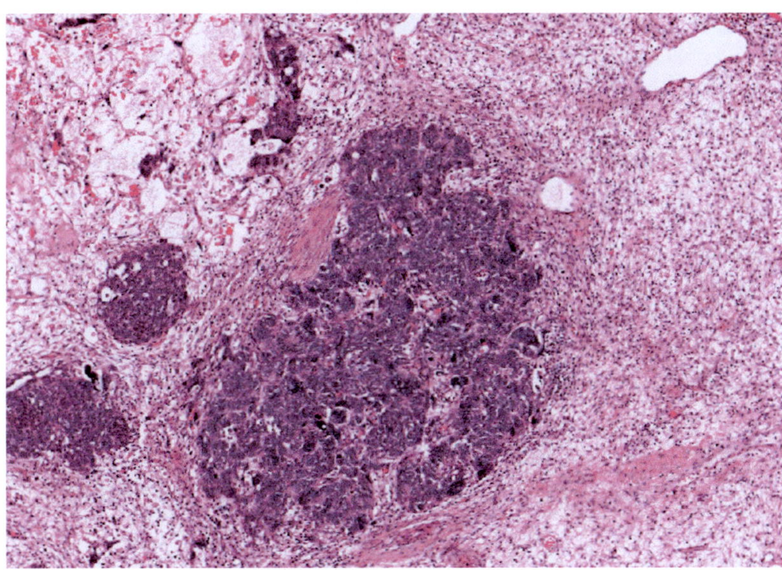

Fig. 4.9 Wilms' tumor with focal anaplasia

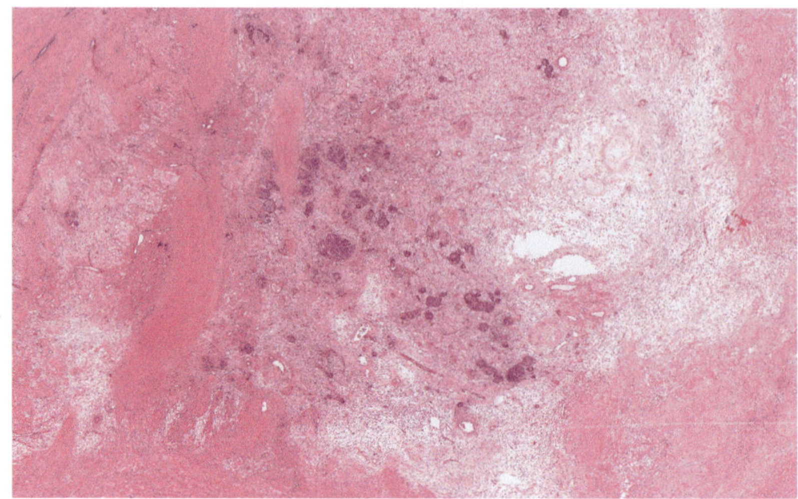

Fig. 4.10 Massive chemotherapy-induced changes with some small foci of viable tumor

respectively) (Dome et al. 2006). While anaplasia is generally a chemotherapy-resistant cell clone and therefore cannot be obliterated or induced by chemotherapy (Sebire et al. 2010), there are rare cases of bilateral tumors treated with prolonged chemotherapy which eventually became anaplastic suggesting that prolonged chemotherapy may induce change to anaplastic clone (Popov et al. 2013). Anaplasia is associated with TP53 mutations and is often (but not always) positive using p53 immunohistochemical staining.

Despite the fact that histological criteria for anaplasia are well established and known for many years, it still represents a serious diagnostic challenge with 39 % and 28 % of cases misdiagnosed in the NWTS and UK trials, respectively (Dome et al. 2006; Sebire et al. 2010). Anaplasia should not be confused with the so-called pseudo-anaplastic changes which are frequently seen in the skeletal muscle tumor's component especially in pretreated tumors, but in such cases, despite sometimes striking nuclear enlargement and pleomorphism, atypical mitoses are not present.

Chemotherapy-induced changes are seen in tumors which have been treated with preoperative chemotherapy, as in the SIOP trials. They include necrosis, fibrosis, haemosiderin deposits and replacement of tumor cells with xanthomatous, foamy histiocytes (Figs. 4.10 and 4.11) (Vujanic and Sandstedt 2010). Other chemotherapy-induced changes include maturation of blastemal, epithelial and stromal components. There is a significant difference in distribution of Wilms' tumor types between primarily operated and cases treated with preoperatively chemotherapy, including blastemal (35.2 % vs. 4.9 %), epithelial (14 % vs. 6.6 %) and stromal (4.9 % vs. 13.7 %) types, respectively (Vujanic et al. 2010). Some tumors may respond to preoperative chemotherapy so well that no viable tumor is found at nephrectomy (completely necrotic-type, low-risk tumor). On the other hand, a small number of tumors (~5 %) with a significant blastemal component show poor or no response to preoperative chemotherapy requiring more aggressive postoperative therapy (Vujanic et al. 2002). Preoperative chemotherapy makes an overall assessment of tumor's histology and its stage more difficult since different components and criteria have to be taken into account, which may result in discrepancies in diagnosis and staging between the institutional pathologists and central pathology review (Vujanic et al. 2009).

4.3.3 Immunohistochemistry

There are no characteristic immunohistochemical features of Wilms' tumor which could be

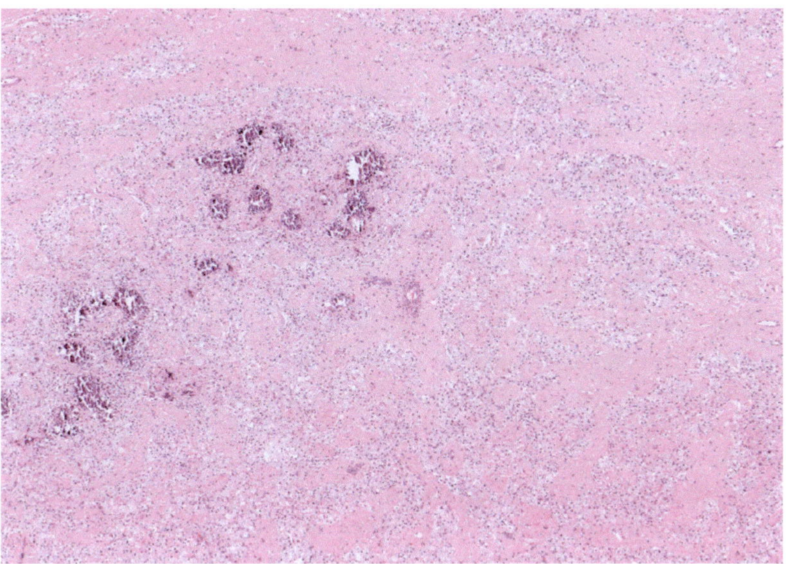

Fig. 4.11 Areas of Wilms' tumor with no viable tumor which is replaced by foamy macrophages (chemotherapy-induced changes)

helpful in the differential diagnosis when necessary. WT1 marker is positive in the blastemal component in ~80 % of cases (nuclear positivity), whereas it is variably and patchy positive in the differentiated epithelial component (Murphy et al. 2004). CD56 is a valuable marker of blastemal cells (Muir et al. 2001). Vimentin is always positive in the blastema, and other markers such as desmin, epithelial markers and CD99 may show variable and focal positivity (Murphy et al. 2004). The epithelial component is positive for CD57 and AE1 (Muir et al. 2001). PAX2 is positive in the epithelial and blastemal components (97 % of cases), stromal (23 %) and anaplastic foci (80 % of cases), but it is also positive in nephrogenic rests, metanephric adenoma and renal cell carcinoma (Davis et al. 2011).

4.3.4 Differential Diagnosis

The diagnosis of Wilms' tumor is usually straightforward in triphasic or even biphasic Wilms' tumors, although their subclassification may be challenging (Vujanic et al. 2009). But monophasic Wilms' tumors may be very difficult to separate from other renal tumors with similar histological features. Pure blastemal Wilms' tumors may be difficult to distinguish from other undifferentiated tumors such as neuroblastoma, primitive neuroectodermal tumor of the kidney (Parham et al. 2001), desmoplastic small round cell tumor (Wang et al. 2007) and synovial sarcoma (Argani et al. 2000a). It is particularly important to consider non-Wilms' tumors in older patients and adults – Wilms' tumor in adults definitely exists, but many of the renal tumors which in the past were labelled as adult Wilms' tumors proved to be some of the mentioned entities. In order to reach the correct diagnosis in such cases, it is critical to apply immunohistochemistry and molecular biology investigations looking for characteristic features. Although blastemal component may show focal CD99 positivity, it is usually not diffuse as in primitive neuroectodermal tumor of the kidney, where genetic studies also show characteristic translocations, t(11;22)(q24;q12) being the most common one (Parham et al. 2001). Desmoplastic small round cell tumor shares many immunohistochemical features with blastemal Wilms' tumor, and the diagnosis should only be made if genetic investigations demonstrate the EWS-WT1 t(11;22)(q13;q12) translocation (Wang et al. 2007). Neuroblastoma usually shows elevated levels of catecholamines, and on histological examination its cells reveal non-overlapping nuclei and coarse 'salt and pepper' chromatin. Both tumors may be positive for neuron-specific enolase and CD56, but WT1 marker is negative in neuroblastoma, and NB84a marker is negative in Wilms' tumor. In the past, in rare cases a rhabdoid tumor could be mistaken for Wilms' tumor, but now it is simple to distinguish between them on immunohistochemistry which shows that INI1 is negative in rhabdoid tumor (Hoot et al. 2004).

Pure epithelial Wilms' tumor may be difficult to distinguish from metanephric adenoma, renal cell carcinoma and hyperplastic perilobar nephrogenic rest. Highly differentiated epithelial Wilms' tumor may be composed of small, well-differentiated and closely packed tubules similar to metanephric adenoma, but the latter can be diagnosed by the lack of capsule between the tumor and renal parenchyma and absent mitotic activity. Renal cell carcinomas in children associated with translocations show distinctive histological features, but papillary renal cell carcinoma (as seen in adults) may be more challenging to diagnose. Immunohistochemistry showing epithelial markers CK7 and CD10 (Muir et al. 2001; Truong and Shen 2011) and cytogenetic abnormalities may be very helpful (Soller et al. 2007).

In the differential diagnosis of pure stromal Wilms' tumors, a clear cell sarcoma of the kidney and mesoblastic nephroma should be considered. In Wilms' tumors treated with preoperative chemotherapy, the stroma may show a striking clear cell sarcoma-like appearance, and extensive sampling may be required in order to find the foci with other Wilms' tumor components.

4.4 Nephrogenic Rests

Nephrogenic rests (NRs) are foci of embryonal cells which are abnormally persistent after 36 weeks of gestation and which are capable of developing into WT. They are found in ~40 % of unilateral and over 90 % of bilateral Wilms' tumors and very rarely in routine infant postmortem examinations. The term nephroblastomatosis is used to describe the presence of multiple nephrogenic rests. Nephrogenic rests are subclassified on the basis of their localisation within the renal lobe into perilobar (PLNRs) and intralobar nephrogenic rests (ILNRs). Both types may be further subclassified as dormant, sclerosing, adenomatous or hyperplastic (Beckwith 1993).

PLNRs and ILNRs have different epidemiological and histological features (Beckwith 1993; Murphy et al. 2004). PLNRs are found at the periphery of the renal lobe; they are usually multifocal and sharply demarcated and consist of blastema and tubules (Fig. 4.12). PLNRs are associated with overgrowth

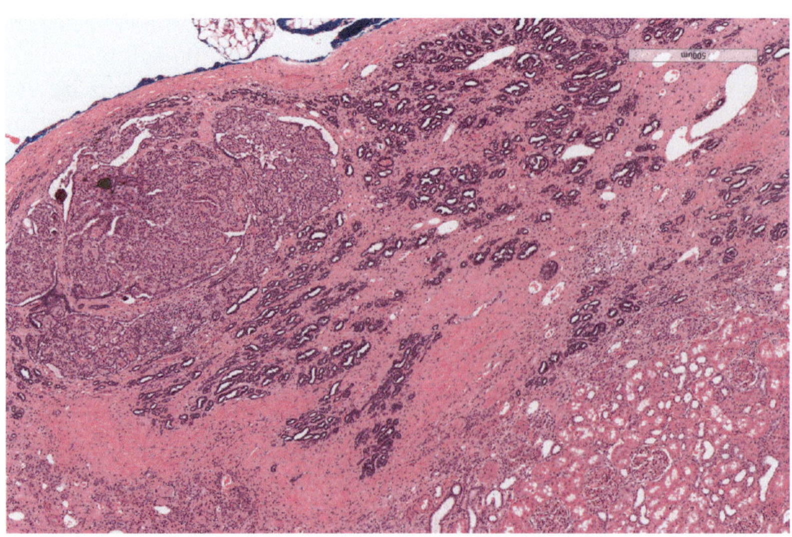

Fig. 4.12 Perilobar nephrogenic rest showing sclerosing and hyperplastic rests

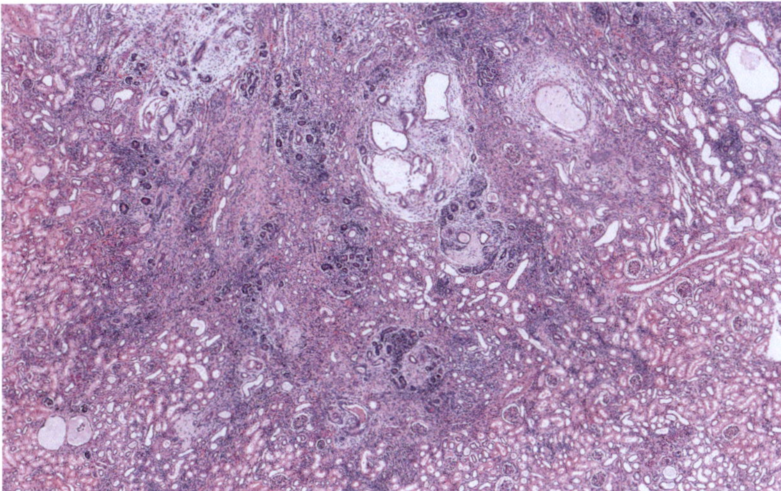

Fig. 4.13 An intralobar nephrogenic rest mixed with normal renal parenchyma

syndromes including hemihypertrophy and Beckwith–Wiedemann syndrome, and they have a lower malignant potential than ILNRs. ILNRs are randomly situated within the renal lobe; show poorly defined, irregular and intermingling margins; and consist of stroma, blastema and tubules (although stroma often predominates) (Fig. 4.13). They are associated with Wilms–aniridia–genital anomaly–mental retardation (WAGR) syndrome and Denys–Drash syndrome (characterised by mesangial glomerular sclerosis and pseudohermaphroditism). Both PLNRs and ILNRs may become hyperplastic and it may be difficult to distinguish them from a WT. However, most NRs regress and do not develop into WT (Beckwith 1993; Murphy et al. 2004). If any type of NR is found in a kidney and/or WT, the child should be considered at increased risk for development of a tumor in the contralateral kidney. The risk is greatest with ILNRs and in children less than 12 months of age (Coppes et al. 1999).

4.5 Cystic Partially Differentiated Nephroblastoma and Cystic Nephroma

Cystic partially differentiated nephroblastoma (CPDN) and cystic nephroma (CN) are related entities which show completely cystic appearance (Joshi and Beckwith 1989). They typically occur in the first 3 years of life, and CN which occurs in the age group of 30+ years with a marked female predominance of 8:1 is now regarded a different entity called mixed epithelial and stromal tumor (Michal et al. 2004).

4.5.1 Macroscopic Features

CN and CPDN both occur as a solitary, unilateral, multilocular cystic lesion measuring 5–10 cm in diameter, with cysts ranging in size from a few mm to 4 cm. They are sharply demarcated from the kidney and may rarely show secondary changes such as necrosis and haemorrhage.

4.5.2 Microscopic Features

CN and CPDN share many histological features (Joshi and Beckwith 1989). The diagnostic criteria for CN include the following: (a) the lesion forms a discrete mass, well demarcated from the non-cystic renal parenchyma; (b) it is composed entirely of cysts and their septa; (c) the septa (which may be of different thickness, but should not form a solid mass) are the only solid portion of the tumor; (d) the cysts are lined by flattened, cuboidal or hobnail epithelium; and (e) the septa are composed of fibrous tissue in which

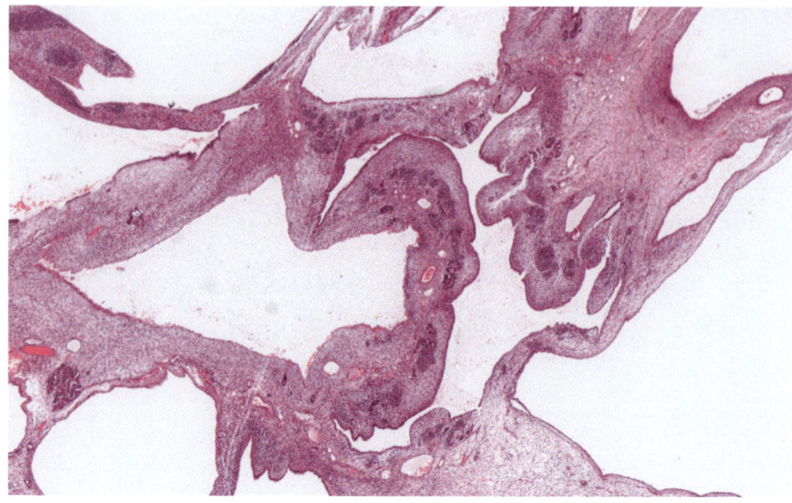

Fig. 4.14 Cystic partially differentiated nephroblastoma showing septa with blastemal elements

well-differentiated tubules may be present (mature tissue such as skeletal muscle may also be present). For the diagnosis of CPDN, in addition to the above criteria, the presence of blastemal cells in any amount, with or without other embryonal stromal or epithelial cell types, is required (Fig. 4.14). Tubules, differentiated glomeruli, striated muscle, cartilage and fat may also be found with blastemal cells in the septa (Joshi and Beckwith 1989).

4.5.3 Differential Diagnosis

The distinction between CN and CPDN is of no prognostic significance as they are both treated with surgical resection only and both have excellent prognosis. But it is important to distinguish them from Wilms' tumor with a prominent cystic component which can be very prominent especially in pretreated tumors but which requires the same treatment as non-cystic Wilms' tumors. The finding of solid areas within the tumor should be sufficient to exclude the diagnosis of CN or CPDN. CN must also be distinguished from polycystic kidney disease and cystic dysplasia.

More importantly, they have to be distinguished from other renal tumors which may have a prominent cystic appearance such as mesoblastic nephroma (Ganick et al. 1981; Truong and Shen 2011) but also clear cell sarcoma of the kidney (CCSK) and rhabdoid tumor of the kidney (RTK) which require much more aggressive postoperative therapy (Argani et al. 2000b; Weeks et al. 1989). Again, the correct diagnosis can be reached if carefully searched for other histological features of these tumors which will be present in the septa and/or tumor's solid areas.

4.6 Mesoblastic Nephroma

Mesoblastic nephroma is a mesenchymal neoplasm with low malignant potential. It is a tumor of early life with ~90 % of cases diagnosed in the first year and never after the age of 3 years. The so-called adult mesoblastic nephromas are now recognised to have represented other tumors such as metanephric stromal tumor (Argani and Beckwith 2000) and mixed epithelial and stromal tumor (Michal et al. 2004). Cellular mesoblastic nephroma shows the characteristic chromosome translocation t(12;15)(p13,q25) which results in ETV6-NTRK3 gene fusion - the same translocation is found in infantile fibrosarcoma, confirming that they represent the same entity (Knezevich et al. 1998)

4.6.1 Macroscopic Features

It appears as a unilateral, solitary mass macroscopically similar to WT. It is usually firm, but necrosis, haemorrhage and cysts are not uncommon features. It is not encapsulated and usually grows near the renal sinus which is often infiltrated.

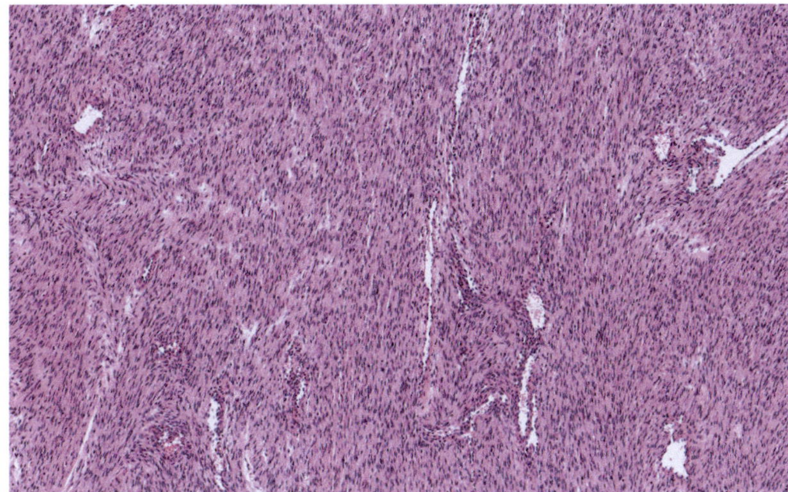

Fig. 4.15 Mesoblastic nephroma, classical type, composed of spindle cells arranged in fascicles

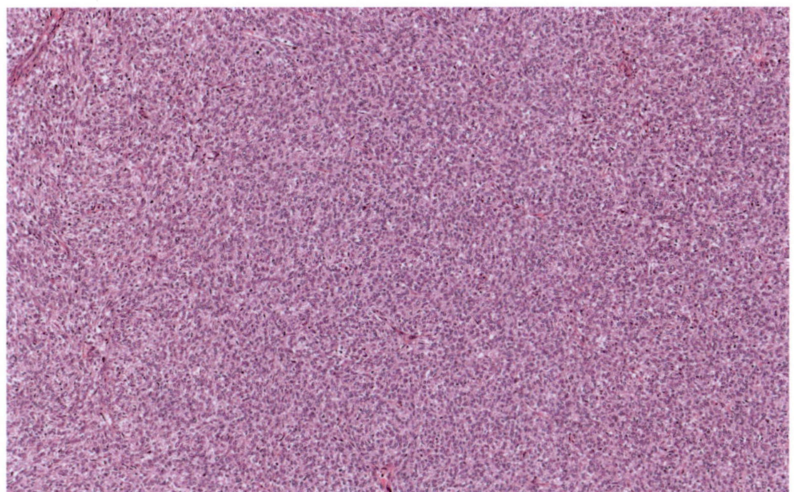

Fig. 4.16 Mesoblastic nephroma, cellular type

4.6.2 Microscopic Features

Histologically, mesoblastic nephromas can be divided into classical, cellular and mixed types, and not infrequently more than one pattern is present. The *classical* type (49 % of cases in the UK series) (England et al. 2011) resembles infantile fibromatosis and is composed of interlacing fascicles of bland, elongated spindle cells with rare mitoses (Fig. 4.15). It contains slit-like thin-walled blood vessels which are scattered throughout the tumor. The tumor shows very infiltrative growth resulting in entrapment of islands of normal renal parenchyma with normal renal tubules which then may be confused with genuine neoplastic tubules which are actually never present in mesoblastic nephromas. The *cellular* type (30 % of cases) consists of densely packed plump, slightly spindled cells with large vesicular nuclei and a moderate amount of cytoplasm (Fig. 4.16). Mitoses are usually frequent. Unlike the classical type, the cellular type has pushing border with the renal parenchyma. The *mixed* type (~20 % of cases) shows the features of the classical and cellular type (Murphy et al. 2004). Mesoblastic nephroma rarely presents in stage I, since in the absence of a capsule, it easily infiltrates the renal sinus and perirenal fat (England et al. 2011; Murphy et al. 2004).

4.6.3 Immunohistochemistry

Mesoblastic nephromas are consistently positive for markers of myofibroblasts (vimentin, smooth muscle actin and fibronectin) and negative for epithelial markers. WT1 can be positive in some cases (Abosoudah et al. 2008).

4.6.4 Differential Diagnosis

In the differential diagnosis, other renal tumors of childhood have to be considered since their treatment and prognosis vary considerably. Some MN may contain cells with prominent nucleoli, very closely resembling the features of a rhabdoid tumor, and rarely MN may have a prominent capillary vascular pattern that mimics the vasculature of a CCSK. Also, it may be difficult to distinguish pure stromal WT and metanephric stromal tumor from MN.

4.7 Clear Cell Sarcoma of the Kidney

CCSK is a malignant mesenchymal neoplasm which comprises about 3–5 % of renal tumors of childhood.

4.7.1 Macroscopic Features

CCSK is always unicentric and unilateral. It varies in weight from 40 to 3,000 g. On cut surface, untreated tumors are homogeneous, firm and light brown. There is usually a distinct tumor–kidney border although there is no capsule. In some cases cysts may be a predominant feature, and in such cases it is important to distinguish CCSK from benign cystic renal lesions or other renal tumors which may also have a marked cystic appearance (Argani et al. 2000b).

4.7.2 Microscopic Features

CCSK shows a broad spectrum of histological patterns which are often found within the same tumor, offering the explanation why it is one of the most commonly misdiagnosed renal tumors of childhood. The classical pattern of CCSK consists of cell cords or nests separated by arborizing blood vessels within the fine septa (*chicken wire* pattern). Tumor cells are uniform in size and distribution, with indistinct borders, and show no overlapping. The nuclei are uniform and pale with finely granular and evenly dispersed chromatin and may appear 'empty'. Nucleoli are small and inconspicuous. 'Clear cells' are a predominant feature in about 20 % of cases, but they can be found in most tumors if adequately sampled. In many tumors, entrapped nephrogenic elements, sometimes with cystically dilated tubules resulting in a cystic appearance, can be seen. However, genuine neoplastic tubules are not a feature of CCSK. In addition to the classical pattern, CCSK may show numerous other patterns including myxoid, sclerosing, cellular, epithelioid, palisading, spindled, storiform and anaplastic patterns (Fig. 4.17a–d) (Argani et al. 2000b).

4.7.3 Immunohistochemistry

There are no diagnostic immunohistochemical markers for CCSK. All CCSKs are vimentin positive and cytokeratin negative, including the epithelioid pattern. WT1 and CD99 markers are also negative (Argani et al. 2000b).

4.7.4 Differential Diagnosis

Due to its numerous histological patterns, CCSK remains the most frequently misdiagnosed renal tumor of childhood. The main differential diagnoses include blastemal WT, rhabdoid tumor of the kidney, PNET, mesoblastic nephroma and metanephric stromal tumor.

The only significant histological factor associated with poor prognosis in tumors that received no preoperative chemotherapy is the presence of necrosis. Favourable survival rate is associated with lower tumor stage, patient's age at diagnosis of 2–4 years of age and treatment with doxorubicin, which improved significantly the overall survival which is now ~70 %, but it varies from 98 % for stage I to 50 % for stage 4 disease (Argani et al. 2000b).

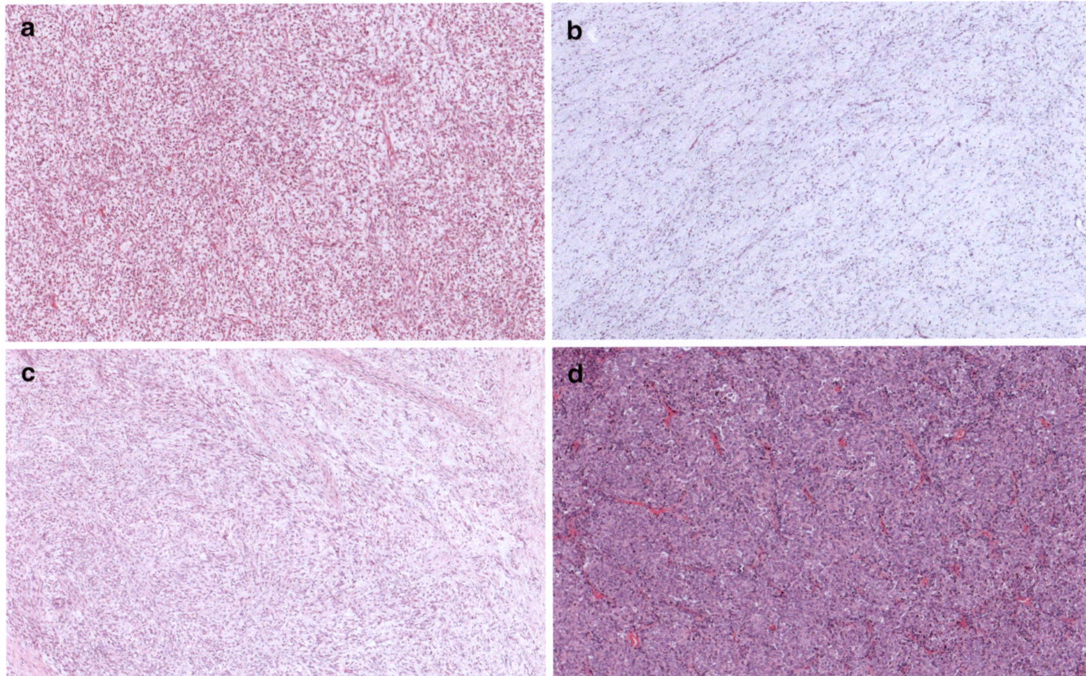

Fig. 4.17 Clear cell sarcoma of the kidney showing different patterns (**a**–**d**)

4.8 Rhabdoid Tumor of the Kidney

Rhabdoid tumor of the kidney (RTK) is a distinctive, highly malignant neoplasm which constitutes about 2 % of paediatric renal tumors. It is a tumor of early childhood with no cases diagnosed after the age of 5 years (Vujanic et al. 1996; Weeks et al. 1989).

4.8.1 Macroscopic Features

RTK is a unilateral and unicentric tumor, sharply demarcated from the renal parenchyma, but satellite nodules are frequently observed as an early manifestation of the aggressiveness of this neoplasm.

4.8.2 Microscopic Features

Classical rhabdoid tumor shows a diffuse pattern of non-cohesive sheets of cells with abundant eosinophilic cytoplasm and large eccentric nuclei with prominent eosinophilic central nucleoli (Fig. 4.18). Tumor cells often have large oval intracytoplasmatic hyaline inclusions composed of whorled masses of intermediate filaments (Fig. 4.20). In addition, there are other patterns which may be present with or without classical pattern including sclerosing, spindled, epithelioid, lymphomatoid and vascular pattern and which may cause diagnostic difficulties (Vujanic et al. 1996; Weeks et al. 1989). Tumor shows a very invasive growth pattern with invasion of blood and lymphatic vessels, the renal parenchyma and the renal sinus.

4.8.3 Immunohistochemistry

RTK shows expression of many markers including vimentin which is virtually always expressed, whereas cytokeratin, epithelial membrane antigen, desmin and neurofilaments are frequently (but not always) co-expressed, and they usually show patchy positivity (Vujanic et al. 1996; Weeks et al. 1989). INI1 staining which is positive in the nuclei of almost all other paediatric tumors is characteristically absent in RT cells (Hoot et al. 2004). INI1 is a marker of

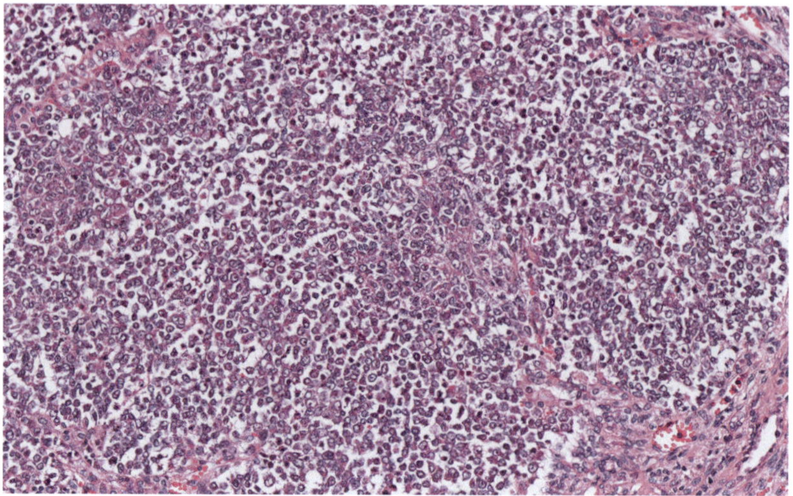

Fig. 4.18 Rhabdoid tumor of the kidney composed of large cells with large nuclei and prominent nucleoli

a common genetic abnormality which is shared with all rhabdoid tumors – the mutation or deletion of the SMARCB1/hSNF5/INI-1 gene located at chromosome 22q11 (Holman and Hornick 2011).

4.8.4 Differential Diagnosis

In the differential diagnosis, a number of other tumors have to be considered including blastemal WT, cellular MN, CCSK, PNET and renal carcinoma (Weeks et al. 1991). However, absent INI1 immunostaining in RTK is regarded as diagnostic and helps in the differential diagnosis which in the past was more challenging. Blastemal elements of WT can rarely contain cytoplasmic inclusions resembling those of RTK, but they may contain the prominent nucleoli which are characteristic of RTK. Cellular MN and RTK occur in the same age period. MN rarely has prominent nucleoli or structures resembling cytoplasmic inclusions, and RTK occasionally shows a spindled pattern either focally or diffusely. The occasional trabecular growth pattern of RTK, and the rare occurrence of prominent nucleoli in CCSK, can sometimes lead to considerable diagnostic difficulty (Vujanic et al. 1996). The presence of classical histological features of CCSK elsewhere in the lesion is a major clue to the accurate diagnosis in such cases.

4.9 Other Tumors

4.9.1 Metanephric Tumors

These tumors comprise a spectrum of recently recognised entities which are classified according to the extent of their epithelial and stromal components. The entities include metanephric stromal tumor, metanephric adenofibroma and metanephric adenoma.

Metanephric stromal tumor is composed entirely of a stromal component (Argani and Beckwith 2000). The median age at diagnosis is 13 months (range 2 days to 13 years), and the majority of previously reported cases of mesoblastic nephroma occurring in children above 3 years of age probably represent metanephric stromal tumors. Histologically, the tumor is unencapsulated but with a very distinctive tumor–kidney border (unlike classical mesoblastic nephroma) and composed predominantly of spindle cells. It shows a nodular appearance resulting from hypo- and hypercellular areas (Fig. 4.19). Other characteristic features include an 'onion-skin' appearance around entrapped renal tubules and blood vessels, angiodysplasia-type changes of intratumoral vessels and juxtaglomerular cell hyperplasia. In about 20 % of cases, foci of heterologous differentiation, in particular glial or cartilaginous nodules, may be found. The diagnosis is based on morphological criteria and CD34 positivity of tumor cells (Argani and

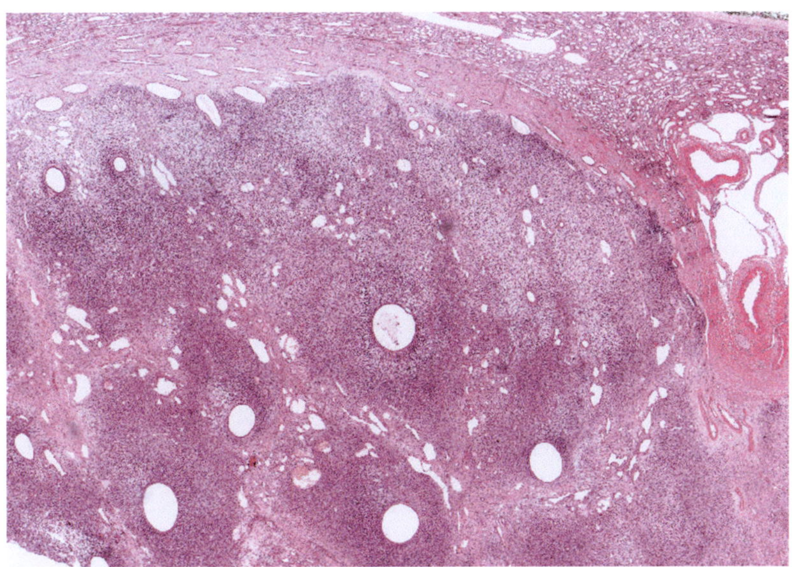

Fig. 4.19 Metanephric stromal tumor showing alternating cellularity and sharp tumor–kidney interface

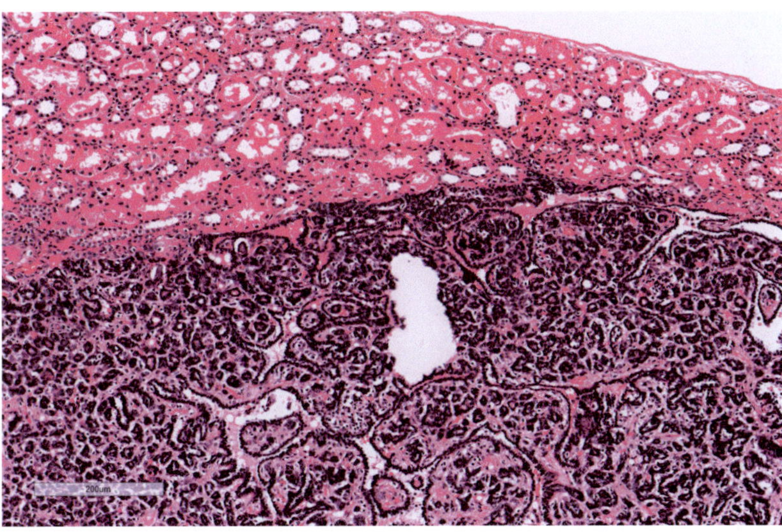

Fig. 4.20 Metanephric adenoma composed of well-differentiated, mature tubules

Beckwith 2000). *Metanephric adenofibroma* is composed of stromal and epithelial components which are present in variable proportions (Arroyo et al. 2001). It has areas histologically indistinguishable from a metanephric adenoma but, in addition, has a spindle cell stromal component showing identical features of metanephric stromal tumors. *Metanephric adenoma* is a purely epithelial lesion composed of small, well-differentiated, closely packed tubules with no nuclear atypia or mitoses (Fig. 4.20) (Davis et al. 1995). It is sharply demarcated from the adjacent renal parenchyma but has no capsule. Age at presentation ranges from 5 to 80 years. Treatment of choice for all metanephric tumors is complete surgical removal and they have an excellent prognosis (Davis et al. 1995).

4.9.2 Renal Cell Carcinomas in Children

Renal cell carcinomas comprise around 1–2 % of renal tumors of childhood but are present in older age than other typical paediatric renal tumors,

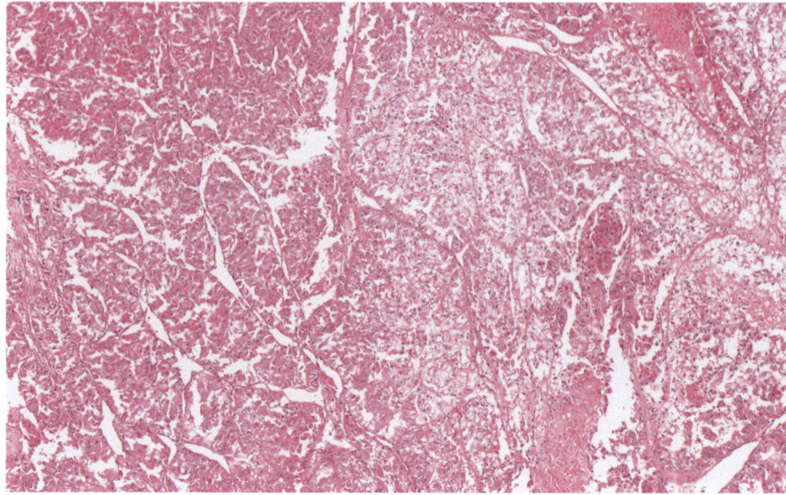

Fig. 4.21 Translocation-associated renal cell carcinoma

usually around the age of 10 years. They show many features not seen in adult renal cell carcinomas such as an association with congenital anomalies or syndromes (found in around one-third of cases) (Selle et al. 2006), different histological types and features (Bruder et al. 2004) and specific translocations involving the *TFE3* gene located at Xp11.2 (Argani and Ladanyi 2005). These translocation-associated renal cell carcinomas comprise nearly 50 % of paediatric renal carcinomas but may rarely be seen in adults, too. Histologically, their typical appearance is a nested pattern, with large cells with granular eosinophilic or clear cytoplasm (Fig. 4.21). Tumor cells show strong nuclear positivity for TFE3 (Argani and Ladanyi 2005). Another translocation-associated renal cell carcinoma in children is t(6;11)-translocation RCC which seems to be less aggressive than Xp11.2-translocation RCC (Argani et al. 2005).

Some of these tumors occur after chemotherapy treatment of neuroblastoma and Wilms' tumors, but there is also a definite association of renal cell carcinoma developing after neuroblastoma, not necessarily after therapy, and renal cell carcinoma following Wilms' tumor (Argani et al. 2006).

Adult-type RCC may also occur in childhood and show similar genetic changes to adult cases (Soller et al. 2007). Renal cell carcinomas with lymph node metastases appear to have a better prognosis in children (Geller and Dome 2004).

Renal medullary carcinoma is a highly aggressive tumor occurring in children and young adults with sickle cell trait or disease (Swartz et al. 2002). It belongs to the family of the so-called INI1-deficient tumors which all show loss of INI1 protein expression, rhabdoid phenotype (Fig. 4.22), and share the same poor prognosis (Hollmann and Horncik 2013). Immunohistochemistry for INI1 is negative, and this is regarded as a diagnostic feature (Hollmann and Horncik 2013; Swartz et al. 2002).

4.9.3 Other Entities

Other renal tumors include very rare tumors which have been recognised on the basis of their characteristic histological features such as juxtaglomerular cell tumor (Martin et al. 2001), ossifying renal tumor of infancy (Hu et al. 2013), anaplastic sarcoma of the kidney (Vujanic et al. 2007) and mixed epithelial and stromal tumor of the kidney (Michal et al. 2004) (originally described as adult mesoblastic nephroma, cystic hamartoma of the renal pelvis and other synonyms). Another group of tumors are those which have been known in other sites but recently recognised in the kidney by the application of molecular biology techniques. This group includes primitive neuroectodermal tumor (Parham et al. 2001), synovial sarcoma (Argani et al. 2000a) and desmoplastic small round cell tumor (Wang et al. 2007).

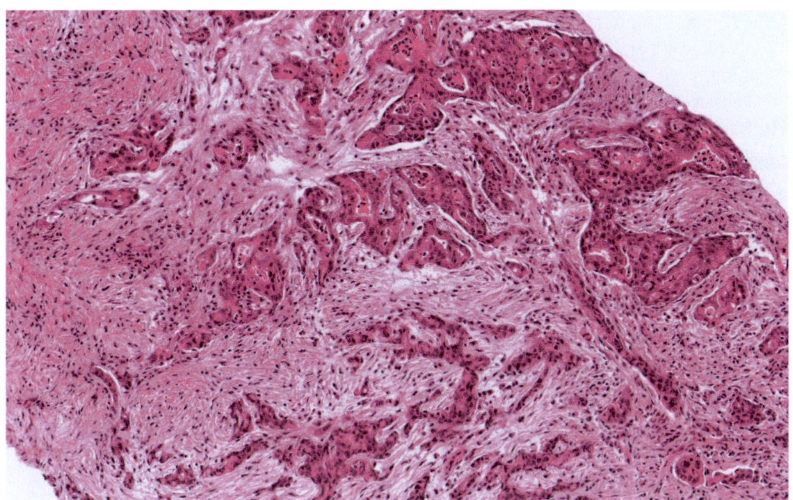

Fig. 4.22 Renal medullary carcinoma

References

Abosoudah I, Ngan BY, Grant R, Weitzman S (2008) WT1 expression and hemihypertrophy in congenital mesoblastic nephroma. J Pediatr Hematol Oncol 30: 768–771

Argani P, Beckwith JB (2000) Metanephric stromal tumor. Report of 31 cases of a distinctive pediatric renal neoplasm. Am J Surg Pathol 24:917–926

Argani P, Ladanyi M (2005) Translocation carcinomas of the kidney. Clin Lab Med 25:363–378

Argani P, Faria PA, Epstein JI et al (2000a) Primary renal synovial sarcoma: molecular and morphologic delineation of an entity previously included among embryonal sarcomas of the kidney. Am J Surg Pathol 24: 1087–1096

Argani P, Perlman EJ, Breslow NE et al (2000b) Clear cell sarcoma of the kidney: a review of 351 cases from the National Wilms Tumor Study Group Pathology Center. Am J Surg Pathol 24:4–18

Argani P, Lae M, Hutchinson B et al (2005) Renal carcinomas with the t(6;11)(p21;q12): clinicopathologic features and demonstration of the specific alpha-TFEB gene fusion by immunohistochemistry, RT-PCR, and DNA PCR. Am J Surg Pathol 29: 230–240

Argani P, Lae M, Ballard ET et al (2006) Translocation carcinomas of the kidney after chemotherapy in childhood. J Clin Oncol 24:1529–1534

Arroyo MR, Green DM, Perlman EJ, Beckwith JB, Argani P (2001) The spectrum of metanephric adenofibroma and related lesions. Clinicopathologic study of 25 cases from the National Wilms Tumor Study Group Pathology Centre. Am J Surg Pathol 25: 433–444

Beckwith JB (1993) Precursor lesions of Wilms tumor: clinical and biological implications. Med Pediatr Oncol 21:158–168

Birch JM, Breslow N (1995) Epidemiologic features of Wilms tumor. Hematol Oncol Clin North Am 9:1157–1178

Breslow N, Olshan A, Beckwith JB, Green DM (1993) Epidemiology of Wilms tumor. Med Pediatr Oncol 21:172–181

Bruder E, Passera O, Harms D et al (2004) Morphologic and molecular characterization of renal cell carcinoma in children and young adults. Am J Surg Pathol 28:1117–1132

Coppes MJ, Arnold M, Beckwith JB et al (1999) Factors affecting the risk of contralateral Wilms tumor development: a report from the National Wilms Tumor Study Group. Cancer 85:1616–1625

Davis CJ Jr, Barton JH, Sesterhenn IA, Mostofi FK (1995) Metanephric adenoma. Clinicopathological study of fifty patients. Am J Surg Pathol 19:1101–1114

Davis JL, Matsumura L, Weeks DA, Troxell ML (2011) PAX2 expression in Wilms tumors and other childhood neoplasms. Am J Surg Pathol 35:1186–1194

Dome JS, Cotton CA, Perlman EJ et al (2006) Treatment of anaplastic histology Wilms' tumor: results from the fifth National Wilms' Tumor Study. J Clin Oncol 24:2352–2358

England RJ, Haider N, Vujanic GM et al (2011) Mesoblastic nephroma: a report from the Children's Cancer and Leukaemia Group. Pediatr Blood Cancer 56:744–748

Faria P, Beckwith JB, Mishra K et al (1996) Focal versus diffuse anaplasia in Wilms tumor–new definitions with prognostic significance: a report from the National Wilms Tumor Study Group. Am J Surg Pathol 20:909–920

Ganick DJ, Gilbert EF, Beckwith JB, Kiviat N (1981) Congenital cystic mesoblastic nephroma. Hum Pathol 12:1039–1043

Geller JI, Dome JS (2004) Local lymph node involvement does not predict poor outcome in pediatric renal cell carcinoma. Cancer 101:1575–1583

Graf N, van Tinteren H, Pritchard-Jones K et al (2011) Is absolute blastemal volume after preoperative chemotherapy in nephroblastoma relevant for prognosis? Pediatr Blood Cancer 57:741–742

Hollmann TJ, Hornick JL (2011) INI1-deficient tumors: diagnostic features and molecular genetics. Am J Surg Pathol 35(10):e47–63. doi: 10.1097/PAS.0b013e3182 2b325b

Hollmann TJ, Horncik JL (2013) INI1-deficient tumors: diagnostic features and molecular genetics. Am J Surg Pathol 35:e47–e63

Hoot AC, Russo P, Judkins AR, Perlman EJ, Biegel JA (2004) Immunohistochemical analysis of hSNF5/INI1 distinguishes renal and extra-renal malignant rhabdoid tumors from other pediatric soft tissue tumors. Am J Surg Pathol 28:1485–1491

Hu J, Wu Y, Qi J, Zhang C, Lv F (2013) Ossifying renal tumor of infancy (ORTI): a case report and review of the literature. J Pediatr Surg 48:e37–e40

Joshi VV, Beckwith JB (1989) Multilocular cyst of the kidney (cystic nephroma) and cystic, partially differentiated nephroblastoma. Terminology and criteria for diagnosis. Cancer 64:466–479

Knezevich SR, Garnett MJ, Pysher TJ et al (1998) ETV6-NTRK3 gene fusions and trisomy 11 establish ahistogenetic link between mesoblastic nephromaand congenital fibrosarcoma. Cancer Res 58:5046–5048

Martin SA, Mynderse LA, Lager DJ, Cheville JC (2001) Juxtaglomerular cell tumor: a clinicopathologic study of four cases and review of the literature. Am J Clin Pathol 116:854–863

Michal M, Hes O, Bisceglia M et al (2004) Mixed epithelial and stromal tumors of the kidney: a report of 22 cases. Virchows Arch 445:359–367

Muir TE, Cheville JC, Lager DJ (2001) Metanephric adenoma, nephrogenic rests, and Wilms' tumor – a histologic and immunophenotypic comparison. Am J Surg Pathol 25:1290–1296

Murphy WM, Grignon DJ, Perlman EJ (2004) Kidney tumors in children. In: Tumors of the kidney, bladder, and urinary structures. Atlas of tumor pathology, 4th Series, Fascicle 1. Armed Forces Institute of Pathology, Washington DC, pp 57–64

Parham DM, Roloson GJ, Feely M, Green DM, Bridge JA, Beckwith JB (2001) Primary malignant neuroepithelial tumors of the kidney: a clinicopathologic analysis of 146 adult and pediatric cases from the National Wilms' Tumor Study Group Pathology Center. Am J Surg Pathol 25:133–146

Perlman EJ (2005) Pediatric renal tumors: practical updates for the pathologist. Pediatr Dev Pathol 8:320–338

Popov SD, Vujanic G, Sebire NJ et al (2013) Bilateral Wilms tumor with p53 related anaplasia. Pediatr Dev Pathol 16:217–223

Sebire NJ, Kelsey A, Pritchard-Jones K et al (2010) Anaplasia in nephroblastoma: findings from the UKW3 and UK SIOP WT 2001 datasets. Pediatr Dev Pathol 13:136(A)

Selle B, Furtwangler R, Graf N, Kaatsch P, Bruder E, Leuschner I (2006) Population-based study of renal cell carcinoma in children in Germany, 1980–2005: more frequently localized tumors and underlying disorders compared with adult counterparts. Cancer 19:1420–1426

Soller MJ, Kullendirf CM, Bekassy AN, Aluments J, Mertens F (2007) Cytogenetic findings in pediatric renal cell carcinoma. Cancer Genet Cytogenet 173: 75–80

Swartz MA, Karth J, Schneider DT, Rodriguez R, Beckwith JB, Perlman EJ (2002) Renal medullary carcinoma: clinical, pathologic, immunohistochemical, and genetic analysis with pathogenetic implications. Urology 60:1083–1089

Truong LD, Shen SS (2011) Immunohistochemical diagnosis of renal neoplasms. Arch Pathol Lab Med 135:92–109

Verschuur AC, Vujanic GM, van Tinteren H, Pritchard-Jones K, de Kraker J, Sandstedt B (2010) Stromal and epithelial predominant Wilms tumours have an excellent outcome: the SIOP 93 01 experience. Pediatr Blood Cancer 55:233–238

Vujanic GM, Sandstedt B (2010) The pathology of Wilms' tumour (nephroblastoma): the International Society of Paediatric Oncology approach. J Clin Pathol 63: 102–109

Vujanic GM, Sandstedt B, Harms D, Boccon-Gibod L, Delemarre JF (1996) Rhabdoid tumour of the kidney: a clinicopathological study of 22 patients from the International Society of Paediatric Oncology (SIOP) nephroblastoma file. Histopathology 28:333–340

Vujanic GM, Sandstedt B, Harms D, Kelsey A, Leuschner I, de Kraker J (2002) Revised International Society of Paediatric Oncology (SIOP) working classification of renal tumors of childhood. Med Pediatr Oncol 38:79–82

Vujanic GM, Kelsey A, Perlman EJ, Sandstedt B, Beckwith JB (2007) Anaplastic sarcoma of the kidney: a clinicopathologic study of 20 cases of a new entity with polyphenotypic features. Am J Surg Pathol 31:1459–1468

Vujanic GM, Sandstedt B, Kelsey A, Sebire NJ (2009) Central pathology review in multicenter trials and studies. Lessons from the Nephroblastoma trials. Cancer 15:1977–1983

Vujanic GM, Kelsey A, Mitchell C, Popov S, Sebire N, Pritchard-Jones K (2010) The effect of pre-operative chemotherapy on histological sub-typing of Wilms' tumour: the UKW3 experience. Pediatr Dev Pathol 13:136(A)

Wang LL, Perlman EJ, Vujanic GM et al (2007) Desmoplastic small round cell tumor of the kidney in childhood. Am J Surg Pathol 31:576–584

Weeks DA, Beckwith JB, Mierau GW, Luckey DW (1989) Rhabdoid tumor of kidney. A report of 111 cases from the National Wilms' Tumor Study Pathology Center. Am J Surg Pathol 13:439–458

Weeks DA, Beckwith JB, Mierau GW, Zuppan CW (1991) Renal neoplasms mimicking rhabdoid tumor of kidney. A report from the National Wilms' Tumor Study Pathology Center. Am J Surg Pathol 15:1042–1054

Weirich A, Leuschner I, Harms D et al (2001) Clinical impact of histologic subtypes in localized non-anaplastic nephroblastoma treated according to the trial and study SIOP-9/GPOH. Ann Oncol 12: 311–319

Treatment of Wilms Tumor in the Children's Oncology Group

5

Conrad Fernandez

Contents

C. Fernandez, MD, FRCPC
Division of Pediatric Hematology and Oncology
Department of Pediatrics and Bioethics,
Dalhousie University, IWK Health Centre,
5850 University Avenue, Halifax, NS
B3K 6R8, Canada
e-mail: Conrad.fernandez@iwk.nshealth.ca

Abstract

The treatment of Wilms tumor (WT) in the Children's Oncology Group (COG) builds upon the pioneering legacy of the National Wilms Tumor Study Group (NWTS) and findings from other successful cooperative groups, in particular SIOP and the UKCSSG. Five successive NWTS trials have used as their foundation a strategy of up-front nephrectomy and subsequent surgical and pathological staging to dictate risk-adapted therapy and have yielded a population of childhood cancer patients with an overall excellent outcome. The current COG renal tumors committee is conducting clinical trials in WT with aims of reducing long-term toxicity for patients who have good risk disease, intensifying therapies for those with poorer risk disease, and banking biological specimens to assist in the discovery of novel pathways that might be exploited. This chapter summarizes the results of the NWTS over four decades and describes the current COG renal trials as they apply to favorable and unfavorable Wilms and nephroblastomatosis.

5.1 Introduction

The Children's Oncology Group (COG) represents more than 200 pediatric oncology institutions in the United States, Canada, Australia, New Zealand, and parts of Europe. The COG approach

K. Pritchard-Jones, J.S. Dome (eds.), *Renal Tumors of Childhood: Biology and Therapy*, Pediatric Oncology,
DOI 10.1007/978-3-662-44003-2_5, © Springer-Verlag Berlin Heidelberg 2014

to treatment of Wilms tumor (WT) finds its primary grounding in the successive trials of the National Wilms Tumor Study (NWTS) group (D'Angio et al. 1976, 1981, 1989; Breslow et al. 1978, 2004; Green et al. 1996, 1998a, b, 2001; Grundy et al. 2005; Kalapurakal et al. 2010). The NWTS was founded from pediatric divisions of the cooperative groups: Acute Leukemia Group B and the Southwest Cancer Chemotherapy Group, the Children's Cancer Study Group, and several independent institutions (Belasco and D'Angio 1981). The NWTS trials first began in the late 1960s, and five large trials have built upon a strategy based in the ascertainment at diagnosis of as much local staging and histological information as possible. This includes baseline diagnostic imaging and, in general, up-front nephrectomy when surgically feasible.

The COG, SIOP, and UKCCSG utilize different prognostic factors to stratify and test therapeutic approaches to WT (Green 2007; Mitchell et al. 2006). The COG default approach of up-front nephrectomy represents the major divergence between the COG and the SIOP/UKCSSG approaches to renal tumors. There are advantages and disadvantages to each approach which will be discussed later in this chapter (Kaste et al. 2008). The major clinical trial groups have learned from each other in applying successful chemotherapeutic strategies to the management of WT. More recently, the COG is testing the hypothesis that further refining these strategies based on molecular findings will enhance outcomes. This chapter will focus on the current treatment approaches to WT including favorable histology, anaplastic, bilateral, and metastatic WT with a brief background describing the evolution of these approaches.

Major advances have been achieved as a consequence of a strong commitment to the international clinical trials process and collaboration of multidisciplinary teams constructed of nursing, diagnostic imaging experts, surgeons, pediatric oncologists, pathologists, and radiation oncologists (Davidoff 2009). The survival rate of children with Wilms has risen from a dismal 20 % 2 years after diagnosis in the 1930s–1940s (Farber 1966) to more than 90 % in 2010 (Davidoff 2009). This chapter will focus on the therapeutic strategies that are currently being used with COG to achieve this remarkable success.

5.2 Staging

The staging system in the COG takes into account preoperative imaging, surgical findings at the time of initial nephrectomy, and pathological review (Table 5.1). While not the subject of this chapter, the COG staging system is also applied to patients found to have clear cell sarcoma of the kidney and rhabdoid tumor of the kidney.

The staging system in current use has evolved from earlier staging systems of NWTS (Farewell et al. 1981). Several important modifications have been incorporated into the current staging system based on findings from the NWTS-5 study. The first change is that of upstaging patients with renal tumors approached by biopsy at diagnosis (Kalapurakal et al. 2010). Historically, these patients have been treated per baseline diagnostic imaging, and the local stage eventually identified when definitive nephrectomy occurred. However, data from NWTS-4 and -5 indicated that local tumor spill is associated with increased risk of recurrence (Kalapurakal et al. 2010; Shamberger et al. 1999). The other major change is the consideration, for therapeutic purposes, of all patients with pulmonary metastases as having disease that merits an approach as a stage IV tumor (Ehrlich et al. 2006; Meisel et al. 1999). The NWTSG had made a distinction for therapeutic purposes between patients with stage IV disease identified by chest X-ray and those identified with smaller pulmonary lesions by the higher-resolution computed tomography (CT) scans (Wilimas et al. 1988). Ehrlich et al. have defined the importance of biopsy of small pulmonary lesions to confirm metastasis (Ehrlich et al. 2006). The current COG AREN0533 study uses CT identification (not chest X-ray) of pulmonary metastases (with biopsy as necessary) to identify stage IV disease and is asking a response-based omission of radiotherapy question for rapid early responders. In addition,

Table 5.1 COG staging system for renal tumors including favorable and unfavorable Wilms tumor, rhabdoid tumor, and clear cell sarcoma of the kidney

Stage I – Tumor limited to kidney, completely resected. The renal capsule is intact. The tumor was not ruptured or biopsied prior to removal. The vessels of the renal sinus are not involved. There is no evidence of tumor at or beyond the margins of resection
Note: For a tumor to qualify for certain therapeutic protocols as stage I, regional lymph nodes must be examined microscopically
Stage II – The tumor is completely resected, and there is no evidence of tumor at or beyond the margins of resection. The tumor extends beyond kidney, as is evidenced by any one of the following criteria: There is regional extension of the tumor (i.e., penetration of the renal capsule or extensive invasion of the soft tissue of the renal sinus, as discussed below) Blood vessels within the nephrectomy specimen outside the renal parenchyma, including those of the renal sinus, contain tumor
Note: Rupture or spillage confined to the flank, including biopsy of the tumor, is no longer included in stage II and is now included in stage III
Stage III – Residual non-hematogenous tumor present following surgery and confined to abdomen
Any one of the following may occur: Lymph nodes within the abdomen or pelvis are involved by tumor. (Lymph node involvement in the thorax or other extra-abdominal sites is a criterion for stage IV) The tumor has penetrated through the peritoneal surface Tumor implants are found on the peritoneal surface Gross or microscopic tumor remains postoperatively (e.g., tumor cells are found at the margin of surgical resection on microscopic examination) The tumor is not completely resectable because of local infiltration into vital structures Tumor spillage occurring either before or during surgery The tumor is treated with preoperative chemotherapy (with or without a biopsy regardless of type – tru-cut, open, or fine needle aspiration) before removal Tumor is removed in greater than one piece (e.g., tumor cells are found in a separately excised adrenal gland; a tumor thrombus within the renal vein is removed separately from the nephrectomy specimen)
Note: Extension of the primary tumor within vena cava into thoracic vena cava and heart is considered stage III, rather than stage IV even though outside the abdomen
Stage IV – Hematogenous metastases (lung, liver, bone, brain, etc.) or lymph node metastases outside the abdominopelvic region are present
Note: The presence of tumor within the adrenal gland is not interpreted as metastasis and staging depends on all other staging parameters present
Stage V – Bilateral renal involvement by tumor is present at diagnosis. An attempt should be made to stage each side according to the above criteria on the basis of the extent of disease

although not specifically stipulated in past staging systems, patients with extension of a renal tumor thrombus into the inferior vena cava (IVC) even as far as the heart have been treated as stage III (Ritchey et al. 1988, 1993). This has now been explicitly added to the COG staging system.

The COG recognizes that attempts at upfront nephrectomy are not always warranted or in the patient's best interest. The decision to pursue delayed nephrectomy is typically based on fulfilling one of two criteria: (a) excess risk for surgical complications for those with clearly unresectable local renal disease at diagnosis (e.g., massive tumors invading organs, extension of tumor thrombus into the IVC, and bilateral tumors) and/or (b) compromise of potential normal renal parenchymal preservation in patients with synchronous bilateral WT or at high risk of metachronous bilateral disease related to underlying syndromic predisposition syndromes (Scott et al. 2006). In these patients, staging may be a limited biopsy or by diagnostic imaging alone.

The main advantage of the COG staging system is that treatment decisions are possible based on up-front diagnostic images and pathological findings of tumors uninfluenced by chemotherapy. Increasingly this includes the risk stratification by molecular prognostic markers obtainable at diagnosis (Kaste et al. 2008). This approach avoids up-front chemotherapy errors where WT is assumed based on diagnostic imaging alone (error rates historically run 1–5 %), in particular for rarer types of unfavorable histology WT or non-WT renal tumors (Miniati et al. 2008; D'Angio 2008; Zoeller et al. 1994). The COG system does allow flexibility with respect to avoiding up-front nephrectomy in patients at clear risk of surgical complications or in which renal parenchymal preservation is paramount. The main disadvantages of the COG staging system are a reported higher rate of surgical complications without up-front chemotherapy (Ritchey et al. 1992; Godzinski et al. 1998) and loss of information with respect to tumor responsiveness (both size and histology) to a trial of chemotherapy (Reinhard et al. 2004a). The SIOP approach appears to result in a more favorable distribution of stages and possible reduction in overall burden of therapy (Pritchard-Jones and Pritchard 2004). Nonetheless, the COG approach remains rooted in primary nephrectomy and staging and subsequent therapy based on these initial findings, following evidence of the excellent outcomes achievable with this strategy.

5.3 Risk Stratification

Risk stratification is key to the determination of subsequent therapeutic regimens for patients with WT. The current risk stratification schema in the COG is supported by central review of all renal tumor cases registered on an overarching renal tumors biology and classification study (AREN03B2). Registration of patients on this study, which reviews pathology, surgical reports, and baseline radiology, is required to be eligible to participate in subsequent COG therapeutic trials and is essential to diminish institutional misclassification (Vujanic et al. 2009). There are three principal aims of the AREN03B2 study. These include (a) accurate risk assignment based on diagnostic imaging and pathological and surgical reviews in addition to molecular markers of loss of heterozygosity for 1 p and 16q and (b) collection and banking of tumor-related tissues for further biological study. In addition to these data points, patients wishing to be considered for the very low-risk strata of observation alone must submit adequate lymph node biopsy samples.

It should be noted that the COG renal tumors committee had adopted central review because of the high rate of misdiagnosis of non-favorable histology WT at local institutions (Dome et al. 2006). This is particularly true for anaplastic and clear cell sarcoma histologies, where up to half of these rarer variants may be misclassified. The cost of missing these is the potential significant undertreatment of a higher-risk lesion.

The factors that are currently being used or tested by the COG for risk stratification include baseline surgical, pathological, and diagnostic imaging staging; tumor histology separating favorable from unfavorable histology (focal or diffuse anaplasia); age of the patient; tumor spill; loss of heterozygosity for 1p and 16 q in favorable histology patients; and rapidity of response of pulmonary metastases to chemotherapy (Breslow et al. 1978, 1985, 1991; Kaste et al. 2008; Shamberger et al. 1999; Lemerle et al. 1976; Sutow et al. 1982; Grundy et al. 1994; Pritchard-Jones et al. 2003; Miller et al. 2005; van den Heuvel-Eibrink et al. 2008). The current risk classification and protocol schema for COG is demonstrated in Table 5.2.

A number of prognostic factors have been identified in other studies that are not routinely incorporated into COG protocols at the present time. Factors not being studied at present encompass histopathological response to prenephrectomy chemotherapy, gain of chromosome 1q as measured by comparative genomic hybridization (Hing et al. 2001; Natrajan et al. 2007), telomerase expression (Dome et al. 2005), and, very recently, global gene classifiers (Huang et al. 2009). Some of these factors are being tested in other cooperative groups (Kaste et al. 2008). Unlike some other childhood cancers, weight or body mass index for age does not appear to predict outcome (Fernandez et al. 2009). There is good evidence

Table 5.2 Risk and treatment protocol classification of patients with Wilms tumor diagnosed within the Children's Oncology Group

Age	Tumor Wt	Stage	LOH (both 1p and 16q)	Rapid response[#]	Risk group	Study
<2 years	<550 g	I	Any	N/A	Very low*	AREN0532
Any	≥550 g	I	None	N/A	Low	AREN03B2
≥2 years	Any	I	None	N/A	Low	AREN03B2
Any	Any	II	None	N/A	Low	AREN03B2
≥2 years	Any	I	LOH	N/A	Standard	AREN0532
Any	≥550 g	I	LOH	N/A	Standard	AREN0532
Any	Any	II	LOH	N/A	Standard	AREN0532
Any	Any	III	None	Any	Standard	AREN0532
Any	Any	III	LOH	Any	Higher	AREN0533
Any	Any	IV	LOH	Any	Higher	AREN0533
Any	Any	IV	None	Yes	Standard[#]	AREN0533
Any	Any	IV	None	No	Higher	AREN0533
Any	Any	V	Any	Any	Bilateral	AREN0534

*Must have had lymph node sampling at the time of nephrectomy to be eligible for the observation only arm.
[#] The standard risk group applies to the Stage IV patients who have a rapid response, as they will receive three drug therapy (DD-4A) and no pulmonary radiotherapy (i.e. the same therapy as standard risk patients). The rapid response status will not be known until Week 6 of therapy, as it is based on their response to chemotherapy. Thus, these patients are enrolled on AREN0533, as are all the Stage IV patients.

that stage- and histology-matched Wilms in older adults has a similar good prognosis as younger children, albeit higher toxicity, if treated with modern chemotherapy regimens (Byrd et al. 1982; Reinhard et al. 2004b; Kalapurakal et al. 2004).

It remains unclear, when the risk factor identified confers a poor prognosis, whether modification of therapy will translate into a patient benefit. As we gain more information about the relevance of the prognostic elements noted above, it is expected that the relative contribution of each of the above elements will be utilized to determine individual patient therapeutic needs.

5.4 Treatment Strategies for Favorable Histology WT

Favorable histology WT is typically triphasic with blastemal, epithelial, and stromal elements, although not all three elements must occur, and is defined by the lack of either focal or diffuse anaplasia. Stage I and II FH WT patients account for approximately 60 % of all children diagnosed with renal tumors. As a consequence of the sheer large number of these children, they make up the largest absolute number of WT patients destined to relapse.

5.4.1 Low-Risk FH WT (Stage I)

In the 1960s, patients with stage I (then called group 1) favorable histology WT were initially treated with 15 months of dactinomycin with abdominal radiation based on a randomized trial of the CCSG (Wolff et al. 1968). The first NWTS (1969–1974) demonstrated that radiation could safely be omitted from the attack on low-stage disease and observed that the combination of vincristine and dactinomycin was active in advanced stage 2 and 3 WT (D'Angio et al. 1976). Based on this promising activity of combination chemotherapy, NWTS-2 (1974–1978) then tested and demonstrated that postoperative chemotherapy with vincristine and dactinomycin was equally effective in treatment periods of 6 months versus 15 months, even when given without radiation. Outcomes achieved showed a terrific 3-year relapse-free survival rates of 90–96 % (D'Angio et al. 1981).

Based on these two studies and the objective to reduce long-term toxicity and complications for patients with good outcomes, NWTS-3 (1979–1985) randomized stage I patients to 6 months (regimen EE) versus 10 weeks (regimen L) of therapy with vincristine and dactinomycin

(D'Angio et al. 1989). Outcomes were not statistically different for the originally treated cohorts, but subset analyses eliminating incorrectly assigned stage II, III, and IV, and unfavorable histology patients showed a more favorable outcome for the longer treatment regimen (EE) [$p=0.05$]. Thus, the shorter 10-week treatment period was not adopted as standard (D'Angio et al. 1989). NWTS-4(1986–1994) was then designed to study a new pulse-intensive schedule of dactinomycin compared to the traditional administration over 5 days. In this study, a new regimen termed EE4A was developed using the pulse-intensive dactinomycin delivered over 18 weeks. EE4A demonstrated a 94.9 % relapse-free survival in favorable histology stage I patients compared to 92.5 % RFS for the longer therapy (Green et al. 1998a, b; Grundy et al. 2005). Overall survival was greater than 98 % in both groups.

In the NWTS-5 trial (1995–2002), no changes were recommended for stage I patients with respect to the EE4A regimen. This trial was designed to determine if LOH 1p and 16q would have an impact upon outcome of uniformly treated patients (Grundy et al. 1994; Coppes et al. 1992). The results demonstrating the prognostic significance of LOH 1- and 16q are shown in Tables 5.3 and 5.4 and underlie the current COG strategy for stage I FH WT patients (Grundy et al. 2005).

In the current COG study, EE4A remains the standard treatment recommended for patients with stage I favorable histology WT unless they have combined LOH 1p and 16 q, in which case three-drug therapy with regimen DD4A (vincristine, doxorubicin, and dactinomycin) without radiotherapy is being tested to determine if this combination reduces relapse compared to historical controls. This strategy has been chosen as more advanced stage patients treated with DD4A appear to have similar outcomes whether or not they have LOH at 1p or 16q, suggesting a benefit to the addition of doxorubicin. Patients with either isolated LOH 1p or16q are not being intensified as the impact is marginal for overall survival and is based on only a very few patients.

Patients with stage I WT without LOH 1p and 16q continue to be followed on AREN03B2 with the collection of biological specimens to ascertain novel prognostic markers that may be used in future risk stratification.

5.4.1.1 Very Low-Risk Favorable Histology WT

Very low-risk favorable histology WT is defined as occurring in children who are less than 2 years of age at diagnosis, with stage I favorable histology WTs and a nephrectomy weight of less than 550 g. Green and Jaffe (Green and Jaffe 1979) postulated that nephrectomy alone may be sufficient for this class of patient and this was supported by a prospective study of no chemotherapy following nephrectomy in eight children (Larsen et al. 1990). The only relapse in this study was a child with hypospadias. A subsequent decision-tree analysis supported an expectation that nearly identical overall survival rates of >95 % are expected for three different strategies for management of this group of patients. These three strategies include standard regimen EE4A (vincristine and dactinomycin for 18 weeks) as is practiced in the COG, vincristine alone for 10 weeks as has been demonstrated to be effective by the UKCCSG, or observation alone (Frazier et al. 2010). All three strategies weigh the potential costs of therapy versus their benefits. The observation-only strategy reduces exposure to and the morbidity of central lines and the short-term potential toxicity of subsequent chemotherapy (hepatotoxicity, neutropenia, vincristine extravasation) for the majority of patients. This is particularly relevant in reducing the risk of severe hepatotoxicity more commonly observed in very young patients (D'Angio 1987; Bisogno et al. 1997; Ludwig et al. 1999). On the other hand, current salvage therapy for relapse following observation alone is recommended to be more intensive than the child would have been exposed to had they received standard therapy. The UKCSSG strategy conveys an intermediate road of limited duration single-agent vincristine (Pritchard-Jones et al. 2003). Participation in an observation-only strategy will be driven by the

Table 5.3 Outcome by LOH 1p and stage for patients with favorable histology Wilms tumor treated on NWTS-5 (Grundy et al. 2005)

Stage	LOH status (1p)	# pts	Relapse-free survival			Overall survival		
			# relapses	4-year RFS (%)	RR (95 % CI) *p*-value	# deaths	4-year OS (%)	RR (95 % CI) *p*-value
I/Age<24 m/Wt<550 g	Loss	10	1	90.0	2.42 (0.30–19.7)	1	90.0	16.5 (1.03–264.0)
	Retain	162	7	95.6	$p=0.41$	1	100.0	$p=0.047$
I/Age≥24 m or Wt≥550 g	Loss	22	2	89.7	1.96 (0.43–8.83)	3	82.4	10.0 (2.01–49.4)
	Retain	221	11	94.2	$p=0.38$	4	98.4	$p=0.005$
II	Loss	74	19	72.9	2.21 (1.32–3.69)	4	94.0	2.21 (0.71–6.85)
	Retain	481	61	86.2	$p=0.003$	12	97.7	$p=0.17$
III	Loss	71	9	86.3	0.94 (0.47–1.89)	4	94.5	1.1 (0.38–3.21)
	Retain	417	57	86.5	$p=0.86$	21	94.4	$p=0.86$
IV	Loss	15	6	59.3	2.07 (0.88–4.89)	3	73.8	1.46 (0.44–4.86)
	Retain	183	40	76.4	$p=0.10$	24	86.1	$p=0.53$
V	Loss	3	0	100.0	0.0 (–)	0	100.0	0.00 (–)
	Retain	65	22	64.8	$p=0.73$	8	87.1	$p=0.85$
Total								
Total (stratified by above categories)	Loss	195	37	79.9	1.56 (1.09–2.22)	15	91.2	1.84 (1.05–3.24)
	Retain	1,529	198	86.2	$p=0.01$	70	95.3	$p=0.03$

Table 5.4 Analysis for the joint effect of LOH 1p and LOH 16q for stage I/II patients with favorable histology Wilms tumor treated on NWTS-5 (Grundy et al. 2005)

		Relapse-free survival			Overall survival		
LOH status	# pts	# relapses	4-year RFS (%)	RR (95 % CI) *p*-value	# deaths	4-year OS (%)	RR (95 % CI) *p*-value
Neither	750	60	91.2	–	14	98.4	–
1p only	60	11	80.4	2.19 (1.15–4.17) $p=0.02$	4	91.2	4.03 (1.20–12.43) $p=0.02$
16q only	114	19	82.5	1.91 (1.14–3.21) $p=0.01$	3	98.1	1.40 (0.40–4.95) $p=0.60$
Both	46	11	74.9	2.88 (1.51–5.49) $p=0.001$	4	90.5	4.25 (1.37–13.19) $p=0.01$

comfort of this balance of risk and benefit carefully considered by physicians and parents.

NWTS-5 planned a prospective study of nephrectomy only for young, small stage I FH WT meeting the VLR criteria (Green et al. 2001). Interim analyses after 2, 3, and 4 years was planned during the projected 5-year study with stringent stopping rules based on a conservative assumption that only 50 % of patients could be salvaged upon relapse. The stopping rule was set at a RFS of less than 90 %, and this was met cut-off in June 1998. The study was thus closed, and remaining VLR children treated with standard EE4A chemotherapy. Seventy-five VLR children were treated with observation only following nephrectomy. Of the 75 children treated with observation alone following nephrectomy, eight patients relapsed at 0.3–2.3 years after diagnosis (median – 4 months) (Green et al. 2001). Lungs were involved in 5 (3 bilateral, 2 unilateral) and the operative bed in 3 patients. Three patients developed disease in the contralateral kidney. The recommended therapy for patients with metachronous tumors was set as the local stage of disease, while patients with local recurrence or metastatic disease were treated with DD4A therapy with radiotherapy directed at the relapse site. The observed salvage rate in this cohort of 11 patients was much higher (91 %) than expected (50 %) and this is stable over many years (Shamberger et al. 2010).

The COG is attempting to replicate these findings in an arm of the therapeutic study for lower- and standard-risk FH WT (AREN0532). Given the greater than expected salvage rate, the opportunity for classification by central review in the current COG set of renal studies, and the more stringent eligibility criteria (children without lymph node biopsies are excluded from the VLR arm), it is hoped that this study will provide definitive evidence for the efficacy of a nephrectomy-only strategy. Of note, in the NWTS-5 study LOH 1p and 16q occurred in only 2 of 141 very low-risk category patients, and this marker will not be used in the current study (Grundy et al. 2005). A secondary aim of the current study is to determine if chemotherapy plays a role in the suppression of development of WTs within nephrogenic rests in the contralateral kidney (Coppes et al. 1999). This question was unanswered in the NWTS5 very low-risk study (Green et al. 2001). The overall risk at 6 years from diagnosis in infants less than 12 months of age for metachronous tumor development is estimated to be approximately 4 % (Coppes et al. 1999). Children diagnosed at age 12–23 months have an even lower risk of 1.5 %. The current COG VLR study has set a stopping rule of 7 % for metachronous relapse accepting slightly higher rates for the prospect of avoiding chemotherapy in the majority.

Histologic (except anaplasia) and molecular features of the tumor are not currently part of the risk stratification strategy for otherwise VLR patient. Of the NWTS-5 surgery-only tumors, an important correlation between pathologic analysis and outcome was the higher frequency of recurrence or metastases in patients whose tumor was incompletely staged due to inadequate sampling of the renal sinus (Green et al. 2001). Preliminary evidence now suggests the feasibility of identifying distinct clusters of patients that appear to correlate with prognosis (Huang et al. 2009; Sredni et al. 2009). These clusters included a subset with epithelial differentiated tubular histology; paucity of nephrogenic rests; lack of LOH 1p, 16 q, and 11p; a unique gene expression profile with no relapses and a second cluster with mixed histology; intralobar nephrogenic rests; and decreased expression of WT1 gene with three relapses. The authors call for prospective validation of this finding which may help to clinically stratify the VLR eligible patients. If validated, this may potentially expand a nephrectomy-only strategy to one that is molecularly defined rather than the imprecise strategy based on age, weight, and stage.

Children who suffer recurrence following observation alone are recommended to have three-drug therapy following regimen DD4A (vincristine, doxorubicin, dactinomycin for 24 weeks) with tumor-directed radiotherapy for those who are not metachronous relapses. For those with metachronous relapse, renal parenchymal sparing surgery is recommended without radiotherapy for those who have negative margins, negative nodes, and no spill. If this strategy confers a high salvage rate as is suggested from NWTS-5, an obvious potential next step is to reduce salvage therapy for other targeted subgroups, perhaps based upon molecular signatures (Sredni et al. 2009).

5.4.2 Low-Risk WT (Stage II)

Stage II favorable histology WT extends beyond the renal capsule but with complete excision. It has followed a different route to the current COG recommended therapy of vincristine and dactinomycin than did stage I FH WT patients. In the original NWTS trial completed in 1974, group II and III (now termed stage II and III) patients were treated with the same randomized questions of single-agent dactinomycin versus single-agent vincristine versus combined chemotherapy (D'Angio et al. 1976). The 4-year relapse-free survival of combined therapy was 79 % with an overall survival of 84 % compared to 56 % RFS and 71 % OS for monochemotherapy ($p=0.01$). All of these patients received abdominal radiotherapy with the dose and fields based on age and group (stage) of the tumor; some received doses as high 4,000 cGy.

NWTS-2 then aimed to improve survival by intensifying chemotherapy by adding doxorubicin to the backbone of vincristine and dactinomycin (regimen D) with radiotherapy. Again all patients received abdominal radiotherapy postoperatively. In this trial, the 3-year RFS improved to 79 % for all group II and III patients, which compared favorably to 65 %, a highly statistically significant outcome (D'Angio et al. 1981). This had a borderline effect on overall survival 84 % for the more intensive arm versus 74 % for the arm with two drugs ($p=0.06$). It was during this time that it was increasingly understood that both radiotherapy and anthracyclines came with potentially severe long-term morbidity and mortality, including bowel obstruction, scoliosis, and renal failure, in addition to cardiotoxicity and second malignancy (Kaste et al. 2008; D'Angio 1987; Jones et al. 1984; Thomas et al. 1988; Green et al. 1990; Meadows et al. 1975; Evans et al. 1991; Attard-Montalto et al. 1992; Cotton et al. 2009).

Thus NWTS 3 undertook to separate group II (now termed stage II) for the next series of doubly randomized studies comparing regimen DD therapy (dactinomycin, vincristine, and doxorubicin) to regimen K (intensive dactinomycin and vincristine, without doxorubicin) for 15 months in patients with or without 2,000 cGy radiotherapy (D'Angio et al. 1989). The 4-year RFS of 88.0 % and overall survival of 92.2 % did not differ significantly between all four arms of treatment suggesting that abdominal radiotherapy and anthracyclines could safely be eliminated from the therapy of stage II FH WT patients. Regimen K without radiotherapy was thus selected as the standard of care.

The efficacy, toxicity, and cost of administration of different regimens of dose intensity and duration of chemotherapy were then tested in NWTS-4 (Green et al. 1998a, b). It had been noted that single-dose dactinomycin was tolerable in other pediatric malignancies such as Ewings sarcoma and rhabdomyosarcoma (Blatt et al. 1981). Stage II Wilms patients in NWTS-4 underwent randomization between pulse-intensive dactinomycin given over 1 day versus the standard 5 days and a second randomization of discontinuation of therapy at 20–24 weeks compared to a then standard duration of 15 months. The dose of pulse-intensive dactinomycin was dropped from 60 to 45 μg/kg after reports of severe liver toxicity (Green et al. 1990). The final results of NWTS-4 supported a finding of no significant difference in outcomes or of hematological or non-hematological toxicity between the pulse-intensive and standard administration schedules of dactinomycin, nor of short- versus long-term therapies. Relapse-free survival was 85–90 % with overall survival at 2 years a superb 97 % with either regimen (Green et al. 1998a, b). Thus, pulse-intensive therapy of short duration was adopted as a strategy to minimize inconvenience, reduce costs, and reduce drug exposure for all patients with stage II FH WT (regimen K4A). Regimen K4A is identical to regimen EE4A. For sake of simplicity, EE4A

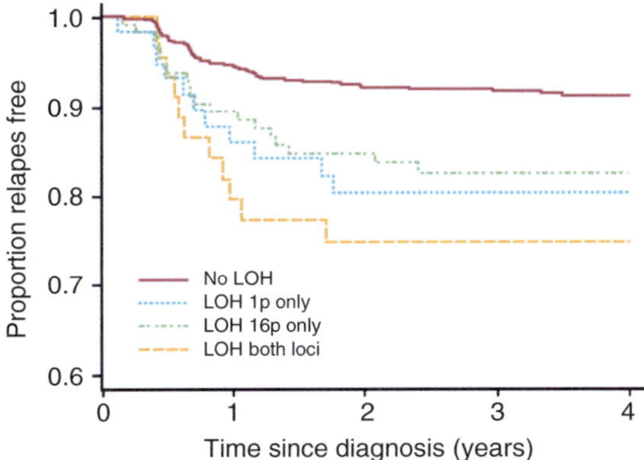

Fig. 5.1 Relapse-free survival by joint loss of heterozygosity at chromosomes 1p and 16q for stage I/II favorable-histology Wilms tumor patients treated on NWTS-5

is the current regimen used for treating patients with stage I and II FH WT.

The aims of NWTS-5 have been described above and focussed on standard treatment with EE4A for stage II patients with the aim of prospectively evaluating the effect of LOH. A higher risk of relapse was demonstrated for stage II FH patients with LOH 1p and with combined LOH 1p and 16q (Grundy et al. 2005) (Fig. 5.1). However, the impact on overall survival was robust only for the combined LOH 1p and 16q. Thus, the current COG AREN0532 protocol is examining the impact of intensifying therapy to DD4A (vincristine, doxorubicin, and dactinomycin) for stage II FH WT patients with combined LOH 1p and 16q alone. No radiotherapy is given to this group of patients. Other unique biological classifiers continue to be sought for the majority of stage II relapsed patients who do not have an identifiable elevated risk factor at diagnosis.

5.4.3 Standard Risk Favorable Histology WT (Stage III)

The evolution of therapy for stage III favorable histology WT shares similar roots as stage II FH WT but diverged following NWTS-3 (Breslow et al. 1991). Stage III FH WT has a clinicopathological definition of residual non-hematogenous tumor confined to the abdomen that is defined by a wider spectrum of possible findings including disease found unresectable beyond the margins of the tumor, WT involving locoregional lymph nodes, spill or rupture, and through implants on the peritoneal surface. It is likely that some of these mechanisms belie a different pathobiological pathway and thus may eventually confer different treatment requirements. At the present time, however, all these routes of spread are considered under the umbrella of stage III for the purpose of treatment recommendations.

The original NWTS study reported aggregate outcomes for group II and III patients treated with abdominal radiotherapy and randomized between combined dactinomycin and vincristine as superior to monochemotherapy ($p=0.004$) (D'Angio et al. 1976). Similarly, NWTS-2 did not separate group II and III FH WT patients in their successful trial of adding doxorubicin to the standard backbone of vincristine, dactinomycin, and radiotherapy (D'Angio et al. 1981). Two important findings in NWTS-2 resulted in a shift of the staging and stratification criteria to include any patient with lymph node metastases as stage III. Previously, patients with periaortic chain involvement were considered by local kidney tumor stage. In addition, unfavorable histology was confirmed to confer a very poor survival (D'Angio et al. 1981; Breslow et al. 1985).

NWTS 3 studied the identical randomized chemotherapy regimen in stage III patients as for stage II FH WT patients, comparing regimen DD (3 drugs) to regimen K (2 drugs) and instead of eliminating radiotherapy randomized patients to a reduced dose of 1,000 cGy compared to the standard of 2,000 cGy. The results were originally reported by D'Angio 1989 and updated as 8- and 16-year relapse-free and overall survival rates in 2000 by Green (D'Angio et al. 1989; Breslow et al. 2004). The subset analysis of NWTS-3 reported by D'Angio demonstrated a benefit for patients with stage III FH WT when doxorubicin was added (Grundy et al. 1989). With the addition of doxorubicin, patients who received 1,000 cGy flank XRT fared as well as those who received 2,000 cGy. The updated outcomes are shown in Table 5.5. Despite the overlapping long-term RR without and without anthracycline therapy, the trend would suggest an

Table 5.5 Long term relapse-free survival and overall survival for stage III patients treated on NWTS-3 (Green 2004)

Regimen	Number	RFS 8 years (%)	RFS 16 years (%)	OS 8 years	OS 16 years
DD1	64	80.4	80.4	88.8	86.2
DD2	61	86.7	86.7	88.2	88.2
K1	65	73.0	73.0	82.3	82.3
K2	70	77.1	75.4	82.6	82.6

DD1: vincristine, doxorubicin, dactinomycin, 1,000 cGy flank XRT
DD2: vincristine, doxorubicin, dactinomycin, 2,000 cGy flank XRT
K1: vincristine, dactinomycin, 1,000 cGy flank XRT
K2: vincristine, dactinomycin, 2,000 cGy flank XRT

Table 5.6 Analysis for the joint effect of LOH 1p and LOH 16q for stage III/IV patients with favorable histology Wilms tumor treated on NWTS-5 (Grundy et al. 2005)

		Relapse-free survival			Overall survival		
LOH status	# pts	# relapses	4-year RFS (%)	RR (95 % CI) *p*-value	# deaths	4-year OS (%)	RR (95 % CI) *p*-value
Neither	500	82	83.0	–	38	91.9	–
1p only	56	6	89.0	0.69 (0.30–1.57) $p=0.37$	2	97.6	0.52 (0.12–2.14) $p=0.36$
16q only	100	15	85.3	0.89 (0.51–1.54) $p=0.67$	7	92.0	0.88 (0.39–1.97) $p=0.76$
Both	30	9	65.9	2.41 (1.20–4.82) $p=0.01$	5	77.5	2.66 (1.04–6.82) $p=0.04$

improved survival with anthracyclines, although not statistically significant. The original findings were used to support the NWTS-4 trial which continued to incorporate anthracyclines for higher-stage disease. The later report is potentially limited by sample size, and evidence of efficacy of anthracyclines from other trials has supported its current use in advanced stage Wilms both in North America and in Europe. Also of note is a significant change in the total dosing of anthracyclines used in earlier NWTS studies, where cumulative doses typically approached 300 mg/m^2. Current anthracycline dosing on the DD4A regimen is limited to 150 mg/m^2. This is hoped to reduce the long-term risk of cardiotoxicity and second malignancy of these therapies (Sorensen et al. 1995; Cotton et al. 2009).

The same randomization as occurred for stage II patients was examined for stage III patients on NWTS-4 in testing long (15 months) versus short (6 months) duration of therapy and pulse-intensive single-day doxorubicin and dactinomycin versus standard 3- or 5-day administration schedules. The results demonstrated equivalent RFS and OS in both randomizations (Table 5.6), and thus pulse-intensive, 6-month DD4A chemotherapy with 1,000 cGy radiation was adopted as standard moving forward (Green et al. 1998a, b).

NWTS-5 studied the effect of LOH status on a standard backbone of DD4A (short) and radiotherapy for stage III FH WT patients. No impact on RFS or OS was noted for patients with isolated 1p or 16q, and thus therapy has not been modified for these patients on the current AREN0532 study (Grundy et al. 2005) (Table 5.7). A small number of stage III patients had combined LOH 1p and 16 q, and these fared significantly more poorly and, thus once identified, are now receiving intensified therapy with a novel chemotherapy (regimen M) on AREN0533 in the COG. It is as yet unknown if this novel regimen is effective at improving either relapse-free or overall survival.

Table 5.7 Relapse-free and overall survival for stage III favorable histology Wilms tumor patients treated with short versus long and pulse-intensive versus standard-duration chemotherapy regimens on NWTS-4 (Green et al. 1998a, b)

Regimen	Number	RFS (%)	OS (%)	Follow-up (years)
DD short	83	93.3[a]	97[a]	4.41
DD long	79	91.4[a]	94[a]	3.82
DD4A short	63	91.8[a]	98[a]	4.59
DD4A long	81	89.5[a]	95.4[a]	4.32
Standard	174	95.3[b]	99.4[b]	4.52
Pulse intensive	175	91.1[b]	98.2[b]	4.72

DD: vincristine/standard dactinomycin and doxorubicin/XRT

DD4A: vincristine/pulse-intensive dactinomycin and doxorubicin/XRT

[a]4 years

[b]2 years

5.4.4 Standard-Risk Favorable Histology WT (Stage IV)

Stage IV WT signifies hematogenous spread of the tumor, most commonly to lung and less so to liver, bone, or brain. Treatment for this group of patients focuses both on local/regional disease control and management of distant metastases with combination chemotherapy and radiation therapy. Note that pulmonary metastases on NWTS 4 and 5 were defined as those metastases visible on chest X-ray, thereby requiring significant tumor burden, whereas current staging classify CT only metastases as stage IV.

Dactinomycin was the first chemotherapy agent to be shown to be active in WT, and Farber provides an excellent account of how the agent was first used in Wilms in the 1950s and 1960 s (Farber 1966) on a backbone of nephrectomy and focal radiotherapy. Vincristine was demonstrated to be active in dactinomycin-refractory Wilms by SWOG in the 1960s (Vietti et al. 1970). NWTS-1 took these observations and tested the additional value of preoperative vincristine in metastatic disease. Vincristine appeared to improve resectability but did not alter the course with respect to survival (D'Angio et al. 1976). NWTS-2 randomized stage IV Wilms patients to vincristine and dactinomycin versus the addition of doxorubicin to the two standard drugs and treated all children with postoperative radiotherapy. This demonstrated the three-drug combination to be very effective and provides the basis for standard therapy to this day. It was noted in this trial that the effect of doxorubicin was most pronounced in the combined grouping of stage II, III, and IV patients rather than stage IV alone (Morgan et al. 1988).

Nonetheless, three-drug therapy (DD-RT) became the baseline approach for favorable histology stage IV WT in NWTS-3, which compared this regimen to a newly devised regimen J, which incorporated cyclophosphamide over a 15-month course of therapy. Abdominal/flank radiation was given based on age-modulated doses with delivered doses as high as 4,000 cGy based on an age over 41 months. Results were promising with >70 % relapse-free survival at 4 years with an overall survival of more than 78 % at 4 years (D'Angio et al. 1989). It was concluded that cyclophosphamide, given in the schedule used in this protocol, did not add any significant benefit. A limitation of this study was the power to detect a difference in the subgroup of stage IV patients who seemed to show a trend of benefit with regimen J with a 77.9 % 4-year RFS and 86.6 % OS at 4 years. Pulmonary, cardiac, and liver toxicities were prominent, especially in high stage patients (observed in 10–20 % of patients) and was a primary contributor overall to 15 % of all the deaths.

As described earlier, NWTS-4 tested pulse-intensive chemotherapy versus standard duration and longer overall duration of 15 months versus 6 months (Green et al. 1998a, b). Like their stage III counterparts, stage IV patients fared very well with no significant difference in RFS or OS for either pulse-intensive or short-duration therapy. Therefore, a 6-month course of DD4A with less dose-intensive radiation therapy was adopted as standard and formed the systemic chemotherapy backbone for the NWTS-5 study. LOH 1p and 16 q alone were associated with no poorer relapse-free or overall survival, but, when both were present, resulted in inferior outcomes with a 65 % RFS and 77 % OS at 4 years compared to over 80 % RFS and over 90 % OS when LOH was absent (Grundy et al. 2005).

The observation that LOH played a role in advanced stage Wilms prompted reconsideration of the role of cyclophosphamide intercalation into the DD4A backbone with the premise that the previous regimen did not give it in a sufficiently high enough dose intensity. The NWTS-3 regimen J also demonstrated a trend towards better outcomes when stage IV patients were examined as a subgroup on NWTS-3. In addition, continuing concern existed, especially about late cardiac, pulmonary toxicity, and second malignancy, and findings of the UKCCSG and SIOP suggesting omission of pulmonary radiation in rapid early responders might be feasible (Cotton et al. 2009; Green 1993; Paulino et al. 2000). Thus, the COG current study for stage IV WT (AREN0533) is testing dose intensification using a novel regimen M in patients with LOH in either stage III or IV FH WT and in those with a slow early radiological response of lung metastases to standard DD4A therapy. It is possible that dose-intensity reduction is feasible on the basis of rapid radiological response of pulmonary metastases based on the findings of European colleagues (Weirich et al. 2004; Mitchell et al. 2000; Pritchard et al. 1995). Regimen M is reserved for the higher-risk patients, and radiotherapy is still provided to metastatic pulmonary disease that persists after 6 weeks of therapy. It is hoped that this strategy both improves outcomes for poor prognosis patients and reduces late effects for those destined to be relapse-free.

5.5 Unfavorable Histology (Anaplasia: Focal and Diffuse)

Anaplasia (focal and diffuse) has been recognized since NWTS-2 to confer a poorer prognosis for patients with otherwise the same stage and age risk factors (D'Angio et al. 1981). In that study, approximately 12 % of patients had unfavorable focal or diffuse anaplasia, and at the time, clear cell sarcoma and rhabdoid sarcomas were categorized under the rubric of unfavorable histology (UH). Anaplasia is now recognized to occur in approximately 5–10 % of all WT (Dome et al. 2006; Bonadio et al. 1985), and clear cell and rhabdoid tumors are managed separately.

The latter tumors were understood to represent quite distinct tumor biology with a different set of clinical presentations and progressions, but all were treated as unfavorable histology tumors until NWTS 3. This was the first study to stratify patients based on histology (D'Angio et al. 1989). All patients with unfavorable histology were randomized between 15 months of intensive treatment with DD (three standard chemotherapy drugs) and regimen J (actinomycin, vincristine, dactinomycin, and cyclophosphamide). All UH patients also received age-adjusted RT to the flank and other involved sites.

NWTS-3 clearly demonstrated that institutional assessment of the UH subtypes was suboptimal. While very accurate in identifying FH Wilms, a substantial proportion of unfavorable subtypes were not identified until central review (10–40 % missed). These findings have been subsequently replicated in the NWTS-4 and 5 (Dome et al. 2006) and support continuing central pathological review.

Neither regimen DD or J demonstrated a significant impact upon outcome either in the stage I–III UH patients or in the stage IV patients. A persistently inferior outcome was present in the relatively small numbers of patients who suffered these disorders; recall that UH then represented CCSK, anaplasia, and rhabdoid tumors combined. Stage I–III UH Wilms had a RFS of 62–7 %, and OS of just 68 % suggesting that almost all who relapsed could not be salvaged. Similarly, stage IV UH patients had identical RFS and OS in the 58 % range (although based on very small numbers). A subset analysis (hampered by small numbers) for focal versus diffuse anaplastic WT demonstrated a significant benefit for regimen J over DD in these focal ($p=0.05$) patients and a trend for the diffuse patients ($p=0.11$).

NWTS-4 examined the role of pulse-intensive therapy and standard versus short therapy in UH patients. In this study, anaplastic patients were reported separately from CCSK and rhabdoid tumors (Green et al. 1994; Seibel et al. 2004). In addition, stage I diffuse anaplastic tumors were

Table 5.8 A 4-year relapse-free survival (%) for patients with diffuse anaplastic Wilms tumor treated on NWTS 3–5 (Dome et al. 2006)

Stage	Regimen DD-RT	Regimen J	Regimen I	Regimen EE4A
I	80 %	100	–	68 %
II	40	72	83	–
III	33	59	65	–
IV	0	17	33	–

DD-RT: vincristine/dactinomycin/doxorubicin/XRT
J: vincristine/dactinomycin/doxorubicin/cyclophosphamide/XRT
I: vincristine/doxorubicin/cyclophosphamide/etoposide/XRT
EE4A: vincristine/dactinomycin

treated as low risk and given regimen EE4A with an outcome comparable to stage I FH WT patients. A retrospective review of a large cohort of these stage I UH WT patients were reviewed and found to have an unexpectedly low relapse-free survival of 68 % (personal communication J Dome). Thus, the current COG study AREN0321 is studying if adding a third drug (doxorubicin) and flank radiation to the EE4A typically delivered to stage I UH patients results in a better outcome.

NWTS 4 study findings suggested that stage I–IV focal anaplastic WT patients do very well irrespective of their treatment (Green et al. 1998a, b). However, patients with stage II–IV diffuse anaplasia benefit substantially from the addition of cyclophosphamide, doubling the 4-year RFS from 27 % without cyclophosphamide to 54.8 % (Faria et al. 1996). It was also described that almost a third of stage III diffuse anaplasia patients relapse in the abdomen at the current radiotherapy dosing of 1,000 cGy.

Despite advances, outcomes for diffuse anaplasia WT remained poor, and NWTS-5 therefore incorporated further intensification with the introduction of regimen I. This new regimen incorporated etoposide as a novel agent in conjunction with higher dose-intensity cyclophosphamide (Dome et al. 2006) than had been previously used. This combination had acceptable toxicity and suggested at least as good, if not better, outcomes than regimen J (Table 5.8).

A retrospective analysis of 81 patients with diffuse stage I disease from NWTS-1–5 shows a 72 % 5-year EFS when treated with EE4A. As a consequence, COG AREN0321 is currently examining if an intensified regimen of DD4A with flank radiation will improve this outcome. More advanced stage II–III diffuse anaplastic WTs are being treated with a novel regimen (revised UH-1) which incorporates carboplatin in a backbone of regimen I therapy. The original UH-1 regimen proved too toxic, and this current version seems to be better tolerated although its benefit has yet to be proven. Stage IV diffuse anaplastic WT outcomes remain extremely poor. On COG AREN0321, these patients are receiving a window-therapy approach with irinotecan based on activity of camptothecins in the xenograft model and activity data of a more hematopoeitically toxic topotecan regimen in heavily pretreated relapsed Wilms patients (Metzger et al. 2007). This strategy also remains under investigation and should not be considered standard of care.

Focal anaplasia remains a rare occurrence. Extrapolation of data for patients with focal anaplasia based on NWTS-5 data suggests suboptimal outcomes for some patients, although the confidence of this observation is limited somewhat by small numbers. Two relapses and 1 death occurred in ten patients with stage I focal anaplasia. Three of 20 patients with stage 2 or 3 focal anaplasia relapsed after treatment with DD4A which is comparable to stage III favorable histology patients. Almost a third of patients with stage IV focal anaplasia relapsed after treatment with DD4A. The current AREN0321 protocol is therefore intensifying treatment for stage I and stage IV focal anaplasia patients but continuing with the DD4A as the primary strategy for stages II and III. The efficacy of this strategy is not yet known.

5.6 Bilateral WT Management

WT may occur in both kidneys either in a metachronous or synchronous fashion. Approximately 5 % of all patients registered on NWTS studies have bilateral WT (BWT) (D'Angio et al. 1976). Anaplastic histology in these patients is noted to be more frequent than in sporadic unilateral WT and may not be congruent between kidneys. The approach for BWT tumors has been highly individualized and incorporates careful decision-making regarding timing for surgical approaches, chemotherapy regimens, and radiation. Historically, cooperative clinical trials groups have collected outcome and treatment data but have not prescribed specific therapeutic regimens. The current COG AREN0534 bilateral study is the first prospective trial with specific interventions stipulated by protocol to support the twin goals of enhancing relapse-free survival while minimizing the likelihood of renal failure secondary to loss of normal renal parenchyma.

The first NWTS trial reported outcomes for bilateral WT patients with a 72 % EFS at 2 years (D'Angio et al. 1976) and an overall outcome of 82 % survival, albeit with a high rate of renal failure primarily secondary to eventual bilateral nephrectomies to achieve disease control (Bishop et al. 1977). Longer-term follow-up showed only a 70 % OS (Montgomery et al. 1991). Subsequently, patients in NWTS 2 and 3 were reported to have outcomes of approximately 40 % complete excision with a very good EFS for this subset, if treated with dactinomycin and vincristine. Patients on these trials were treated by the local stage of each kidney, as best as that could be ascertained. Patients appeared to do better with complete excision (82 %) compared to biopsy (57 %) although there was inadequate power to demonstrate statistical significance (Blute et al. 1987). BWT patients treated on NWTS-4 continued to pose challenges for relapse. A summary of combined outcomes for NWTS-3 and -4 BWT demonstrated an approximately 65 % 10-year RFS and an 82 % OS but with a significant rate of renal failure (P Grundy, personal communication); no further improvement was achieved on NWTS-5. Similar outcomes have been reported in SIOP despite preoperative chemotherapy (Coppes et al. 1989). Contributing factors to poor outcomes have been identified to be factors such as initial under-staging related to difficulties in surgical approach to the hilum, higher rates of anaplasia, delayed nephrectomy, and death secondary to complications of renal failure. Some patients with delayed nephrectomy did so to try to optimize response to chemotherapy preoperatively but when histology was examined had rhabdomyomatous differentiation (a histology destined never to regress in size) (Shamberger et al. 1999, 2006). Of note, on NWTS-4, a not insignificant minority of BWT had diffuse anaplasia (27/188) ultimately identified; however, none of these were found at baseline on needle biopsy, just 3 of 9 on wedge biopsy and 10 of 18 with partial or complete nephrectomy (Hamilton et al. 2006). Patients were typically treated for very long periods (months) prior to definitive resection and identification of anaplasia (Hamilton et al. 2006).

Review of data from St. Jude's Research Hospital by Paulino demonstrates a significantly reduced risk of relapse in synchronous BWT when using three-drug therapy with DD4A (8 %) versus 42 % with dactinomycin and vincristine alone (Paulino et al. 1996). Preservation of renal parenchyma is a critical goal of therapy in BWT, whether in the setting of synchronous or at high risk of metachronous disease. Therefore, maximization of shrinkage of the tumor prior to definitive therapy is a logical strategy. The European experience provides an excellent baseline for expectations of preoperative chemotherapy with an expected 48 % reduction in tumor volume by 4 weeks, the availability of a postoperative histology classification system that can be used to stratify therapies, and confidence with respect to tolerability in utilizing intensive vincristine, dactinomycin, and doxorubicin therapy (VAD) that would give good drug exposure prior to nephrectomy (Weirich et al. 2004; Graf et al. 2000; Boccon-Gibod et al. 2000; Beckwith et al. 1996; Tournade et al. 2001).

These elements of surgical strategies to optimize renal parenchymal sparing, intensive but limited chemotherapy to maximize response, early biopsy to determine the etiology of non-response with respect to volume reduction of tumor, and postoperative histology-driven follow-on therapy are all incorporated into the current COG BWT AREN0534 study. In this protocol, up-front biopsy of tumor is discouraged to avoid upstaging local disease by tumor spill. Initial therapy is a dose-intensive vincristine, dactinomycin, and doxorubicin for 6 weeks that allow exposure to two doses each of dactinomycin and doxorubicin before the 6-week imaging point. For those who have resectable disease at 6 weeks, resection is encouraged. If there has been a greater than 50 % reduction in size (PR) but the tumor remains unresectable, continuation of therapy with VAD is recommended. However, for those who do not have a PR, open biopsy to ascertain the presence of necrosis, rhabdomyomatous differentiation, or anaplasia as an etiology for non-response is required. The protocol strongly encourages proactive biopsy or resection of tumor to avoid very long periods without definitive surgery as has been past practice. Follow-up chemotherapy and radiotherapy are dictated by the experience of SIOP based on local stage and histological response (Reinhard et al. 2004a; de Kraker et al. 2004).

5.7 Nephroblastomatosis Management

Nephrogenic rests are normal metanephric tissue that should not persist after 36 weeks gestation but, when they do, may give rise to WT (Perlman et al. 2006). They are commonly found in Wilms nephrectomy specimens (up to 40 % in one series) and occur as two predominant subtypes – perilobar (PLNR) or intralobar (INLR) nephrogenic rests (Beckwith et al. 1990). Rests are categorized by their developmental phase as incipient/dormant, hyperplastic, or regressing (sclerosing) rests. They may occur in four categories: perilobar, intralobar, combined, or universal. Of 282 evaluable unilateral WT specimens, 28.4 % were definitely rest-positive, and an additional 12.4 % were probably positive, with equal prevalence of PLNRs and ILNRs. Median age at diagnosis of WT was 36 months with PLNRs, 16 months with ILNRs, and 12 months if both types were present. PLNRs are highly associated with synchronous bilateral WTs especially in the setting of BWS and hemihypertrophy, while ILNRs are more commonly seen with metachronous contralateral WTs in the setting of aniridia or Denys-Drash syndrome (Beckwith et al. 1990; Green et al. 1993). The recognition of these histological subtypes is potentially important in appreciating the presence of an undiagnosed syndrome and may be useful in determining management, follow-up, and prediction of renal outcome (Breslow et al. 2000).

Nephroblastomatosis is defined as the presence of multiple or diffuse nephrogenic rests. Included in the category of hyperplastic perilobar nephroblastomatosis is the extensive involvement of the cortical tissue of one or both kidneys by hyperplastic nephroblastic tissue (Vicens et al. 2009).

Hyperplastic perilobar rests are associated with progression to WT (Perlman et al. 2006). Treatment for this entity has varied widely over time as progression to WT is variable, the incidence rare with only small case series, and no formal cooperative group studies have been performed. Thus, the ideal clinical management of these patients is uncertain (de Chadarevian et al. 1977; Heideman et al. 1985; Regalado et al. 1997; Prasil et al. 2000; Cozzi et al. 2004, 2006).

Perlman et al. have reviewed the NWTS experience over 40 years and reported clinicopathological features in the largest series to date of 52 patients (Perlman et al. 2006). The majority underwent an initial renal biopsy (33) and 19 a unilateral nephrectomy, the latter of whom only 2 had WT confirmed histologically. Biopsy made the distinction between WT and HPLNR extremely difficult unless the interface between the lesion and the normal kidney was preserved. The majority of these patients received adjuvant chemotherapy (EE4A) for a variable length of time depending upon the study era. Many demonstrated a waxing and waning course in the first year of therapy. Of those who had a biopsy only, 57 % developed WT (Perlman et al. 2006). Of those who had an up-front nephrectomy followed by adjuvant chemotherapy, the majority never developed a WT despite most being bilateral. However, of all those who were diagnosed with a WT, just under half developed more than one (13–116 months – mean 42 months from diagnosis). A significant proportion of the whole cohort had anaplastic WT (15 % of the whole group and 33 % of those who developed WT).

The management of these DHLPN patients should be multidisciplinary with close collaboration of radiologist, pathologists, surgeons, and pediatric oncologists with judicious sampling and intervention with stage-and disease specific chemotherapy. The chemotherapy protocols applicable to favorable and unfavorable histology by stage should be applied when WT is identified. Therapy for DHLPN without WT must be considered weighing the risks of chemotherapy versus the apparent excess incidence of WT in those who are untreated. Typically, clinicians have used EE4A therapy for isolated DHLPN with the aim of reducing the number of cells capable of malignant transformation, but the duration has been individualized based in part on radiological response (such as darkening on T2-weighted MRI imaging) (Gylys-Morin et al. 1993).

Patients with nodular HPLN have insufficient evidence available to guide one as to therapy and the approach must be individualized. As their total nephrogenic rest burden is far lower than DHLPN, observation alone may be indicated. It should be noted that many of these cases occurred in the setting of Beckwith-Wiedemann syndrome (Regalado et al. 1997; Lonergan et al. 1998), and thus, strategies that can preserve renal parenchyma are essential.

5.8 Dosing of Chemotherapy in Infants

Review of data from the first two NWTS trials revealed that infants had a significantly greater risk of developing severe complications and toxic deaths than older children (Breslow et al. 1978; Jones et al. 1984). Excess neurotoxicity and life-threatening toxicity have been recognized in infants in leukemia as well (Jones et al. 1984; Woods et al. 1981). This excess toxicity is attributed to the relatively greater body surface area (BSA) of infants in proportion to their body weight (BW). As a consequence, calculation of chemotherapy dosing based on BSA delivers nearly twice as much chemotherapy as would calculations based on body weight. In addition, the metabolism of drugs is less vigorous in immature infants.

In NWTS-2, the toxic death rate was almost 10 % in the first cohort of infants treated at full-dose chemotherapy, while a 50 % dose reduction reduced this rate to zero (Jones et al. 1984). In view of this finding, NWTS-3 recommended 50 % dose reduction for infants. Concerns with respect to jeopardizing cure rates by this reduction were alleviated on review of stage-matched outcomes (excluding mesoblastic nephromas known to have a preponderance in infancy and an excellent outcome (van den Heuvel-Eibrink et al. 2008)). Infants with reduced chemotherapy doses had identical 4-year RFS and OS outcomes as did older children (Corn et al. 1992). Thus, this dose reduction has continued to be adopted for infants in subsequent trials and remains the standard.

5.9 Future Directions

The COG approach to WT remains grounded in up-front nephrectomy, if feasible, with baseline staging, histology, and increasingly molecular classifiers determining initial approach to management. The current COG studies are examining the effectiveness of dose intensification for those patients with a historically poor outcome, and dose reduction for those with good outcomes where toxicity may contribute to long-term poorer outcomes in morbidity and mortality. Further refinement of the care of children with WT will be contingent upon identification of risk stratifiers at diagnosis that have adequate reliability and specificity to guide appropriate therapy. In addition, as the molecular characterization of these tumors improves, it is very likely that these markers will be incorporated into risk stratification and serve as platforms for the development of biologically targeted therapies especially in children with a high risk of relapse.

Continued close collaborations with the incorporation of validated risk factors and response data from other cooperative groups will be essential in maximizing outcomes for children with WT. The management of

WT remains a multidisciplinary effort with improvements in outcomes linked to refinements in surgical, radiotherapeutic, and pediatric oncological care.

5.10 Late Breaking Updates

Since the submission of this chapter, a number of relevant publications have been released and the status of the current COG therapeutic trials has changed. The therapeutic studies AREN0321, AREN0532 and AREN0533 have all closed to accrual. The only therapeutic study that remains open for new patients is the bilateral WT study (AREN0534), and this will likely close in the next year. Data from AREN0532 have not yet been released by the Data Safety Monitoring Committee.

A portion of the data has been released for AREN0533. This has been presented at the American Society of Clinical Oncology (ASCO) Meeting in Chicago 2014 in abstract form and demonstrates that the estimated 3-year EFS for the 163 patients with Slow Incomplete Response when CT lung metastases were assessed at Week 6 and subsequently treated with regimen M ($N=163$) is 88 % (95 % CI: 81, 93 %). The estimated 3-year overall survival for these 163 patients with SIR at Week 6 and subsequently treated with regimen M ($N=163$) is 92 % (95 % CI: 86, 96 %). These data compare favorably with historical controls.

A portion of data has also been released for AREN0321 and was presented at the 2014 ASCO meeting and the 2014 International Society of Pediatric Oncology (SIOP) meeting in Toronto. For stage II–IV anaplastic WT, the estimated 3-year event-free survival (EFS) for these patients is 69 % (95 % CI: 56–80 %). This EFS observed in 66 patients is on the boundary of concluding that Regimen UH-1/Revised UH-1 results are better than those expected from NWTS-5. This apparent improvement was associated with considerable toxicity including death as a first event. If adopting Regimen Revised UH-1, physicians are urged to closely monitor and promptly adjust for cardiac, hepatic and pulmonary toxicity. For malignant rhabdoid tumor, the EFS with Regimen UH-1 does not appear to be significantly improved compared to NWTS-5. Further investigation is recommended for these very difficult to treat tumors.

References

Attard-Montalto SP, Kingston JE, Eden OB, Plowman PN (1992) Late follow-up of lung function after whole lung irradiation for Wilms' tumour. Br J Radiol 65:1114–1118

Beckwith JB, Kiviat NB, Bonadio JF (1990) Nephrogenic rests, nephroblastomatosis, and the pathogenesis of Wilms' tumor. Pediatr Pathol 10:1–36

Beckwith JB, Zuppan CE, Browning NG, Moksness J, Breslow NE (1996) Histological analysis of aggressiveness and responsiveness in Wilms' tumor. Med Pediatr Oncol 27:422–428

Belasco J, D'Angio GJ (1981) Wilms' tumor. CA Cancer J Clin 31:258–270

Bishop HC, Tefft M, Evans AE, D'Angio GJ (1977) Survival in bilateral Wilms' tumor–review of 30 National Wilms' Tumor Study cases. J Pediatr Surg 12:631–638

Bisogno G, de Kraker J, Weirich A et al (1997) Veno-occlusive disease of the liver in children treated for Wilms tumor. Med Pediatr Oncol 29:245–251

Blatt J, Trigg ME, Pizzo PA, Glaubiger D (1981) Tolerance to single-dose dactinomycin in combination chemotherapy for solid tumors. Cancer Treat Rep 65: 145–147

Blute ML, Kelalis PP, Offord KP, Breslow N, Beckwith JB, D'Angio GJ (1987) Bilateral Wilms tumor. J Urol 138:968–973

Boccon-Gibod L, Rey A, Sandstedt B et al (2000) Complete necrosis induced by preoperative chemotherapy in Wilms tumor as an indicator of low risk: report of the international society of paediatric oncology (SIOP) nephroblastoma trial and study 9. Med Pediatr Oncol 34:183–190

Bonadio JF, Storer B, Norkool P, Farewell VT, Beckwith JB, D'Angio GJ (1985) Anaplastic Wilms' tumor: clinical and pathologic studies. J Clin Oncol 3:513–520

Breslow NE, Palmer NF, Hill LR, Buring J, D'Angio GJ (1978) Wilms' tumor: prognostic factors for patients without metastases at diagnosis: results of the National Wilms' Tumor Study. Cancer 41:1577–1589

Breslow N, Churchill G, Beckwith JB et al (1985) Prognosis for Wilms' tumor patients with nonmetastatic disease at diagnosis–results of the second National Wilms' Tumor Study. J Clin Oncol 3:521–531

Breslow N, Sharples K, Beckwith JB et al (1991) Prognostic factors in nonmetastatic, favorable histology Wilms' tumor. Results of the Third National Wilms' Tumor Study. Cancer 68:2345–2353

Breslow NE, Takashima JR, Ritchey ML, Strong LC, Green DM (2000) Renal failure in the Denys-Drash and Wilms' tumor-aniridia syndromes. Cancer Res 60:4030–4032

Breslow NE, Ou SS, Beckwith JB et al (2004) Doxorubicin for favorable histology, Stage II-III Wilms tumor: results from the National Wilms Tumor Studies. Cancer 101:1072–1080

Byrd RL, Evans AE, D'Angio GJ (1982) Adult Wilms tumor: effect of combined therapy on survival. J Urol 127:648–651

Coppes MJ, de Kraker J, van Dijken PJ et al (1989) Bilateral Wilms' tumor: long-term survival and some epidemiological features. J Clin Oncol 7:310–315

Coppes MJ, Bonetta L, Huang A et al (1992) Loss of heterozygosity mapping in Wilms tumor indicates the involvement of three distinct regions and a limited role for nondisjunction or mitotic recombination. Genes Chromosomes Cancer 5:326–334

Coppes MJ, Arnold M, Beckwith JB et al (1999) Factors affecting the risk of contralateral Wilms tumor development: a report from the National Wilms Tumor Study Group. Cancer 85:1616–1625

Corn BW, Goldwein JW, Evans I, D'Angio GJ (1992) Outcomes in low-risk babies treated with half-dose chemotherapy according to the Third National Wilms' Tumor Study. J Clin Oncol 10:1305–1309

Cotton CA, Peterson S, Norkool PA et al (2009) Early and late mortality after diagnosis of wilms tumor. J Clin Oncol 27:1304–1309

Cozzi F, Schiavetti A, Cozzi DA et al (2004) Conservative management of hyperplastic and multicentric nephroblastomatosis. J Urol 172:1066–1069; discussion 1069–1070

Cozzi F, Schiavetti A, Zani A, Cozzi DA (2006) Management of hyperplastic nephroblastomatosis. Pediatr Blood Cancer 46:263

D'Angio GJ (1987) Hepatotoxicity with actinomycin D. Lancet 2:104

D'Angio GJ (2008) Pre- or postoperative therapy for Wilms' tumor? J Clin Oncol 26:4055–4057

D'Angio GJ, Evans AE, Breslow N et al (1976) The treatment of Wilms' tumor: results of the national Wilms' tumor study. Cancer 38:633–646

D'Angio GJ, Evans A, Breslow N et al (1981) The treatment of Wilms' tumor: results of the Second National Wilms' Tumor Study. Cancer 47:2302–2311

D'Angio GJ, Breslow N, Beckwith JB et al (1989) Treatment of Wilms' tumor. Results of the Third National Wilms' Tumor Study. Cancer 64:349–360

Davidoff AM (2009) Wilms' tumor. Curr Opin Pediatr 21:357–364

de Chadarevian JP, Fletcher BD, Chatten J, Rabinovitch HH (1977) Massive infantile nephroblastomatosis: a clinical, radiological, and pathological analysis of four cases. Cancer 39:2294–2305

de Kraker J, Graf N, van Tinteren H et al (2004) Reduction of postoperative chemotherapy in children with stage I intermediate-risk and anaplastic Wilms' tumour (SIOP 93-01 trial): a randomised controlled trial. Lancet 364:1229–1235

Dome JS, Bockhold CA, Li SM et al (2005) High telomerase RNA expression level is an adverse prognostic factor for favorable-histology Wilms' tumor. J Clin Oncol 23:9138–9145

Dome JS, Cotton CA, Perlman EJ et al (2006) Treatment of anaplastic histology Wilms' tumor: results from the fifth National Wilms' Tumor Study. J Clin Oncol 24:2352–2358

Ehrlich PF, Hamilton TE, Grundy P, Ritchey M, Haase G, Shamberger RC (2006) The value of surgery in directing therapy for patients with Wilms' tumor with pulmonary disease. A report from the National Wilms' Tumor Study Group (National Wilms' Tumor Study 5). J Pediatr Surg 41:162–167

Evans AE, Norkool P, Evans I, Breslow N, D'Angio GJ (1991) Late effects of treatment for Wilms' tumor. A report from the National Wilms' Tumor Study Group. Cancer 67:331–336

Farber S (1966) Chemotherapy in the treatment of leukemia and Wilms' tumor. JAMA 198:826–836

Farewell VT, D'Angio GJ, Breslow N, Norkool P (1981) Retrospective validation of a new staging system for Wilms' tumor. Cancer Clin Trials 4:167–171

Faria P, Beckwith JB, Mishra K et al (1996) Focal versus diffuse anaplasia in Wilms tumor–new definitions with prognostic significance: a report from the National Wilms Tumor Study Group. Am J Surg Pathol 20:909–920

Fernandez CV, Anderson J, Breslow NE et al (2009) Anthropomorphic measurements and event-free survival in patients with favorable histology Wilms tumor: a report from the Children's Oncology Group. Pediatr Blood Cancer 52:254–258

Frazier AL, Shamberger RC, Henderson TO, Diller L (2010) Decision analysis to compare treatment strategies for Stage I/favorable histology Wilms tumor. Pediatr Blood Cancer 54:879–884

Godzinski J, Tournade MF, de Kraker J et al (1998) Rarity of surgical complications after postchemotherapy nephrectomy for nephroblastoma. Experience of the International Society of Paediatric Oncology-Trial and Study "SIOP-9". International Society of Paediatric Oncology Nephroblastoma Trial and Study Committee. Eur J Pediatr Surg 8:83–86

Graf N, Tournade MF, de Kraker J (2000) The role of preoperative chemotherapy in the management of Wilms' tumor. The SIOP studies. International Society of Pediatric Oncology. Urol Clin North Am 27:443–454

Green DM (1993) Effects of treatment for childhood cancer on vital organ systems. Cancer 71:3299–3305

Green DM (2007) Controversies in the management of Wilms tumour – immediate nephrectomy or delayed nephrectomy? Eur J Cancer 43:2453–2456

Green DM, Jaffe N (1979) The role of chemotherapy in the treatment of Wilms' tumor. Cancer 44:52–57

Green DM, Norkool P, Breslow NE, Finklestein JZ, D'Angio GJ (1990) Severe hepatic toxicity after treatment with vincristine and dactinomycin using single-dose or divided-dose schedules: a report from the National Wilms' Tumor Study. J Clin Oncol 8:1525–1530

Green DM, Breslow NE, Beckwith JB, Norkool P (1993) Screening of children with hemihypertrophy, aniridia, and Beckwith-Wiedemann syndrome in patients with Wilms tumor: a report from the National Wilms Tumor Study. Med Pediatr Oncol 21:188–192

Green DM, Beckwith JB, Breslow NE et al (1994) Treatment of children with stages II to IV anaplastic Wilms' tumor: a report from the National Wilms' Tumor Study Group. J Clin Oncol 12:2126–2131

Green DM, Breslow NE, Evans I, Moksness J, D'Angio GJ (1996) Treatment of children with stage IV favorable histology Wilms tumor: a report from the National Wilms Tumor Study Group. Med Pediatr Oncol 26: 147–152

Green DM, Breslow NE, Beckwith JB et al (1998a) Effect of duration of treatment on treatment outcome and cost of treatment for Wilms' tumor: a report from the National Wilms' Tumor Study Group. J Clin Oncol 16:3744–3751

Green DM, Breslow NE, Beckwith JB et al (1998b) Comparison between single-dose and divided-dose administration of dactinomycin and doxorubicin for patients with Wilms' tumor: a report from the National Wilms' Tumor Study Group. J Clin Oncol 16: 237–245

Green DM, Breslow NE, Beckwith JB et al (2001) Treatment with nephrectomy only for small, stage I/ favorable histology Wilms' tumor: a report from the National Wilms' Tumor Study Group. J Clin Oncol 19:3719–3724

Green DM (2004) The treatment of stages I-IV favorable histology Wilms' tumor. J Clin Oncol 22(8):1366–1372

Grundy P, Breslow N, Green DM, Sharples K, Evans A, D'Angio GJ (1989) Prognostic factors for children with recurrent Wilms' tumor: results from the Second and Third National Wilms' Tumor Study. J Clin Oncol 7:638–647

Grundy PE, Telzerow PE, Breslow N, Moksness J, Huff V, Paterson MC (1994) Loss of heterozygosity for chromosomes 16q and 1p in Wilms' tumors predicts an adverse outcome. Cancer Res 54:2331–2333

Grundy PE, Breslow NE, Li S et al (2005) Loss of heterozygosity for chromosomes 1p and 16q is an adverse prognostic factor in favorable-histology Wilms tumor: a report from the National Wilms Tumor Study Group. J Clin Oncol 23:7312–7321

Gylys-Morin V, Hoffer FA, Kozakewich H, Shamberger RC (1993) Wilms tumor and nephroblastomatosis: imaging characteristics at gadolinium-enhanced MR imaging. Radiology 188:517–521

Hamilton TE, Green DM, Perlman EJ et al (2006) Bilateral Wilms' tumor with anaplasia: lessons from the National Wilms' Tumor Study. J Pediatr Surg 41:1641–1644

Heideman RL, Haase GM, Foley CL, Wilson HL, Bailey WC (1985) Nephroblastomatosis and Wilms' tumor. Clinical experience and management of seven patients. Cancer 55:1446–1451

Hing S, Lu YJ, Summersgill B et al (2001) Gain of 1q is associated with adverse outcome in favorable histology Wilms' tumors. Am J Pathol 158:393–398

Huang CC, Gadd S, Breslow N et al (2009) Predicting relapse in favorable histology Wilms tumor using gene expression analysis: a report from the Renal Tumor Committee of the Children's Oncology Group. Clin Cancer Res 15:1770–1778

Jones B, Breslow NE, Takashima J (1984) Toxic deaths in the second National Wilms' Tumor Study. J Clin Oncol 2:1028–1033

Kalapurakal JA, Nan B, Norkool P et al (2004) Treatment outcomes in adults with favorable histologic type Wilms tumor-an update from the National Wilms Tumor Study Group. Int J Radiat Oncol Biol Phys 60: 1379–1384

Kalapurakal JA, Li SM, Breslow NE et al (2010) Intraoperative spillage of favorable histology Wilms tumor cells: influence of irradiation and chemotherapy regimens on abdominal recurrence. A report from the National Wilms Tumor Study Group. Int J Radiat Oncol Biol Phys 76:201–206

Kaste SC, Dome JS, Babyn PS et al (2008) Wilms tumour: prognostic factors, staging, therapy and late effects. Pediatr Radiol 38:2–17

Larsen E, Perez-Atayde A, Green DM, Retik A, Clavell LA, Sallan SE (1990) Surgery only for the treatment of patients with stage I (Cassady) Wilms' tumor. Cancer 66:264–266

Lemerle J, Tournade MF, Marchant RG et al (1976) Wilms' tumor: natural history and prognostic factors: a retrospective study of 248 cases treated at the Institut Gustave-Roussy 1952–1967. Cancer 37: 2557–2566

Lonergan GJ, Martinez-Leon MI, Agrons GA, Montemarano H, Suarez ES (1998) Nephrogenic rests, nephroblastomatosis, and associated lesions of the kidney. Radiographics 18:947–968

Ludwig R, Weirich A, Abel U, Hofmann W, Graf N, Tournade MF (1999) Hepatotoxicity in patients treated according to the nephroblastoma trial and study SIOP-9/GPOH. Med Pediatr Oncol 33:462–469

Meadows AT, D'Angio GJ, Evans AE, Harris CC, Miller RW, Mike V (1975) Oncogenesis and other late effects of cancer treatment in children. Radiology 114: 175–180

Meisel JA, Guthrie KA, Breslow NE, Donaldson SS, Green DM (1999) Significance and management of computed tomography detected pulmonary nodules: a report from the National Wilms Tumor Study Group. Int J Radiat Oncol Biol Phys 44:579–585

Metzger ML, Stewart CF, Freeman BB 3rd et al (2007) Topotecan is active against Wilms' tumor: results of a multi-institutional phase II study. J Clin Oncol 25:3130–3136

Miller MA, Karacay B, Breslow NE et al (2005) Prognostic value of quantifying apoptosis factor

expression in favorable histology wilms tumors. J Pediatr Hematol Oncol 27:11–14
Miniati D, Gay AN, Parks KV et al (2008) Imaging accuracy and incidence of Wilms' and non-Wilms' renal tumors in children. J Pediatr Surg 43:1301–1307
Mitchell C, Jones PM, Kelsey A et al (2000) The treatment of Wilms' tumour: results of the United Kingdom Children's cancer study group (UKCCSG) second Wilms' tumour study. Br J Cancer 83:602–608
Mitchell C, Pritchard-Jones K, Shannon R et al (2006) Immediate nephrectomy versus preoperative chemotherapy in the management of non-metastatic Wilms' tumour: results of a randomised trial (UKW3) by the UK Children's Cancer Study Group. Eur J Cancer 42:2554–2562
Montgomery BT, Kelalis PP, Blute ML et al (1991) Extended followup of bilateral Wilms tumor: results of the National Wilms Tumor Study. J Urol 146:514–518
Morgan E, Baum E, Breslow N, Takashima J, D'Angio G (1988) Chemotherapy-related toxicity in infants treated according to the Second National Wilms' Tumor Study. J Clin Oncol 6:51–55
Natrajan R, Little SE, Sodha N et al (2007) Analysis by array CGH of genomic changes associated with the progression or relapse of Wilms' tumour. J Pathol 211:52–59
Paulino AC, Wilimas J, Marina N et al (1996) Local control in synchronous bilateral Wilms tumor. Int J Radiat Oncol Biol Phys 36:541–548
Paulino AC, Wen BC, Brown CK et al (2000) Late effects in children treated with radiation therapy for Wilms' tumor. Int J Radiat Oncol Biol Phys 46:1239–1246
Perlman EJ, Faria P, Soares A et al (2006) Hyperplastic perilobar nephroblastomatosis: long-term survival of 52 patients. Pediatr Blood Cancer 46:203–221
Prasil P, Laberge JM, Bond M et al (2000) Management decisions in children with nephroblastomatosis. Med Pediatr Oncol 35:429–432; discussion 433
Pritchard J, Imeson J, Barnes J et al (1995) Results of the United Kingdom Children's Cancer Study Group first Wilms' Tumor Study. J Clin Oncol 13:124–133
Pritchard-Jones K, Pritchard J (2004) Success of clinical trials in childhood Wilms' tumour around the world. Lancet 364:1468–1470
Pritchard-Jones K, Kelsey A, Vujanic G, Imeson J, Hutton C, Mitchell C (2003) Older age is an adverse prognostic factor in stage I, favorable histology Wilms' tumor treated with vincristine monochemotherapy: a study by the United Kingdom Children's Cancer Study Group, Wilm's Tumor Working Group. J Clin Oncol 21:3269–3275
Regalado JJ, Rodriguez MM, Toledano S (1997) Bilaterally multicentric synchronous Wilms' tumor: successful conservative treatment despite persistence of nephrogenic rests. Med Pediatr Oncol 28:420–423
Reinhard H, Semler O, Burger D et al (2004a) Results of the SIOP 93-01/GPOH trial and study for the treatment of patients with unilateral nonmetastatic Wilms Tumor. Klin Padiatr 216:132–140
Reinhard H, Aliani S, Ruebe C, Stockle M, Leuschner I, Graf N (2004b) Wilms' tumor in adults: results of the Society of Pediatric Oncology (SIOP) 93-01/Society for Pediatric Oncology and Hematology (GPOH) Study. J Clin Oncol 22:4500–4506
Ritchey ML, Kelalis PP, Breslow N, Offord KP, Shochat SJ, D'Angio GJ (1988) Intracaval and atrial involvement with nephroblastoma: review of National Wilms Tumor Study-3. J Urol 140:1113–1118
Ritchey ML, Kelalis PP, Breslow N et al (1992) Surgical complications after nephrectomy for Wilms' tumor. Surg Gynecol Obstet 175:507–514
Ritchey ML, Kelalis PP, Haase GM, Shochat SJ, Green DM, D'Angio G (1993) Preoperative therapy for intracaval and atrial extension of Wilms tumor. Cancer 71:4104–4110
Scott RH, Stiller CA, Walker L, Rahman N (2006) Syndromes and constitutional chromosomal abnormalities associated with Wilms tumour. J Med Genet 43:705–715
Seibel NL, Li S, Breslow NE et al (2004) Effect of duration of treatment on treatment outcome for patients with clear-cell sarcoma of the kidney: a report from the National Wilms' Tumor Study Group. J Clin Oncol 22:468–473
Shamberger RC, Anderson JR, Breslow NE, et al (2010) Long-term outcomes for infants with very low risk Wilms tumor treated with surgery alone in National Wilms Tumor Study-5. Ann Surg 251:555–558
Shamberger RC, Guthrie KA, Ritchey ML et al (1999) Surgery-related factors and local recurrence of Wilms tumor in National Wilms Tumor Study 4. Ann Surg 229:292–297
Shamberger RC, Haase GM, Argani P et al (2006) Bilateral Wilms' tumors with progressive or nonresponsive disease. J Pediatr Surg 41:652–657; discussion 652–657
Sorensen K, Levitt G, Sebag-Montefiore D, Bull C, Sullivan I (1995) Cardiac function in Wilms' tumor survivors. J Clin Oncol 13:1546–1556
Sredni ST, Gadd S, Huang CC et al (2009) Subsets of very low risk wilms tumor show distinctive gene expression, histologic, and clinical features. Clin Cancer Res 15:6800–6809
Sutow WW, Breslow NE, Palmer NF, D'Angio GJ, Takashima J (1982) Prognosis in children with Wilms' tumor metastases prior to or following primary treatment: results from the first National Wilms' Tumor Study (NWTS-1). Am J Clin Oncol 5:339–347
Thomas PR, Tefft M, D'Angio GJ, Norkool P (1988) Acute toxicities associated with radiation in the second National Wilms' Tumor Study. J Clin Oncol 6:1694–1698
Tournade MF, Com-Nougue C, de Kraker J et al (2001) Optimal duration of preoperative therapy in unilateral and nonmetastatic Wilms' tumor in children older than 6 months: results of the Ninth International Society of Pediatric Oncology Wilms' Tumor Trial and Study. J Clin Oncol 19:488–500
van den Heuvel-Eibrink MM, Grundy P, Graf N et al (2008) Characteristics and survival of 750 children

diagnosed with a renal tumor in the first seven months of life: a collaborative study by the SIOP/GPOH/SFOP, NWTSG, and UKCCSG Wilms tumor study groups. Pediatr Blood Cancer 50:1130–1134

Vicens J, Iotti A, Lombardi MG, Iotti R, de Davila MT (2009) Diffuse hyperplastic perilobar nephroblastomatosis. Pediatr Dev Pathol 12:237–238

Vietti TJ, Sullivan MP, Haggard ME, Holcomb TM, Berry DH (1970) Vincristine sulfate and radiation therapy in metastatic Wilms' tumor. Cancer 25:12–20

Vujanic GM, Sandstedt B, Kelsey A, Sebire NJ (2009) Central pathology review in multicenter trials and studies: lessons from the nephroblastoma trials. Cancer 115:1977–1983

Weirich A, Ludwig R, Graf N et al (2004) Survival in nephroblastoma treated according to the trial and study SIOP-9/GPOH with respect to relapse and morbidity. Ann Oncol 15:808–820

Wilimas JA, Douglass EC, Magill HL, Fitch S, Hustu HO (1988) Significance of pulmonary computed tomography at diagnosis in Wilms' tumor. J Clin Oncol 6:1144–1146

Wolff JA, Newton WA Jr, Krivit W, D'Angio GJ (1968) Single versus multiple dose dactinomycin therapy of Wilms's tumor. A controlled co-operative study conducted by the Children's Cancer Study Group A (formerly Acute Leukemia Co-operative Chemotherapy Group A). N Engl J Med 279:290–294

Woods WG, O'Leary M, Nesbit ME (1981) Life-threatening neuropathy and hepatotoxicity in infants during induction therapy for acute lymphoblastic leukemia. J Pediatr 98:642–645

Zoeller G, Pekrun A, Lakomek M, Ringert RH (1994) Wilms tumor: the problem of diagnostic accuracy in children undergoing preoperative chemotherapy without histological tumor verification. J Urol 151:169–171

Treatment of Wilms Tumor: The SIOP Approach

6

Rhoikos Furtwängler and Kathy Pritchard-Jones

Contents

Abstract

Retrospective studies before 1950 showed a remarkable gain of survival at institutions with structured diagnostic and perioperative care. Irradiation pre-, intra- and postoperatively as well as chemotherapy were used, and pretreatment prior to surgery was widely accepted. However, the optimum timing of nephrectomy was the subject of lively debate between institutions. The improving imaging modalities and thus reliable radiologic diagnosis of nephroblastoma prepared the ground for systematic preoperative treatment. SIOP's nephroblastoma studies starting from 1971 proved the decrease of ruptures and stage III tumors by preoperative irradiation. After demonstrating the equality of preoperative dactinomycin- and vincristine-based chemotherapy with irradiation in the following study, postoperative treatment burden was reduced from trial to trial and adjusted to the individual risk. With an overall survival reaching 81.5 % in the late 1970s during SIOP 5, the subsequent trials were focusing on reducing side effects and long-term sequelae whilst maintaining survival. Nowadays less than 20 % of patients with a localised WT who are treated according to SIOP-2001 protocol receive irradiation. Thirty-seven percent of all patients with localised WT can be cured with a 4-week pre- and 4-week post-nephrectomy dactinomycin and vincristine course only. The 5-year EFS and OS for all patients with localised

R. Furtwängler (✉)
Specialist in Pediatric Oncology and Hematology, Saarland University Hospital, Pediatric Hematology and Oncology, Building 9, D-66421 Homburg, Saarland, Germany
e-mail: rhoikos.furtwaengler@uniklinikum-saarland.de

K. Pritchard-Jones
Department of Developmental Biology and Cancer, Institute of Child Health, University College London, 30 Guilford Street, London, WC1N 1EH, UK
e-mail: k.pritchard-jones@ucl.ac.uk

K. Pritchard-Jones, J.S. Dome (eds.), *Renal Tumors of Childhood: Biology and Therapy*, Pediatric Oncology, DOI 10.1007/978-3-662-44003-2_6, © Springer-Verlag Berlin Heidelberg 2014

nephroblastoma reach 87 and 94 %, respectively. However, patients having a local stage III, metastasis or high-risk histology WT need intensified treatment including additional doxorubicin and often etoposide, cyclophosphamide and carboplatin.

WT and nephroblastomatosis can also occur bilaterally or in combination. Under these circumstances WT patients must be treated in a multidisciplinary, chemo-response-dependent manner, aiming to preserve renal parenchyma as much as reasonably possible.

6.1 Delayed Versus Upfront Surgery: A Discussion Originating in the Early Twentieth Century

In the late nineteenth century, several clinicians, including luminary Sir William Osler described renal tumors of childhood. A description from 1872 included a bilateral case (Eberth 1872). In 1886, Hoisholt, a German pathologist living in San Francisco, introduced the name 'Mischgeschwulst der Niere' whilst describing a pulmonary metastasised nephroblastoma in an 18-year-old boy and hypothesising its embryonic genesis (Hoisholt 1886). The first comprehensive monograph from the eponym giving surgeon Max Wilms bore the same name (Wilms 1899). Treatment at the beginning of the twentieth century was complete nephrectomy if possible and had an appalling 25 % perioperative mortality. As nowadays, the most frequent symptom was painless enlargement of the abdomen though modern imaging modalities were lacking and differential diagnosis was difficult. Nevertheless, several authors in the 1930s were in favour of preoperative irradiation for the purpose of shrinking the tumor. A pre- and postoperative irradiation concept was developed (Ladd 1938). However every hospital, rather every physician had his own way to treat WT. Patients were seen by multiple doctors and students. In consequence, they underwent repetitive physical examinations possibly contributing to preoperative rupture and hence abdominal dissemination of tumor cells. A remarkable increase of survival was achieved by structuring the perioperative care as reported in a retrospective study by Robert E. Gross and Edward BD Neuhauser about their experience from 1930 to 1950. Restricted and cautious physical exam, sufficient transfusion, intravenous liquids and structured surgery, using a transabdominal approach carried out by experienced surgeons, led to elimination of deaths on the table and increased OS from 15 % in the 1914–1930 period to 32 % in the 1931–1939 period. Systematic postoperative irradiation with usually 20–40 Gy, starting whilst still sleeping from surgery's anaesthesia, increased OS to 48 % in the 1940–1947 period. Reasoning any delay that puts off nephrectomy would increase the chance of metastasis, and irradiation would cause liquefaction of the tumor mass thus enhancing haematogenous metastasis, the authors favoured upfront surgery (Gross and Neuheuser 1950). However, combined pre- and postoperative treatment was in use, but nobody had yet done randomised prospective trials of preoperative treatment.

6.2 Preoperative Treatment: The SIOP Approach in Localised Unilateral Nephroblastoma

In 1970, the SIOP investigators, based in Europe, decided to investigate the two main approaches to WT treatment in a randomised trial. Already in this study, centres from all over Europe including, amongst others, Scandinavia, Western Europe, France, Germany, Yugoslavia and Poland cooperated. Between September 1971 and October 1974, 398 patients were registered in the *SIOP 1* study (Lemerle et al. 1976). Due to the better survival for infants, the higher incidences of mesoblastic nephroma in patients younger than 6 months and the increasing frequency of renal cell carcinoma in the adolescent, patients aged less than 1 year or older than 15 years were not eligible for preoperative treatment. Hundred and thirty-seven patients with a unilateral, localised disease were eligible for randomisation to preoperative irradiation with

Table 6.1 Pretreatment trials in the SIOP studies: patient numbers, survival estimates, ruptures, stage distributions and *p* values in relation to trial arms

The SIOP studies pretreatment trials		DFS/OS (%)	Ruptures (n=)	Stage (%) I	II	III
SIOP 1	**Irradiation 20 Gy** ($n = 73$)	52/83 %	3	**43 %**	45 %	12 %
		n. s./n. s.	**$p = 0.001$**	**$p = 0.025$**		
Randomized	Upfront surgery ($n = 64$)	44/71 %	20	22 %	44 %	**34 %**
SIOP 2	**Irradiation 20 Gy + A** ($n = 86$)	–	4	**51 %**	22 %	27 %
		–	**$p = 0.0025$**	**$p < 0.005$**		
Choice	Upfront surgery[a] ($n = 52$)	–	10	28 %	35 %	**37 %**
SIOP 5	Irradiation 20 Gy + A ($n = 76$)	67/83 %	7	53 %	31 %	16 %
		n. s./n. s.	n. s.	**Equivalent**		
Randomized	**1 cycle AV (4 weeks)** ($n = 88$)	77/89 %	5	43 %	36 %	21 %
SIOP 9	2 cycles AV (8 weeks)[b] ($n = 189$)	83/87 %	6	62 %	22 %	16 %[c]
		n. s./n. s.	n. s.	**Equivalent**		
Randomized	1 cycle AV (4 weeks) ($n = 193$)	84/92 %	2	64 %	22 %	14 %[c]

DFS disease-free survival, *OS* overall survival, *A* dactinomycin, *AV* dactinomycin and vincristine induction protocol
[a]Significantly smaller tumors in the upfront surgery group
[b]Significantly decreased tumor volume in the long arm group without impact on stage or rupture rate
[c]Including stages III and IIN+

20 Gy combined with postoperative 15 Gy irradiation and dactinomycin versus upfront surgery combined with postoperative 30 Gy irradiation and dactinomycin. Even though overall survival and disease-free survival (Table 6.1) were equal, a significant higher rate of ruptures (32 %) in the upfront surgery group compared to 4 % ruptures in the irradiation group was found (p=0.001). Moreover, rupture was correlated with relapse: the disease-free survival was 27 % with a rupture compared to 51 % without (p=0.01). In contrast, patients who had preoperative irradiation more frequently had local stage I and hence reduced treatment. The consecutive *SIOP 2* trial (1974–1976) validated these results in a nonrandomised fashion in 132 patients. Interestingly patients who underwent upfront nephrectomy had smaller tumors in this study due to the physician's choice of treatment, but nevertheless they had significantly more ruptures. SIOP 1 and SIOP 2 have hence shown that preoperative irradiation reduces tumor ruptures and increases the proportion with a favourable local stage, thereby reducing total treatment burden, especially reducing the need for total abdominal irradiation with its sequelae.

After the NWTSG had shown the increased effectiveness of dactinomycin and vincristine (AV) combination treatment in the postoperative treatment in NWTS1 (D'Angio et al. 1976), AV was naturally interesting as a possible substitute

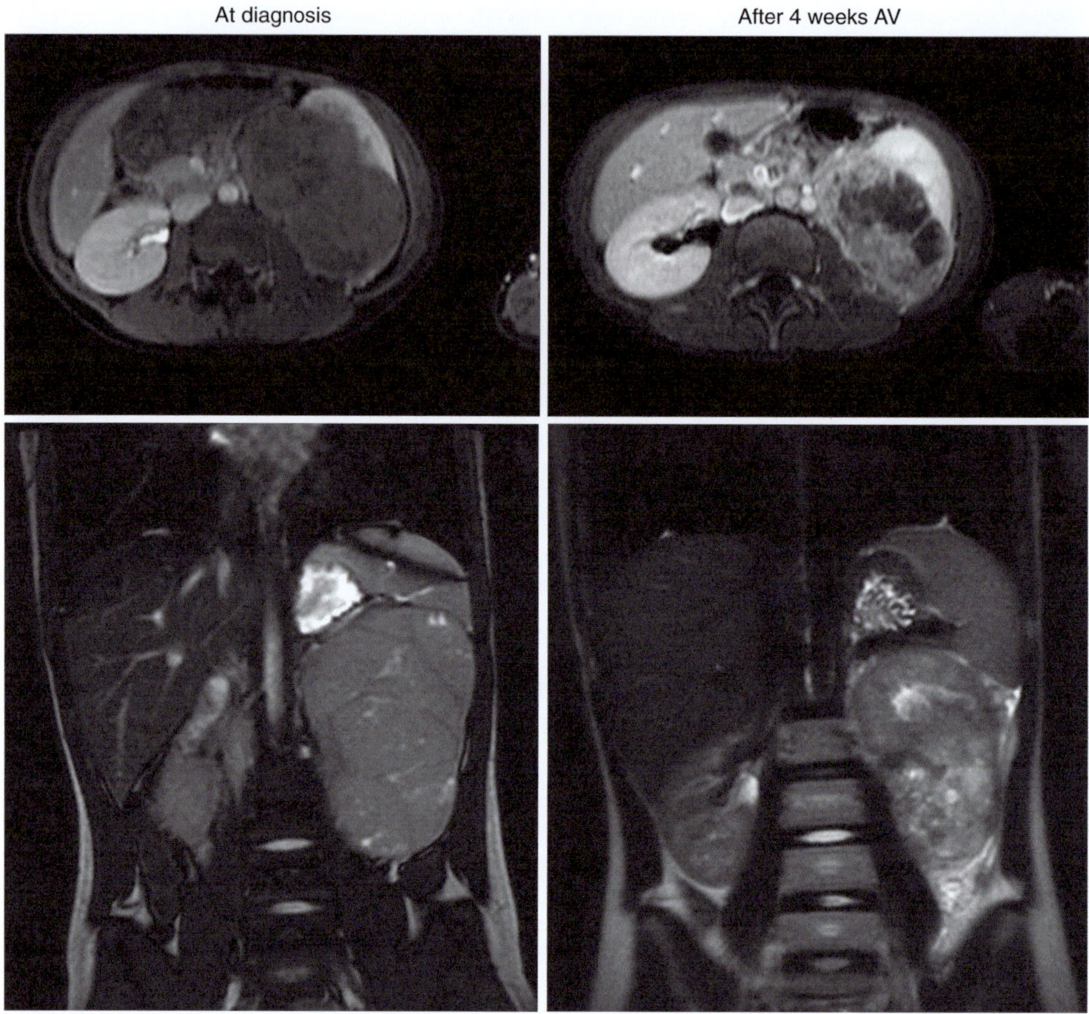

Fig. 6.1 Tumor response to 4-week AV pretreatment: in >50 % of nephroblastoma patients the tumor volume shrinks to less than 50 % of the initial volume after 4 weeks of AV pretreatment

for preoperative irradiation. From 1977 to 1979, the *SIOP 5* study (Lemerle et al. 1983) therefore addressed the effectiveness of preoperative AV randomised against preoperative irradiation (Table 6.1). Postoperative irradiation for patients with stage I had already been successfully omitted in SIOP 1 and SIOP 2 if patients had been irradiated preoperatively; hence, a careful attempt was made to evaluate an irradiation-free treatment in nephroblastoma and to investigate whether or not chemotherapy could replace irradiation. One hundred and sixty-four out of 397 registered patients were randomly assigned to 20 Gy irradiation (group R) or 4 weeks of AV (group C: 3 × 15 μg/kg dactinomycin week 1 & 3, 1 × 1.5 mg/m^2 vincristine weekly). The rate of ruptures in group C and R and the stage distribution were similar. However in group R, tumors had significantly more regressive changes in the histologic pattern, suggesting higher sensitivity to irradiation. Survival was equivalent in both groups (Table 6.1). In conclusion, the currently used preoperative combination chemotherapy of AV for 4 weeks was established. This caused a volume reduction of more than half in >50 % of patients (Fig. 6.1) (Tournade et al. 2001). Fractioned dose dactinomycin was changed to single dose, after its safety had been proved

(DeCamargo et al. 1993). Single-dose dactinomycin reduces the treatment costs in line with increasing patients and patients' parent convenience and compliance without increasing hepatic toxicity and without impairing treatment success. The following *SIOP 6* study affirmed the established pretreatment and focused on stratification of postoperative treatment (Chapter 6.3).

Reports about patients having prolonged pretreatment, for example, due to bilateral renal tumors, suggested further reduction of tumor volume in case of treatment prolongation. The aim of the *SIOP 9* study (Tournade et al. 2001) therefore was to determine the optimal preoperative treatment duration by investigating whether an additional 4-week course AV would lead to less ruptures and more stage I tumors. From 1989 to 1993, the preoperative treatment of 382 eligible patients was randomised between the standard 4-week one-cycle arm and the 8-week two-cycle experimental arm. The proportion of stage I was virtually the same (64 % vs. 62 %), and the rates of tumor ruptures were 1 % in the 4 weeks group versus 3 % in the 8-week group. However, the second AV cycle led to further significant decrease in tumor volume. Interestingly tumor histology and volume response correlated: only 17 % of stromal or epithelial predominant type WT had ≥40 % volume reduction, whilst 72 % of mixed and regressive WT and 54 % of blastemal predominant WT tumors showed >40 % volume reduction (Weirich et al. 2001). The 5-year OS and -DFS were equivalent in both groups (Table 6.1); hence, 4-week AV remained the gold standard practice given in both *SIOP 93-01* and *SIOP 2001* studies to the vast majority of patients meeting the eligibility criteria for unilateral localised tumors (Table 6.2).

Table 6.2 SIOP eligibility criteria for standard 4-week AV preoperative treatment

Eligibility criteria	Rationale
Two types of high-resolution imaging (US, CT or MRI) showing typical nephroblastoma features	To exclude neuroblastoma, nephroblastomatosis and other malign or benign tumors/infections (for details see chapters 3 and 8)
Age >6 months and <16 years	Due to high rate of CMN and RCC in the respective age groups, upfront surgery is indicated
No metastasis	Patients need intensified treatment for stage IV: 6-week AVD
Unilateral tumor	Prolonged response adapted treatment is needed to save as much as possible renal parenchyma in stage V patients
Normal catecholamine levels in sera and/or urine	To exclude neuroblastoma
No other medical or social impairment contradicting chemotherapy	

6.3 Postoperative Treatment

Even though preoperative treatment was the primary aim in the 1970s *SIOP 1* study, it investigated the postoperative treatment too. Treatment was given according to the local tumor stage, defined at the time of nephrectomy (see chapter 4). Patients with a stage I tumor received chemotherapy but no postoperative irradiation if they had already received preoperative irradiation. Stage II and stage III patients from both preoperative groups had postoperative chemotherapy and irradiation (15 or 30 Gy, respectively). Chemotherapy consisted of a single course 5 × 15 μg dactinomycin, and then patients were randomly assigned to no further treatment or six additional courses of 5 × 15 μg dactinomycin. However, the significant increase in survival for patients with dactinomycin and vincristine combination treatment in NWTS 1 prompted the SIOP study committee to stop the randomisation. Disease-free (DFS) and overall survival (OS) were equivalent in both groups (see Table 6.3). In the consecutive *SIOP 2* study (1974–1976), the postoperative treatment was based on the effective combination of dactinomycin and vincristine. Survival for patients randomised to 15 or 9 months of treatment was equivalent (Voute et al. 1978) supporting the shorter postoperative maintenance treatment.

Table 6.3 Simplified postoperative treatment overview of published SIOP studies

The SIOP studies		Postoperative treatment	DFS (%)	OS (%)	Duration
SIOP 1	I (*n* = 58)	20 Gy irradiation (pre-or ostop) & A	49 %	92 %	2 month
Stage	II & III (*n* = 160)	Irradiation (15y/30 Gy) & 1 × A	54 %	86 %	2 month
			n.s.	n.s.	
	R	Irradiation (15y/30 Gy) & 7 × A	58 %	82 %	16 month
SIOP 2	I	AV	–	–	11 month
Stage	II & III	Irradiation (15y/30 Gy) & AV	–	–	10 month
	R	Irradiation (15y/30 Gy) & AV	–	–	16 month
SIOP 5	AV	Stage I: 6× AV			
Preop-	(*n* = 80)	Stage II & III: 30 Gy irradiation & 6× AV	76 %	89 %	12 month
therapy			n.s.	n.s.	
	20 Gy Irradiation	Stage I: 6× AV	67 %	83 %	
	(*n* = 80)	Stage II & III: 15 Gy irradiation & 6× AV			12 month
SIOP 6	**I** (*n* = 145)	**3× AV**	92 %	98 %	5 month
			Equiv.	Equiv.	
	R (*n* = 158)	6× AV	88 %	94 %	10 month
SH & stage	**II N0** (*n* = 64)	20 Gy irradiation & 6× AV	72 %[b]	89 %	10 month
			Equiv.	Equiv.	
	R (*n* = 59)	**No irradiation & 6× AV**	78 %	85 %	
	II N1 & III (*n* = 43)	Irradiation 30 Gy & 6× intensified[a] AV	49 %	74 %	11 month
			$p < .03$		
	R (*n* = 40)	**Irradiation 30 Gy & AVD** (6 × VD & 5 × AV)	74 %	87 %	10 month
SIOP 9	**LH I** (*n* = 5)	No further treatment	100 %	100 %	1–2month
	UH & SH I (*n* = 244)	3 × AV	88 %	93 %	5–6 month
Histo-logy & stage	**SH IIN0** (*n* = 75)	AVD(5× VD & 5× AV)	84 %	88 %	8–9 month
	SH IIN1 & III (*n* = 56)	Irradiation 15 Gy & AVE (5×VE & 5× AV)	71 %	85 %	8–9 month
	UH II-III (*n* = 14)	Irradiation 30 Gy & AVDI (5× VD, 5× AV & 5× IV)	71 %	71 %	10–11 month
SIOP 93-01	**FH Stage I** (*n* = 200)	1× AV	87 %	95 %	2 month
			Equiv.		
	R (*n* = 210)	3× AV	88 %		5 month

Survival in respect to study and treatment arm

y years, *DFS* disease-free survival (predominantly 24–36 months of follow-up), *OS* overall survival (usually 60 months of follow-up), *R* randomisation, *N* lymph node involvement, *Gy* gray, *A* dactinomycin, *V* vincristine, *D* anthracycline (doxorubicin/epirubicin), *I* ifosfamide, *C* cyclophosphamide, *LH* low-risk histology, *SH* standard histology, *UH* unfavourable histology

[a] 2 additional vincristine each course

[b] Stopping rule! Equivalent in Dunnet and Gent test: $p < 0.05$

The following SIOP 5 study had no postoperative experimental arm. However, a secondary objective of the study was to investigate whether cure without irradiation was feasible in a large group of patients. Therefore, patients with local stage I received the established dactinomycin and vincristine treatment without irradiation. Patients having a local stage II or III had additional 15 or 30 Gy irradiation depending on whether they had already been irradiated preoperatively (Table 6.3). The 4-year overall and relapse-free survival reached 86 and 71 %, respectively, for the whole cohort (Lemerle et al. 1983). Forty-three percent of patients after preoperative chemotherapy had a localised stage I, and only one out of those 38 patients had a local recurrence. Patients having a local stage I could hence be treated effectively without any irradiation.

SIOP 6 from 1980 to 1986 was the first SIOP study focusing on postoperative treatment and a major step in the direction of elaborating risk adapted postoperative treatment (Table 6.3). Additionally to the established staging, stratification for localised nephroblastoma was now based on lymph node involvement and histology (favourable (FH)/unfavourable histology (UH)). Three randomised questions were addressed.

The respectable survival rate of >85 % in stage I patients in earlier studies shifted investigators' focus from gain of survival to treatment reduction. Hence in the first randomised question, the shortened experimental 17 weeks of AV arm proved to be equivalent to the 38-week standard arm in terms of DFS and OS (see Table 6.3) (Tournade et al. 1993). Prompted by SIOP investigators who had found lymph node invasion to correlate positively with abdominal relapse, analysing data from SIOP 1 and SIOP 2 (Jereb et al. 1980), the second randomised question investigates whether irradiation can be omitted in stage II N0 FH patients. Unfortunately six consecutive patients in the non-irradiation arm suffered from abdominal relapse, and randomisation was stopped. Despite this, the 5-year OS and the 2-year DFS were equivalent (Dunnet and Gent analysis for equivalence, $p<0.05$), and this together with similar results in NWTS 3 suggested omitting irradiation in the next study (Tournade et al. 1993). The third question demonstrated a gain of disease-free survival in stages III and IIN1 FH patients when receiving AV plus doxorubicin compared to intensified AV (Table 6.3). The stimulus to treat patients needing intensified treatment (stages III and IIN1 and unfavourable histology) with additional doxorubicin came from NWTS 2 results, which had demonstrated improved survival in stage III patients treated with doxorubicin (D'Angio et al. 1981). The small group of unfavourable histology tumors including clear cell sarcoma of the kidney, malignant rhabdoid tumor of the kidney and anaplastic tumors (Beckwith and Palmer 1978) was treated in a distinct group as study patients. They had intensified treatment too and the resulting 5-year OS was 58 %. Finally SIOP and NWTSG investigators had identified a small group of patients having multicystic or fibroadenomatous type nephroblastoma with excellent survival in retrospective analyses on earlier data (Delemarre 1977; Delemarre et al. 1984; Joshi and Beckwith 1989). The 38 patients with this subtype had an excellent 97 % 5-year OS and 2-year DFS confirming the observation made (Tournade et al. 1993). There was no recurrence in this group if patients had a stage I tumor. In consequence, the postoperative treatment for this group of patients was omitted in the following SIOP 9 study.

SIOP 9 registered 1,095 patients from 1983 to 1989 (Tournade et al. 2001) and had a randomised question concerning the duration of preoperative treatment. Postoperative treatment was based on the regimens investigated in SIOP 6. However, some smaller changes had been made in the protocol. Patients with the above-mentioned low-risk histology nephroblastoma in stage I had no postoperative treatment, and all survived without relapse (Boccon-Gibod et al. 2000). Patients with a stage IIN1 FH tumor received an intensified intravenous treatment with additional anthracycline (AVD with epi- or doxorubicin), but irradiation was omitted, and DFS rose 10 % compared to the historical comparison (Table 6.3). An acceptable 6.6 % abdominal recurrence rate supported the concept of reduced irradiation. In consequence, only 18 % of all patients were irradiated in SIOP 9. The standard risk histology group with higher risk (stages IIN1 and III) was treated as established in SIOP 6 and confirmed its results.

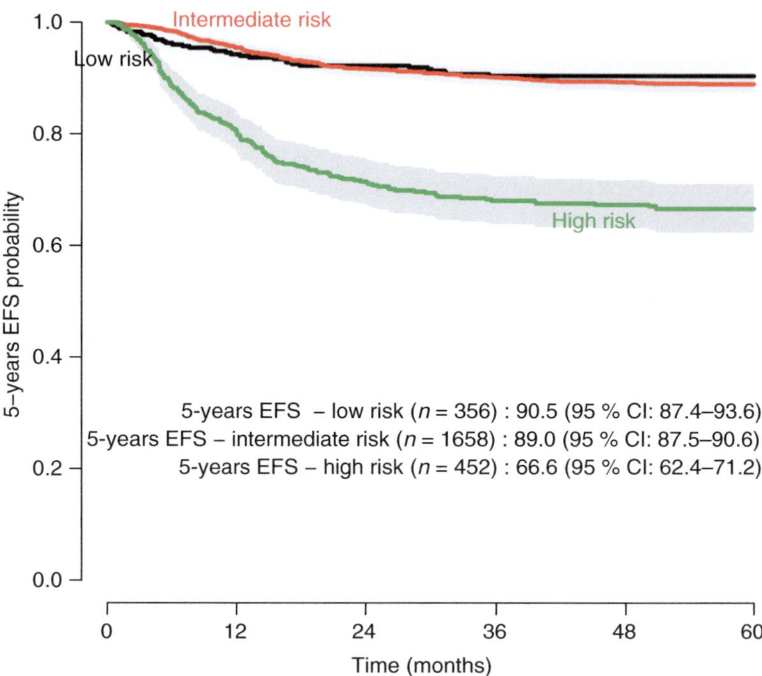

Fig. 6.2 Event-free survival of localised Wilms tumor according to histologic subtype after preoperative chemotherapy in the SIOP-93-01 trial

Patients with UH (anaplasia) had had a very poor survival so far. The treatment was extended and intensified by adding ifosfamide to AVD and brought a slight yet insignificant gain in survival to 71 %. Survival rates for the different risk groups are shown in Table 6.3. The group of stage I standard-risk patients treated with the established 17-week-AV maintained excellent disease-free survival of 88 %.

This largest of all risk groups was also the focus in *SIOP 93-01*. From July 1993 to June 2000, 1,940 patients having a childhood kidney tumor were registered, 410 of whom with stage I intermediate/standard-risk or anaplastic histology. They were randomly assigned to receive 8 or 17 weeks of postoperative AV treatment (Table 6.3). DFS proved to be equivalent for both groups in the exact non-inferiority test ($p=0.008$) (DeKraker et al. 2004) establishing that less than 3 months of minimal postoperative chemotherapy treatment is adequate for a major group of patients with stage I non-anaplastic Wilms tumor. Starting with SIOP 93-01, SIOP's histologic classification has discriminated three categories of low-, intermediate- and high-risk histology (Fig. 6.2) (Vujanic et al. 2002). Former favourable histology subtypes, such as cystic partially differentiated and fibroadenomatous-like structure nephroblastomas together with highly differentiated epithelial nephroblastomas, were allotted to the low-risk group (Delemarre et al. 1992). Anaplastic tumors, together with the non-Wilms CCSK and MRTK, formed the high-risk group, and all others were part of the intermediate-risk group type. Low-risk patients with stage I continued to receive no postoperative treatment and had no relapse in the GPOH (Gesellschaft für Pädiatrische Onkologie und Hämatologie – Austria, Switzerland and Germany) cohort (Reinhard et al. 2004). Postoperative treatment for the intermediate-risk stage IIN0 and IIN+ and III risk groups was the established postoperative treatment from SIOP 6/9. Event-free survival was 92 % for stage IIN0 and 82 % for stages IIN1 and III in the GPOH cohort (Reinhard et al. 2004). Similar results were achieved in the entire trial population (Graf et al. 2012). Whilst analysing the intermediate cohort according to the histologic subtypes (see chapter 4), SIOP investigators found improved survival rates for stromal and epithelial predominant subtypes (Fig. 6.3), whilst blastemal predominant subtypes had inferior survival compared to the rest of the intermediate-risk histologies (Weirich et al.

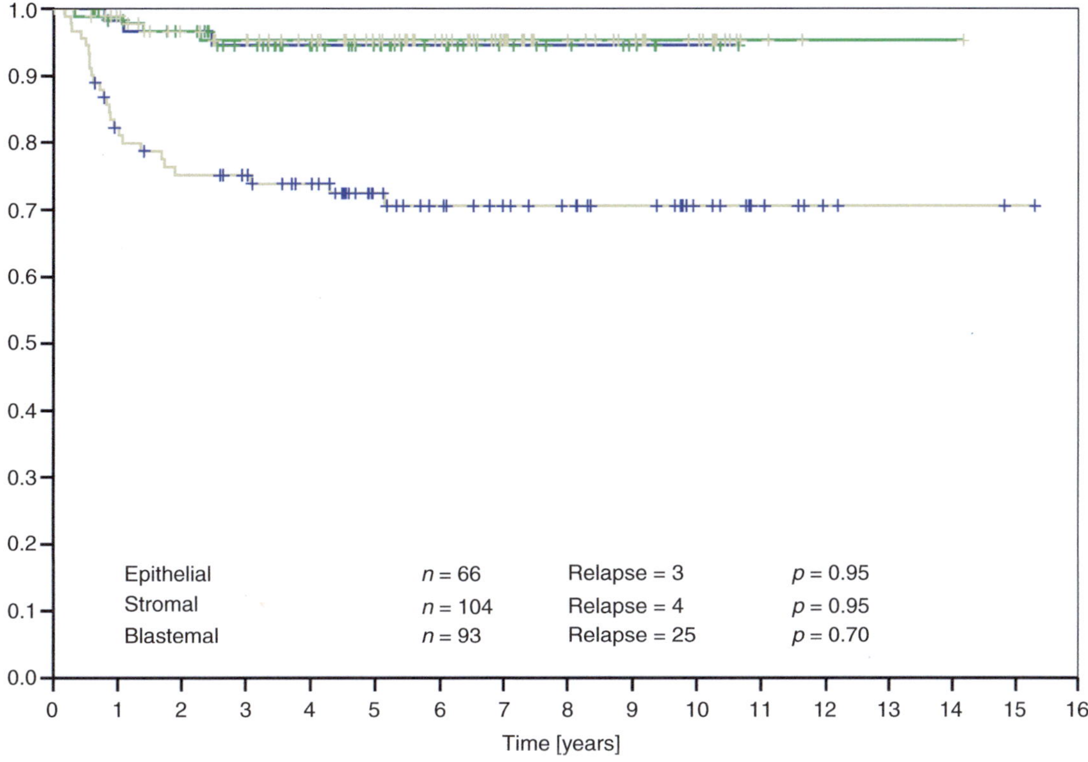

Fig. 6.3 Epithelial stromal blastemal: disease-free survival of pretreated patients from SIOP 9/GPOH, 93-01/GPOH and 2001/GPOH having a localised unilateral blastemal, epithelial or stromal predominant nephroblastoma $p=5$ year – EFS

2001). This suggests a central role of blastema in the pathogenesis of recurrence. Since blastema in pretreated tumors has proven resistance to standard AV preoperative chemo, patients with blastemal predominant tumors after pretreatment were moved to high-risk tumor stratum in the subsequent SIOP WT 2001 study.

Treatment for anaplastic (high-risk) nephroblastoma in SIOP 93-01 was changed to a 34-week combination of six courses of carboplatin and etoposide alternated with six courses of anthracycline and ifosfamide. These drugs had proven effectiveness as salvage treatment. The EFS for the whole group of anaplastic tumors rose to 78 % (Reinhard et al. 2004). Several definitions for diffuse and focal anaplasia had been used, but they were not able to discern different risk groups at that time. Hence, in SIOP 93-01 any kind of anaplasia was treated according to the high-risk protocol. However, retrospective analysis of SIOP 6 and SIOP 9 data then showed a significant difference in overall survival for the newly defined focal and diffuse anaplasia subtypes of 75 % versus 51 %, respectively ($p=0.03$) (Vujanic et al. 1999). This is also true for EFS in SIOP 93-01/GPOH patients with 91 % versus 68 %, respectively. Consequently in SIOP WT 2001, focal anaplasia was allotted to the intermediate-risk group.

6.4 SIOP 2001 and Résumé

The aim of the SIOP WT 2001 trial is to determine in a randomised fashion whether anthracyclines are needed in postoperative chemotherapy for stage II and III intermediate-risk tumors, excluding blastemal type from randomisation to the reduced therapy experimental arm. Since IIN1 had been treated together with stage III for two decades, IIN1 has now been included in stage III. Furthermore, some slight changes in the

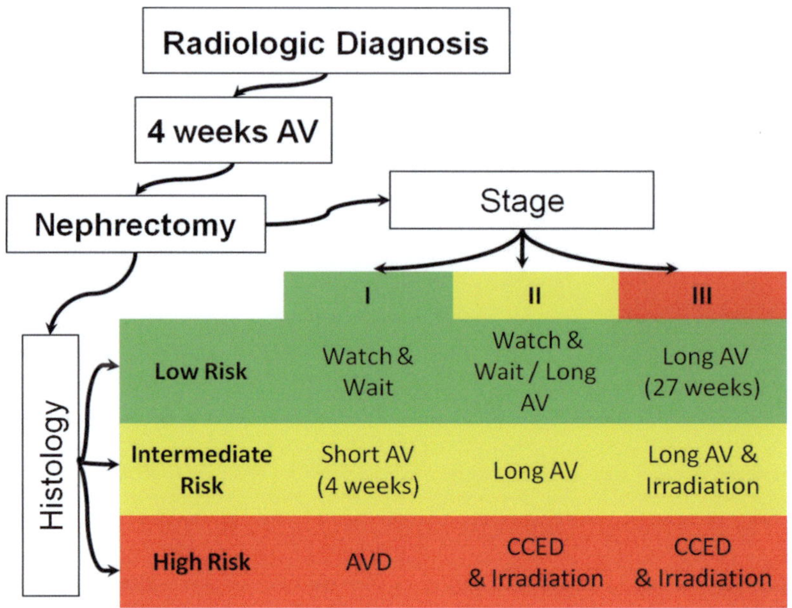

Fig. 6.4 SIOP 2001 treatment flow chart

postoperative treatment were introduced for patients with stage I tumors and high-risk histology (either diffuse anaplasia or blastemal type) who will now receive AVD for 27 weeks. A summarised overview of the current treatment is given in Fig. 6.4 and of the outcome by tumor stage for all localised WT patients treated with preoperative chemotherapy in the SIOP 93-01 and SIOP 2001 trials combined in Fig. 6.5.

Over the last four decades, SIOP investigators consolidated the concept of pretreatment of renal tumors before nephrectomy with the goal of rendering possible safer surgery with fewer complications (e.g. tumor ruptures) and 'downstaging' the tumor. Tumor stage and the in vivo histologic response are assessed at delayed nephrectomy, leading to less overall burden of therapy for the whole population and refined histologic response stratification (Vujanic et al. 2002). The often-discussed risk of erroneously treating a benign tumor remains minimal (Table 6.4). Needle biopsy can be used safely as routine or a defined measure to exclude other histology as shown by the United Kingdom Children's Cancer Study Group (Vujanic et al. 2003). Initial imaging can be centrally reviewed. The national paediatric radiologists can hence guide treatment together with the national oncologist regularly assuring quality and helping in difficult cases as carried out by the GPOH (Schenk et al. 2006). Postoperative treatment could be reduced to 4 weeks for the largest subgroup of stage I and omitted in low-risk patients. Open international collaboration and a protocol that sticks to the 'as-simple-as-possible' principle convinced many paediatric oncology centres not only all over Europe but also in America, Asia and Africa to adopt a preoperative chemotherapy approach. Further optimisation of treatment will need molecular genetics for risk classification. However, data and results from NWTS/COG and SIOP (see chapters 9 and 10 for further details) indicate the likely genetic heterogeneity in Wilms tumor and the likely need for a panel of genes to provide a powerful stratification. The results of ongoing analyses on material systematically collected during the SIOP WT 2001 trial will be integrated into planning of the next protocol. At the moment two major approaches for future stratification are emerging from the pooled data: total residual "resistant" blastema as powerful negative predictor and a panel of molecular biomarkers. While it is hoped that Wilms Tumor will have defining molecular characeristics that

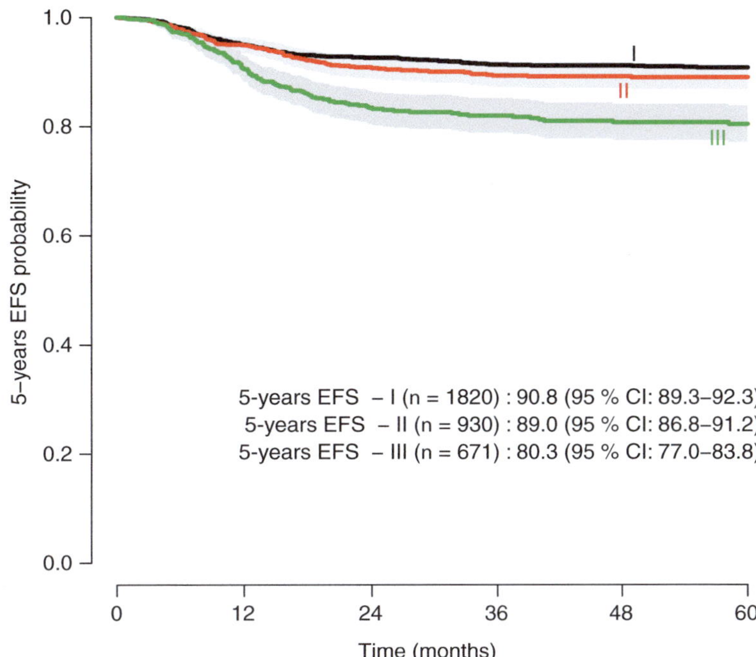

Fig. 6.5 EFS by stage of WT patients with localised disease treated with preoperative chemotherapy as per protocol, data from SIOP9301 and SIOP2001 trials combined

Table 6.4 Rate of patients treated preoperatively with benign lesions

Benign lesions treated preoperatively	
SIOP 6	1.5 %
SIOP 9	1.6 %
SIOP 93-01	1.8 %
SIOP 2001[a]	1 %

[a]Only GPOH data

can lead to a sophisticated and robust diagnostic test for high-risk subtype, the more subjective assessment of residual "resistant" blastema could be implemented easily in a broad number of industrial and developing countries.

6.5 Stage IV Treatment

Fifteen to eighteen percent of nephroblastoma patients have metastasis at diagnosis. They are most frequently located in the lungs (~95 %) or in the liver (~9 %). Rarer sites are bones, CNS and extra-abdominal lymph nodes. Although clinical good response to preoperative treatment had been seen for a while, the early studies did not investigate this subset of patients for a response-adapted approach. At the end of the 1970s, a group of six SIOP centres decided to build on their joint experience of seeing frequent good response of metastatic disease to chemotherapy and ran a prospective trial accompanying the SIOP 6 study (DeKraker et al. 1990). Dr. DeKraker and colleagues hypothesised that patient having a complete remission of their pulmonary metastases after preoperative treatment can achieve a continuous complete remission without pulmonary irradiation. They aimed to reduce the risk of the severe potential sequelae of pulmonary irradiation such as pulmonary fibrosis and congestive heart failure in survivors. Hoping to maximise the complete metastatic response rate, preoperative AV chemotherapy was intensified by addition of an anthracycline, which had been a highly effective anti-Wilms tumor drug in NWTS 2 (D'Angio et al. 1981). Patients thus received 6-week preoperative AVD (100 mg/m^2 doxorubicin), and response was assessed by chest x-ray at time of nephrectomy. Patients with residual metastases underwent metastasectomy if possible. Both groups were spared from irradiation if complete metastatic remission could be achieved by chemotherapy with or without surgical resection.

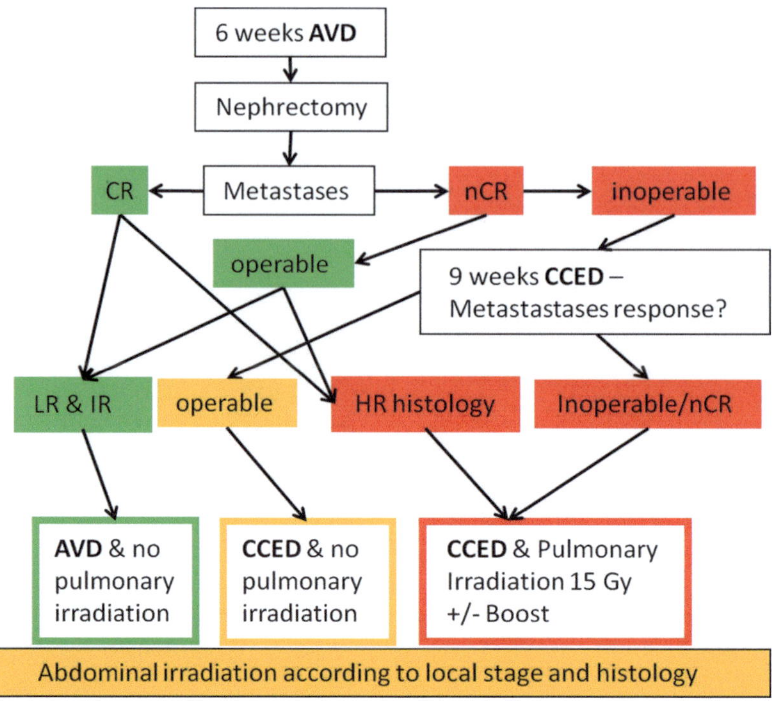

Fig. 6.6 Stage IV nephroblastoma treatment flow chart SIOP 2001. *AVD* dactinomycin, vincristine and doxorubicin, *CCED* cyclophosphamide, carboplatin, etoposide, doxorubicin, *CR* complete remission, *nCR* non-complete remission, *LR* low-risk histology, *IR* intermediate-risk histology, *HR* high-risk histology, *Gy* gray

Only those patients with multiple inoperable metastases received 15 Gy pulmonary irradiation. Postoperative treatment consisted of AVD and irradiation to the tumor bed in abdominal stages II and III. Seventy-five percent (27/36) achieved a complete remission after preoperative treatment, and 5 patients more achieved CR after surgery. Only 4 pulmonary recurrences occurred, though relatively short mean follow-up of 4 years might have masked some later recurrences. However, the vast majority had been cured without irradiation to the lungs. As a consequence, this concept became the basis of the treatment recommendations in SIOP 9.

In SIOP 9, this concept was now applied to any site of metastasis. Preoperative and perioperative procedures remained as stated above, though postoperative treatment was given according to local stage and histology, with the good responders completing 27 weeks of postoperative AVD chemotherapy and the poor responders or high-risk histology patients receiving alternative, intensified chemotherapy drugs and doses. The 2-year EFS and the 2-year OS of all 151 patients with metastatic disease, including high-risk CCSK and MRTK, having a minimal follow-up of 2.5 years, were 66.4 and 74.3 %, respectively (DeKraker et al. 1997). After the maintained success in SIOP 9, this concept was carried on in the following SIOP 93-01 study. In this study the 5 Year EFS/OS for 244 patients with unilateral stage IV WT was 73% and 82% respectively. 148 patients had achieved a CR after preoperative treatment. Their 5 year EFS/OS was 77% and 88% respectively, thus proving the concept of omitting pulmonary irradiation in good responders. Risk factors for relapse included multiple unresectable metastases, high-risk histology and local stage III (Verschuur et al. 2012). In SIOP WT 2001, additionally to the established concept, patients lacking complete response after 6-week AVD and inoperable metastasis could avoid irradiation, if they showed a complete remission of their metastasis to 9 weeks of four-drug treatment

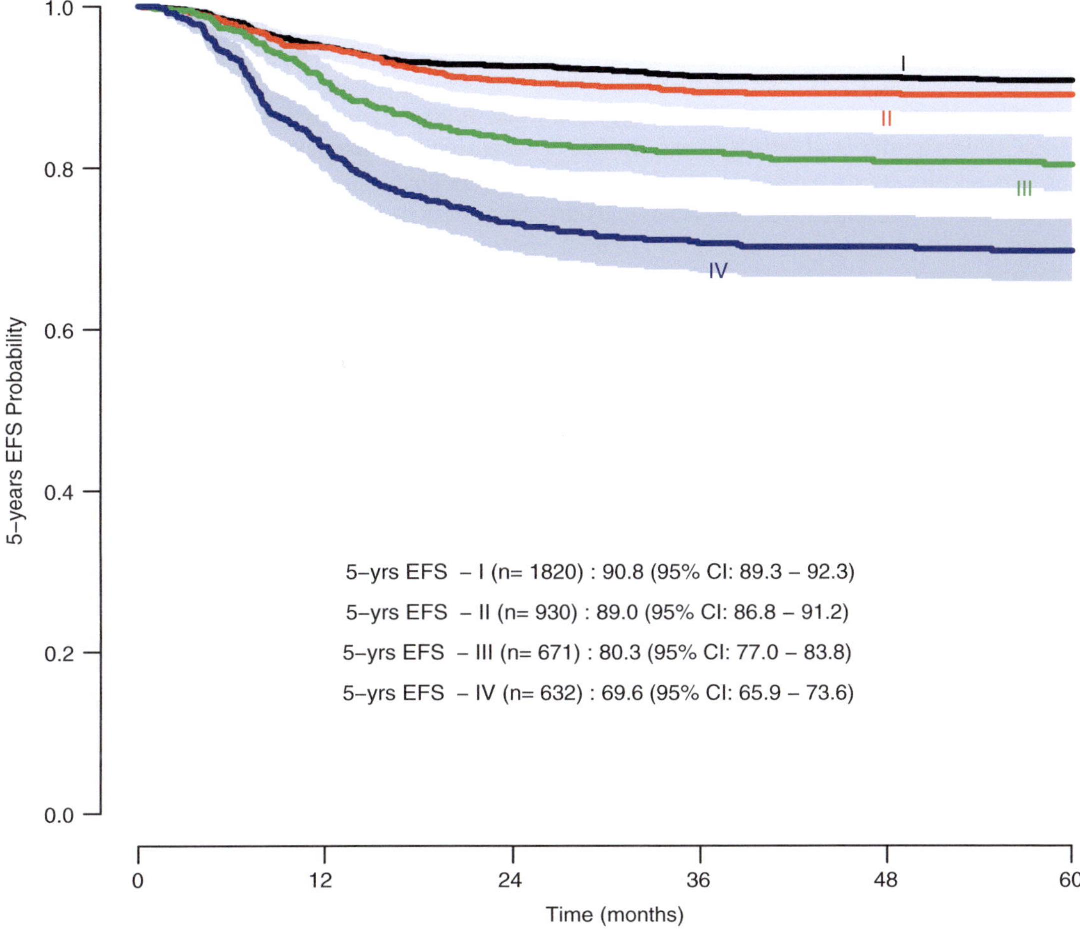

Fig. 6.7 EFS by stage of all WT patients treated with preoperative chemotherapy as per protocol, data from SIOP9301 and SIOP2001 trials combined

(CCED). The SIOP 2001 treatment concept is shown in Fig. 6.6, and the event-free survival of all stage IV patients from SIOP 93-01 and SIOP 2001 combined compared to localised WT is shown in Fig. 6.7. Here the added challenge was how to define 'complete metastatic response', since children were variably staged in the thorax using two-view chest radiograph or chest CT scan, the latter picking up smaller lesions and also being more sensitive to detection of residual abnormalities. Despite the challenge of how to handle so-called 'CT-only' lung disease, it seems clear that children with an abnormality detected on a CT chest have a worse outcome than children with no evidence of lung lesions but do somewhat better than 'true' metastatic disease visible on a plain chest radiograph (Smets et al. 2012).

6.6 Stage V Treatment

Bilateral renal tumors occur in 5–8 % of all childhood renal tumor patients (Coppes et al. 1989). A retrospective study analysing all 67 stage V patients from SIOP 1, SIOP 2 and SIOP 5 included 42 metachronous patients. The 10-year OS was 64 % and stage III as well as age at diagnosis >2 years correlated with survival (Coppes et al. 1989). However due to improved imaging modalities, smaller lesions, including presumed small nephrogenic rests, can now be diagnosed preoperatively, and inspection of the contralateral side is no longer crucial (Furtwängler et al. 2014). The combination of nephroblastoma and nephroblastomatosis or bilateral nephroblastomatosis is diagnosed radiologically almost as frequently as bilateral nephroblastoma nowadays. Nephroblastomatosis predisposes for the development of nephroblastoma (Bergeron et al. 2001). Therefore, clinicians should treat all of these situations as bilateral disease with consideration of nephron-sparing surgery whilst aiming for complete tumor excision. Such cases confront the clinician with the challenge of balancing effective tumor control by radical surgery whilst maintaining renal function.

It is possible to achieve further tumor regression by additional courses of AV, as shown in SIOP 9 (Tournade et al. 2001), thus rendering renal salvage procedures secure and effective. Preoperative treatment must therefore be response dependent. After every course of 4-week AV, the response must be assessed by imaging (see Fig. 6.8). MRI is recommended due to the better assessment of kidney and tumor and reduced radiation exposure. In case of good response to the given treatment, the course can be repeated. In case of poor response, treatment can be intensified with an additional dose of doxorubicin. A renal salvage procedure can be considered at every stage of preoperative treatment if deemed feasible. It should first be carried out on the kidney with the smaller tumor, for further courses might make salvage procedures feasible on the larger tumor side too (Godzinski et al. 1998).

Long duration preoperative treatment due to insufficient response to allow nephron-sparing surgery or extensive nephroblastomatosis might favour the development of anaplasia (Perlman et al. 2006; Furtwängler et al. 2014). Fine-needle biopsies are often discussed as a diagnostic tool in the setting of bilateral renal lesions. Unfortunately they are not able to exclude anaplasia, as small samples easily miss foci of (diffuse) anaplasia which can be located at any place in a tumor (Hamilton et al. 2006). Hence, the optimal time of surgery is a controversial topic, and every bilateral case needs careful monitoring and treatment planning by an experienced multidisciplinary team. If one simply goes by size reduction, unnecessary intensified treatment might be given to lower-risk stromal-predominant tumors, which tend to show less decrease in tumor volume than others (Verschuur et al. 2012). Patients from the GPOH usually had 1 to 3 preoperative cycles, usually without doxorubicin and rarely underwent unilateral complete nephrectomy. Though it is remarkably shorter than the average 16.3 weeks reported by the NWTS4 (Horwitz et al. 1996), it does not jeopardise renal parenchyma. Furthermore, 52 % had two functioning kidneys after the end of treatment. The reasonable survival of 75 % 5-year RFS and 88 % 5-year OS for the whole cohort of non-metastsized bilateral WT (mean FU: 8.6 years; *GPOH cases only*) underlines the effectiveness of this approach (Furtwängler et al. 2014). Two to three cycles of preoperative treatment are therefore sufficient to enable bilateral nephron-sparing surgery in most of the cases.

Postoperative treatment is given according to the highest local stage and the highest-risk histology of either side, though the minimum recommended post-op chemotherapy is 'long-AV' followed by monthly AV to a total of 1 year. Though most of the recurrences are located in the abdomen and irradiation is effective in bilateral nephroblastomas, it should be limited to cases with residual tumor. Patients need extended follow-up of renal function and for relapse on a frequent schedule, with ultrasound by an experienced and consistent operator, every 2–3 months, especially if intralobar nephrogenic rests were found or the patient was very young at diagnosis (Coppes et al. 1983).

6.7 Nephroblastomatosis

Nephroblastomatosis can occur on one or more often on both sides as solitary nephrogenic rest, or multiple nephrogenic rests or as diffuse nephroblastomatosis leading to remarkable expansion of the kidney. It does not metastasise and can be discerned by localisation into perilobar and intralobar

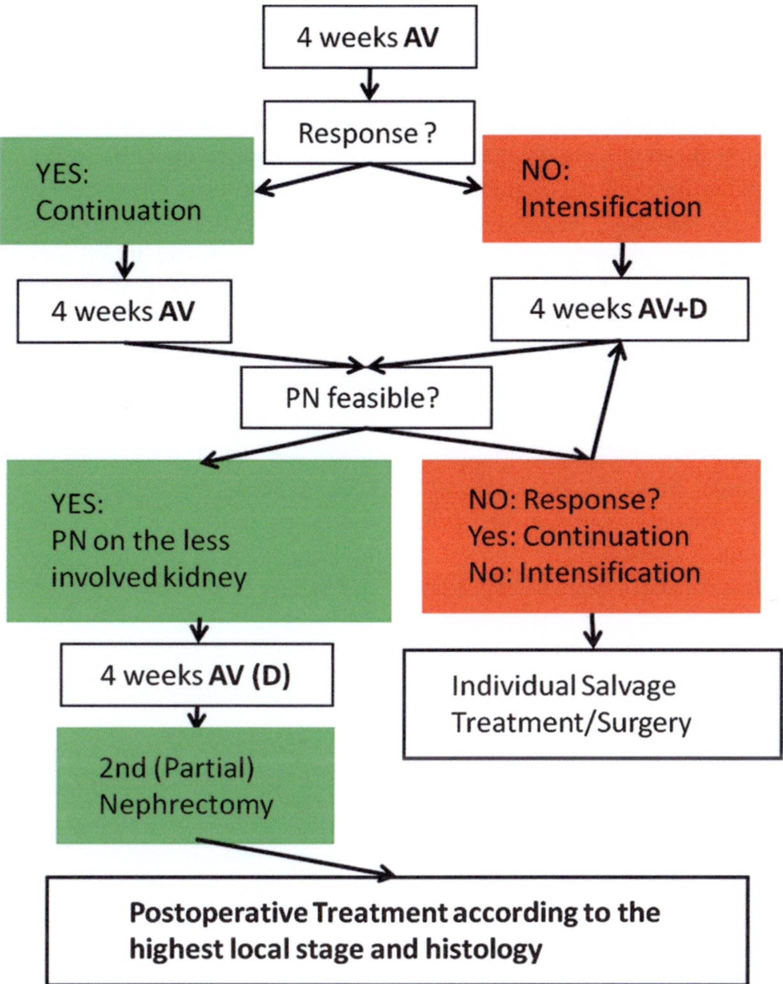

Fig. 6.8 Treatment of stage V flow chart according to SIOP WT 2001 recommendation

nephrogenic rests and by histology (see chapter 4). In the GPOH (90 million inhabitants), 2–5 patients with clinically relevant nephroblastomatosis per year are reported to the national coordinator (Graf et al. 2001). Mean age at diagnosis is 1.4 years (Furtwängler et al. 2008). Treatment can be initiated in case of obvious findings on imaging (Rohrschneider et al. 1998), but it is often impossible to discern larger nephrogenic rests from nephroblastoma. Likewise fine-needle biopsy cannot exclude blastemal predominant nephroblastoma securely (Perlman et al. 2006). In cases where diagnosis remains uncertain, preoperative treatment for nephroblastoma must be initiated, with frequent response assessment. Nephron-sparing surgery should be considered, especially in bilateral cases.

Patients with nephrogenic rests are registered in the SIOP studies, but no intervention study has been carried out yet. Several retrospective reports (Bergeron et al. 2001; Perlman et al. 2006) and case studies have proven the effectiveness of AV in the treatment of nephroblastomatosis, and the combination of AV with anthracycline seems to be even more effective, whilst single drug treatment is ineffective (Coppes et al. 1999; Bergeron et al. 2001; Perlman et al. 2006). Treatment duration has been reported to last more than 4 years, but the current SIOP WT 2001 recommendation is 12 months. Often dramatic volume response is seen initially, but small sclerosing nephrogenic rests can remain, and close follow-up is needed. A regrowing lesion developing a sphere rather than ellipsoid and heterogeneous texture must be investigated to exclude nephroblastoma before treatment can be carried on; ~50 % of the treated nephroblastomatosis develop progressions. Progressive nephroblastomatosis usually develops nephroblastoma (Bergeron et al. 2001; Perlman et al. 2006; Furtwängler et al. 2014). Reports of an increased risk for anaplasia especially in patients with prolonged treatment (Perlman et al. 2006; Furtwängler et al. 2014) suggest an earlier surgical approach to persistent/growing lesions if feasible.

Treatment recommendations are mainly based on the chemosensitivity of nephroblastomatosis to AV. Treatment duration depends on response. After 4 weeks of standard induction (2× dactinomycin 45 μg/kg, 4× vincristine 1.5 mg/m^2) and response in the first US/MRI courses of single-dose AV (1× A & 1× V) are repeated every second week until week 16 as long as a response is seen. Then single-dose AV is given every third week until complete resolution of all lesions. Maintenance treatment is given every fourth week up to 1 year.

Recently two patients with bilateral nephroblastomatosis from the GPOH showed a good response to 13-cis-retinoic-acid in a 2 weekly on-off schedule (dose), as established for neuroblastoma maintenance, in combination with AV and as single drug after progression under AV treatment. However, one of the patients developed a nephroblastoma later (Witt et al. 2009). 13-cis-Retinoic-acid might be of interest for upcoming protocols.

6.8 The UK Experience in Preoperative Treatment of Wilms Tumor

Between 1991 and 2001, the UK investigators of the Children's Cancer Study Group ran a randomised trial to address the question of which initial treatment approach to Wilms tumor gave the least overall burden of treatment whilst maintaining the best outcomes for the whole population of localised tumors (Mitchell et al. 2006). There was a reduced prevalence of tumor rupture in the group treated with preoperative chemotherapy (Powis et al. 2013) and a significant shift towards a more favourable stage distribution and thus less overall use of anthracyclines and radiotherapy. There was no difference in either event-free or overall survival between the two treatment arms. Although only 39 % of eligible patients were randomised, the subsequent report of all patients with localised non-anaplastic Wilms tumor registered in the trial gave similar results, of 83.2 % 5-year EFS and 92.9 % 5-year OS, with approximately equal numbers being treated by immediate nephrectomy or preoperative chemotherapy (Pritchard-Jones et al. 2012). Overall, 47 % of non-anaplastic Wilms tumors received doxorubicin and 27 % radiotherapy as part of their first-line therapy. During the lifetime of the UKW3 trial, the UK clinical teams developed a strong preference for adopting a universal preoperative chemotherapy approach to the treatment of renal tumors in childhood and joined with colleagues in the SIOP Renal Tumors Study Group to design the SIOP WT 2001 trial.

References

Beckwith JB, Palmer N (1978) Histopathology and prognosis of Wilms' tumor. Results of the NWTS. Cancer 41:1937–1948

Bergeron C, Iliescu C, Thiesse P, Bouvier R, Dijoud F, Ranchere-Vince D, Basset T, Chapuis JP, Buclon M, Frappaz D, Brunat-Mentigny M, Philip T (2001) Does nephroblastomatosis influence the natural history and relapse rate in Wilms' tumour? A single centre experience over 11 years. Eur J Cancer 37:385–391

Boccon-Gibod L, Rey A, Sandstedt B, Delemarre J, Harms D, Vujanic G, De Kraker J, Weirich A, Tournade MF (2000) Complete necrosis induced by preoperative chemotherapy in Wilms tumor as an indicator of low risk. Report of the international society of pediatric oncology (SIOP) nephroblastoma trial and study 9. Med Pediatr Oncol 34:183–190

Coppes MJ, de Kraker J, van Dijken PJ, Perry HJ, Delemarre JF, Tournade MF, Lemerle J, Voûte PA (1989) Bilateral Wilms' tumor: long term survival and some epidemiological features. J Clin Oncol 7:310–315

D'Angio GJ, Evans A, Brelsow N, Beckwith B, Bishop H, Feigl P, Goodwin W, Leape L, Sinks LF, Sutow W,

Tefft M, Wolff J (1976) The treatment of Wilms' tumor: results of the National Wilms' Tumor Study. Cancer 38:633–646

D'Angio GJ, Evans A, Brelsow N, Beckwith B, Bishop H, Farewell V, Goodwin W, Leape L, Palmer N, Sinks LF, Sutow W, Tefft M, Wolff J (1981) The treatment of Wilms' tumor: results of the Second National Wilms Tuomr Study. Cancer 47:2302–2311

DeCamargo B, Franco EL for the GBTTW (1993) A randomized clinical trial of single dose versus fractioned dose dactinomycin in the treatment of Wilms' tumor. Cancer 73:3081–3086

DeKraker J, Lemerle PA, Zucker JM, Tournade MF, Carli M for the SIOP Nephroblastoma Trial and Study Committee (1990) Wilms' tumor with pulmonary metastases at diagnosis: the significance of primary chemotherapy. J Clin Oncol 8:1187–1190

DeKraker J, Tournade MF, Weirich A, Ludwig R, Zucker JM, Burgers JMV, Delemarre JFM, Carli M, Godzinski J (1997) Wilms tumour stage IV a report from the SIOP 9 study. Med Pediatr Oncol 29:370, O-189 [Abstract]

DeKraker J, Graf N, Pein F, Sandstedt B, Godzinski J, Tournade MF for the SIOP Nephroblastoma Trial committee (2004) Reduction of postoperative chemotherapy in children with stage I intermediate-risk and anaplastic Wilms' tumour (SIOP93-01 trial): a randomised controlled trial. Lancet 364:1229–1235

Delemarre JFM (1977) The multicystic type of nephroblastoma. In: Abstracts IXth SIOP meeting, Philadelphia [Abstract]

Delemarre JFM, Sandstedt B, Tournade MF (1984) Nephroblastoma with fibroadenomatous-like structures. Histopathology 8:55–62

Delemarre JFM, Rey A, Harms D, Sandstedt B, Vujanic G, Tournade MF (1992) Epithelial type of nephroblastoma: to be considered as a nephroblastoma with favourable histology? Med Pediatr Oncol 20:435 [Abstract]

Eberth CJ (1872) Myoma sarcomatodes renum. Virchows Arch 55:518–520

Furtwängler R, Schmolze M, Leuschner I, von Schweinitz D, Alkassar M, Graf N, GPOH Nephroblastoma Study Group (2008) Bilateral renal tumours –the GPOH experience. In: Abstracts of the 40th annual conference of the SIOP, Berlin [Abstract]

Furtwangler R, Schmolze M, Graber S, Leuschner I, Amann G, Schenk JP, et al (2014) Pretreatment for Bilateral Nephroblastomatosis is an Independent Risk Factor for Progressive Disease in Patients with Stage V Nephroblastoma. Klin Padiatr 226(3):175–181.

Godzinski J, Tournade MF, Weirich A, de Kraker J, Ludwig R, Gauthier F, Habrand JL, Rey A, Boutard P, Core C, Karten J, Kolmannskog S, de Lumley L, Rubie H for the SIOP Wilms' Tumour Committee (1998) Prognosis for the bilateral Wilms' tumour patients after non-radical surgery: the SIOP-9 experience. Med Pediatr Oncol 31:241 [Abstract]

Graf N, Aliani S, Weirich A, Harms D, Rohrschneider W, Bürger D for the GPOH Nephroblastoma Study Committee 2001 (2001) Treatment and follow-up of 30 children with nephroblastomatosis registered in the SIOP 93-01/GPOH study. Med Pediatr Oncol 37:237 (P115) [Abstract]

Graf N, van Tinteren H, Bergeron C, Pein F, van den Heuvel-Eibrink MM, Sandstedt B, Schenk JP, Godzinski J, Oldenburger F, Furtwängler R, de Kraker J (2012) Characteristics and outcome of stage II and III non-anaplastic Wilms' tumour treated according to the SIOP trial and study 93-01. Eur J Cancer 48(17):3240–3248. doi:10.1016/j.ejca.2012.06.007, Epub 2012 Jul 12

Gross RE, Neuheuser EBD (1950) Treatment of mixed tumors of the kidney. Pediatrics 6:843–852

Hamilton TE, Green DM, Perlman EJ, Argani P, Grundy P, Ritchey ML, Shamberger RC (2006) Bilateral Wilms' tumor with anaplasia: lessons from the National Wilms' Tumor Study. J Pediatr Surg 41:1641–1644

Hoisholt AW (1886) Mischgeschwulst der Niere (Chondromyosarcom). Virchows Arch 104:118–121

Horwitz JR, Ritchey ML, Moksness J, Breslow NE, Smith GR, Thomas PRM, Haase G, Shamberger RC, Beckwith JB (1996) Renal salvage procedures in patients with synchronous bilateral Wilms' tumors: a report from the National Wilms' Tumor Study Group. J Pediatr Surg 31:1020–1025

Jereb B, Tournade MF, Lemerle J, Voute PA, Delemarre JF, Ahstrom L, Flamant R, Gerard-Marchant R, Sandstedt B (1980) Lymph node invasion and prognosis in nephroblastoma. Cancer 45:1632–1636

Joshi V, Bechwith JB (1989) Multilocular cyst of the kidney (cystic nephroma) and cystic partially differentiated nephroblastoma. Cancer 64:466–479

Ladd WE (1938) Embryoma of the kidney (Wilms tumor). Ann Surg 108:885–902

Lemerle J, Voute PA, Tournade MF, Delemarre JFM, Jereb B, Ahstrom L, Flamant R, Gerard-Marchant R (1976) Preoperative versus postoperative radiotherapy, single versus multiple courses of actinomycin D in the treatment of Wilms tumor. Cancer 38:647–654

Lemerle J, Voute PA, Torunade MF, Rodary C, Delemarre JFM, Sarrazin D, Burgers JMV, Sandstedt B, Mildenberger H, Carli M, Jereb B, Moorman-Voestermans CGM (1983) Effectiveness of preoperative chemotherapy in Wilms' tumor: results of an International Society of Paediatric Oncology (SIOP) trial. J Clin Oncol 1:604–609

Mitchell C, Pritchard-Jones K, Shannon R, Hutton C, Stevens S, Machin D, Imeson J, Kelsey A, Vujanic GM, Gornall P, Walker J, Taylor R, Sartori P, Hale J, Levitt G, Messahel B, Middleton H, Grundy R, Pritchard J (2006) Immediate nephrectomy versus pre-operative chemotherapy in the management of non-metastatic Wilms' tumour; results of a randomised trial (UKW3) by the UK Children's Cancer Study Group. Eur J Cancer 42(15):2554–2562

Perlman EJ, Faria P, Soares A, Hoffer F, Sredni S, Ritchey M, Shamberger RC, Green D, Beckwith JB (2006) Hyperplastic perilobar nephroblastomatosis: long-term survival of 52 patients. Pediatr Blood Cancer 46:203–221

Powis M, Messahel B, Hobson R, Gornall P, Walker J, Pritchard-Jones K (2013) Surgical complications after immediate nephrectomy versus preoperative chemotherapy in non-metastatic Wilms' tumour: findings from the 1991–2001 United Kingdom Children's Cancer Study Group UKW3 trial. J Pediatr Surg 48(11):2181–2186. doi:10.1016/j.jpedsurg.2013.07.001

Pritchard-Jones K, Moroz V, Vujanic G, Powis M, Walker J, Messahel B, Hobson R, Levitt G, Kelsey A, Mitchell C; on behalf of the Children's Cancer and Leukaemia Group (CCLG) Renal Tumours Group (2012) Treatment and outcome of Wilms' tumour patients: an analysis of all cases registered in the UKW3 trial. Ann Oncol 23(9):2457–2463

Reinhard H, Semler O, Bürger D, Bode U, Flentje M, Göbel U, Gutjahr P, Leuschner I, Maaß E, Niggli F, Scheel-Walter HG, Stöckle M, Thüroff JW, Tröger J, Weirich A, von Schweinitz D, Zoubek A, Graf N (2004) Results of the SIOP 93-01/GPOH trial and study for the treatment of patients with unilateral nonmetastatic Wilms tumor. Klin Padiatr 216: 132–140

Rohrschneider WK, Weirich A, Rieden K, Darge K, Tröger J, Graf N (1998) US, CT and MR imaging characteristics of nephroblastomatosis. Pediatr Radiol 28:435–443

Schenk JP, Schrader C, Zieger B, Furtwängler R, Leuschner I, Ley S, Graf N, Troeger J (2006) Reference radiology in nephroblastoma: accuracy and relevance for preoperative chemotherapy. Rofo 178:38–45 [German]

Smets AM, van Tinteren H, Bergeron C, De Camargo B, Graf N, Pritchard-Jones K, de Kraker J (2012) The contribution of chest CT-scan at diagnosis in children with unilateral Wilms' tumour. Results of the SIOP 2001 study. Eur J Cancer 48(7):1060–1065

Tournade MF, Com-Nogué C, Voute PA, Lemerle J, DeKranker J, Delemarre JFM, Burgers JMV, Habrand JL, Moorman CGM, Bürger D, Rey A, Zucker JM, Carli M, Jereb B, Bey P, Gauthier B (1993) Results of the sixth international society of pediatric oncology 6 Wilms' tumor trial and study: a risk-adapted therapeutic approach in Wilms' tumor. J Clin Oncol 11:1014–1023

Tournade MF, Com-Nogué C, DeKraker J, Ludwig R, Rey A, Burgers JMB, Sandstedt B, Godzinski J, Carli M, Potter R, Zucker JM for the SIOP (2001) Optimal duration of preoperative therapy in unilateral and nonmetastatic Wilms tumor in children older than 6 months: results of the ninth international society of pediatric oncology Wilms tumor trial and study. J Clin Oncol 19:488–500

Verschuur AC, Vujanic GM, Van Tinteren H, Jones KP, de Kraker J, Sandstedt B (2010) Stromal and epithelial predominant Wilms tumours have an excellent outcome: the SIOP 93 01 experience. Pediatric blood & cancer 55(2):233–238

Verschuur A, Van Tinteren H, Graf N, Bergeron C, Sandstedt B, De Kraker J (2012) Treatment of pulmonary metastases in children with stage IV nephroblastoma with risk-based use of pulmonary radiotherapy. Journal of Clinical Oncology 30(28):3533–3539

Voute PA, Tournade MF, Lemerle J et al (1978) Results of the studies conducted by the SIOP from 1971–78. Concerning Wilms tumor. In: 10th meeting of the SIOP, Brussels [Abstract]

Vujanic GM, Harms D, Sandstedt B, Weirich A, DeKraker J, Delemarre JFM (1999) New definitions of focal and diffuse anaplasia in Wilms' tumour: the SIOP experience. Med Pediatr Oncol 32:317–323

Vujanic GM, Sandstedt B, Harms D, Kelsey A, Leuschner I, de Kraker J for the SIOP Nephroblastoma Scientific Committee (2002) Revised international society of paediatric oncology (SIOP) working classification of renal tumors of childhood. Med Pediatr Oncol 38:79–82

Vujanic GM, Kelsey A, Mitchell C, Rosemary SS, Gornall P (2003) The role of biopsy in the diagnosis of renal tumors of childhood: results of the UKCCSG Wilms tumor study 3. Med Pediatr Oncol 40:18–22

Weirich A, Leuschner I, Harms D, Vujanic GM, Tröger J, Abel U, Graf N, Shcimdt D, Ludwig R, Voute PA (2001) Clinical impact of histologic subtypes in localized non-anaplastic nephroblastoma treated according to the trial and study SIOP-9/GPOH. Ann Oncol 12:311–319

Wilms M (1899) Die Mischgeschwülste der Niere. A Georgi, Leipzig

Witt O, Hämmerling S, Stockklausner C, Schenk JP, Günther P, Behnisch W, Hamad B, Al Mulla NA, Kulozik A (2009) 13-cis retinoic acid treatment of a patient with chemotherapy refractory nephroblastomatosis. J Pediatr Hematol Oncol 31:296–299

7 Treatment of Relapsed Wilms Tumor

Filippo Spreafico and Marcio H. Malogolowkin

Contents

F. Spreafico (✉)
Department of Hematology and Pediatric Onco-Hematology, Fondazione IRCCS Istituto Nazionale dei Tumori, Pediatric Unit, Milano, Italy
e-mail: Filippo.Spreafico@istitutotumori.mi.it

M.H. Malogolowkin, MD
Hematology-Oncology-Transplant Children's Hospital of Wisconsin, Medical College of Wisconsin, Milwaukee, Wisconsin, USA
e-mail: mmalogol@mcw.edu

7.1 Introduction

The outlook for children with newly diagnosed Wilms tumors (WT) has improved dramatically with the advent of multimodal therapy, which includes surgery, chemotherapy, and for some, radiation therapy, with survival rates currently approaching 90 % (Lemerle et al. 1983; D'Angio et al. 1981, 1976). Although the overall relapse rate for children with WT has decreased to less than 15 %, the overall long-term survival for patients with recurrent disease remains at approximately 50 % (Grundy et al. 1989; Pinkerton et al. 1991; Pein et al. 1998; Kremens et al. 2002; Tannous et al. 2000). Due to the small numbers of relapsed patients, advancements in the treatment of these patients have remained a challenge. Investigators from different cooperative groups have evaluated the role of different therapeutic strategies in an attempt to improve the outcomes of patients with recurrent WT. Therapy for these patients depends on characteristics of their primary disease, extent of previous therapy, and time from initial diagnosis to relapse.

K. Pritchard-Jones, J.S. Dome (eds.), *Renal Tumors of Childhood: Biology and Therapy*, Pediatric Oncology, DOI 10.1007/978-3-662-44003-2_7, © Springer-Verlag Berlin Heidelberg 2014

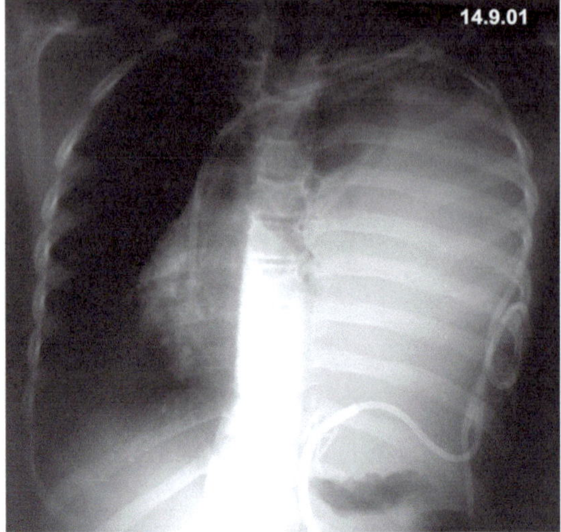

Fig. 7.1

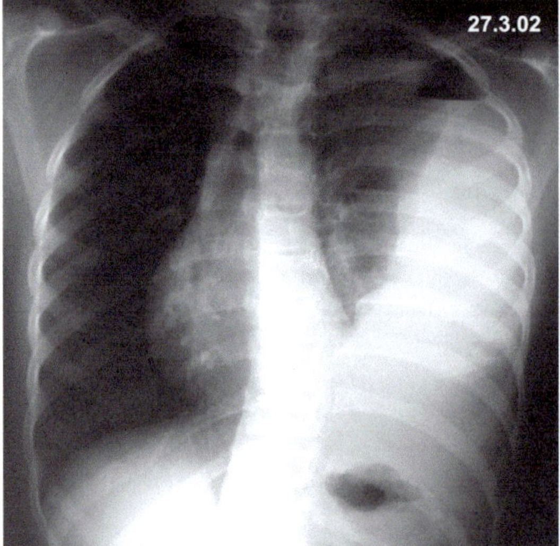

Fig. 7.2

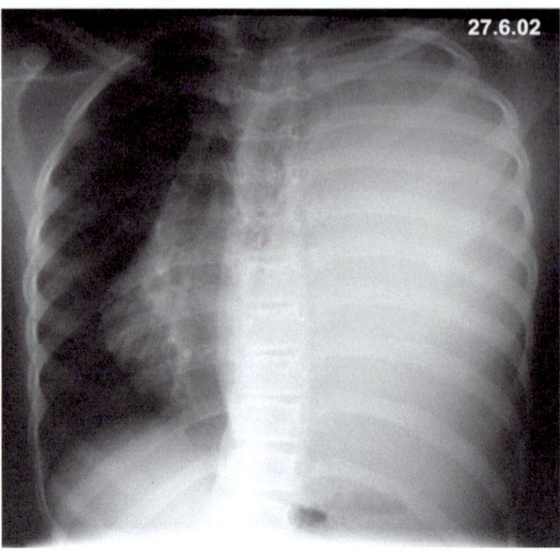

Fig. 7.3

7.2 Risk Stratification

A number of potential prognostic features influencing outcome post-recurrence have been analyzed, but it is difficult to separate whether these factors are independent of each other. Moreover, the prognostic factors appear to be changing over time as therapy for primary and recurrent WT evolves.

Grundy and coworkers provided a comprehensive analysis of prognostic indicators after relapse on National Wilms Tumor Studies (NWTS)-2 and NWTS-3 (Grundy et al. 1989). The time to recurrence was strongly predictive of survival, with those patients who relapsed early (0–5 months from nephrectomy) having worse outcome than those who relapsed later than 6 months. Other adverse factors were anaplastic histology, advanced tumor stage, and relapse outside the lung. Interestingly, the more recent experience from NWTS-5 showed that time to recurrence and site of recurrence were no longer prognostically significant (Malogolowkin et al. 2008; Green et al. 2007). Gender was predictive of outcome, with males faring worse than females. In addition, the group of patients treated initially with two drugs fared better than patients treated initially with three drugs, indicating that initial treatment remains a powerful prognostic factor.

The International Society of Pediatric Oncology (SIOP) identified adverse factors for relapsed WT including initial stage 4 disease, unfavorable histology, time to recurrence 6 months or less after diagnosis, and recurrence in multiple organs or a previously irradiated field (Pein et al. 1999). The German group analyzed a cohort of 170 relapsed patients and in accordance with the previous studies initial stage III or IV, high-risk histology (according to the SIOP classification (Vujanic et al. 2002)), early event, and combined site of relapse emerged as relevant prognostic indicators (Reinhard et al. 2008).

The explanation for the different prognosis between pulmonary and abdominal relapses may be that many of the abdominal recurrences occur in irradiated fields, whereas most lung recurrences developed in nonirradiated sites. Furthermore, it is sometimes difficult to extrapolate the precise recurrence site in the published reports, with "lung relapses" category including not only pulmonary parenchymal relapses but also those involving the mediastinum. Abdominal recurrence generally involves the original tumor bed (kidney area), but can correspond to retroperitoneal lymph nodes, liver, peritoneum, or contralateral kidney disease. Most "recurrences" in the contralateral kidney probably represent second primary tumors rather than true relapses. For these reasons, the site of relapse should deserve more analysis before being definitively considered for patient risk grouping.

However, it is likely that factors originally identified as predictors of survival, like combined site of relapse or recurrence-free interval, can lose their significance when more aggressive and effective regimens, like the ones adopted in recent years, are applied at relapse. Furthermore, the changes in initial disease therapy, now evolving towards less intense treatment, may influence outcome at recurrence. The more conservative upfront use of radiation in the recent era may have allowed for increased use at relapse, contributing to the improved patient outcome. Worthy of note is the fact that some stage I or II tumors also received radiation therapy in past years.

In conclusion, features that seem clearly associated with a worse outcome after relapse are anaplastic or SIOP high-risk histology and initial chemotherapy including doxorubicin. On the other hand, it is less clear whether time to recurrence remains prognostically significant with contemporary therapy.

Based on current data, three risk categories for recurrent Wilms tumor can be schematically identified:

1. *Standard risk*: defined as patients with favorable histology WT with relapse after therapy with only vincristine and/or actinomycin D. These patients are expected to have event-free survival (EFS) estimates in the 70–80 % range, as the results reported for the NWTS-5 or United Kingdom Children's Cancer and Leukemia Group (UKCCLG) recurrent protocols (Green et al. 2007; Hale et al. 2008). These situations account for 30 % of recurrences.
2. *High risk*: defined as patients with favorable histology WT with relapse after therapy with three or more agents (at least including doxorubicin). These patients, accounting for 45–50 % of the children with WT who relapse, are expected to have survival rates in the 40–50 % range (Malogolowkin et al. 2008).
3. *Very high risk*: defined as patients with recurrent anaplastic – regardless of adoption of primary chemotherapy or primary surgery- or post-chemotherapy blastemal-type WT. These patients are expected to have survival rates in the 10 % range (Reinhard et al. 2008; Dome et al. 2006). This group accounts for 10–15 % of all WT relapses.

7.3 Principles of Treatment

7.3.1 Surgery

In general, the discussion on indications, timing, and modality of surgery in children with recurrent WT has been rarely addressed, and it is more difficult to standardize a surgical approach for recurrent tumor. Most of the information we gather on surgery and radiation are extrapolated from unselected groups of patients or case discussions. Surgical removal of operable recurrent tumors is probably helpful, but has not been examined prospectively.

The lack of data on surgical excision of lung metastases in relapsed patients precludes precise interpretation of its potential role. Because the lungs are the most frequent site of first recurrence, more information on the therapeutic role of surgical resection of pulmonary metastases, and on which techniques to adopt, might be important. The only systematic evaluation – retrospectively acquired – is the one by the NWTS group, which suggested that surgical removal of all pulmonary metastases is unlikely to improve post-relapse survival compared with treatment with whole-lung radiation therapy and chemotherapy (Green et al. 1991). However, in the retrospective analysis by Dome et al., patients who underwent a complete surgical resection of recurrent tumor had a higher probability of survival than did patients who had a partial resection or no surgery (Dome et al. 2002).

The German data on surgical aspects for liver metastases or recurrences suggested that complete surgical resection of liver recurrences improves survival. Fuchs et al. reported that in children with a recurrence in the liver, those with a complete resection survived, whereas the patients with an incomplete resection all died (Fuchs et al. 2008). Patients who achieved a complete remission following chemotherapy and/or hepatic resection did not receive radiation therapy to the liver. Overall, it is tempting to speculate that surgery plays an important role in treating recurrent disease, but we cannot exclude the possibility that patients who underwent a complete surgical resection had less aggressive disease.

7.3.2 Radiation Therapy

The radiosensitivity of WT has been well documented since 1950, when Gross and Neuhauser (Gross and Neuhauser 1950) demonstrated the benefits of routine postoperative radiation to the renal fossa in patients with WT. Since then the cooperative groups (NWTS, SIOP, and UKCCG) have defined the interrelationship between adjuvant radiation therapy and chemotherapy, progressively limiting the indications for and intensity of radiation without negatively impacting survival rates. Differently then for newly diagnosed patients, the indication and doses of radiation for children with relapsed WT have not been investigated in a uniform fashion. The administration of radiation to a previously unirradiated field is less controversial and is frequently associated with a higher probability of survival.

Uniform guidelines for radiation therapy were developed for the NWTS-5 relapse study and included higher doses when compared with those used at initial diagnoses, even if the primary therapy did not include radiotherapy (Malogolowkin et al. 2008; Green et al. 2007). Although the outcomes of patients entered onto this study improved in comparison to the historical controls, due to the non-randomized design of this study, the role of radiation therapy for the treatment of relapse remained undetermined. The indication for the use of radiotherapy and the appropriate doses to be delivered for patients with relapsed WT who previously received radiation therapy remains controversial. Treatment plans for these patients should be done in conjunction with the radiation oncologist and taking into consideration the response to chemotherapy, extent of surgical resection, and consideration for the use of high-dose chemotherapy with stem cell rescue.

7.3.3 Chemotherapy

A general principle for the treatment of relapsed WT is to use agents not used for primary therapy. Phase 2 trials demonstrated efficacy of ifosfamide (52 % objective responses) (Tournade et al. 1988), etoposide (42 % responses) (Pein et al. 1993), and carboplatin (52 % responses) (De Camargo et al. 1994) either as single agents or as combinations (Pinkerton et al. 1991; Pein et al. 1994). More recently, investigators at St. Jude Children's Research Hospital (Memphis) documented the activity of topotecan (48 %) responses in favorable histology WT (Metzger et al. 2007).

The treatment of recurrent WT has improved dramatically during the past two decades. In a review of 54 cases involved in consecutive trials at St. Jude Children's Hospital, Dome et al. underline that outcome has improved noticeably since around the mid-1980s, when cyclophosphamide, ifosfamide, platinum compounds, and etoposide became available (Dome et al. 2002). The introduction of these drugs led to disease-free survival (DFS) rates for children with recurrent WT ranging between 50 and 70 %. Nevertheless, the best combination, dose intensity, and duration of chemotherapy agents remain poorly explored.

7.4 Standard-Risk Recurrent Patients

Children with low-stage favorable histology WT have an excellent survival with minimal therapy; therefore, the number of patients matching the criteria for the definition of standard-risk recurrent tumors is very small accounting for approximately 30 % of all recurrences, making the study of these patients a challenge. There is a paucity of reports focusing on this patient population. Recently, Green et al. reported on the outcome of 58 patients who relapsed after immediate nephrectomy (stages I and II), initial chemotherapy with vincristine and actinomycin D, and no radiation therapy (low-risk) and were registered on stratum B of the NWTS-5 relapse protocol (Green et al. 2007). Relapsed treatment included surgical excision, when feasible; radiation therapy; and alternating courses of vincristine-doxorubicin-cyclophosphamide and etoposide-cyclophosphamide. For 31 patients, the lung was the only site of relapse. The 4-year event-free survival and overall survival were 71.1 and 81.8 %, respectively, for all patients and 67.8 and 81.0 % for those who relapsed only to their lungs. The most frequent toxicities were hematological. This survival rate appears to be improved compared to a crude survival rate of 57.9 % among 19 children with stage I or II, favorable histology WT who relapsed after treatment on the United Kingdom Children's Cancer Study Group Wilms Tumor 1 protocol (Dome et al. 2002), or to the 47.8 % 5-year overall survival rate for children with relapsed stage I or II favorable or anaplastic histology reported by investigators from Saint Jude Children's Research Hospital (Malogolowkin et al. 2008).

7.5 High-Risk Relapsed Wilms Tumors

More recent experiences on *high-risk* recurrent WT, in series ranging between 11 and 60 cases, seem to support the rationale for dose-intense strategies, though there is not yet consensus on whether or not high-dose chemotherapy with autologous stem cell rescue (ASCR) can account for the improvement in outcome. Table 7.1 summarizes the results of these studies.

7.6 Conventional-Dose Chemotherapy

Abu-Gosh et al. reported on 11 cases treated with ifosfamide, carboplatin, and etoposide (ICE) chemotherapy, obtaining a 63.6 % EFS and OS at 3 years, although almost all received additional therapies, including surgery, radiation, or other chemotherapy drugs (Kung et al. 1995). Doses for ifosfamide were 1,800 mg/m^2/day × 5 days, carboplatin 400 mg/m^2/day × 2 days, and etoposide 100 mg/m^2/day × 5 days. The ICE regimen was demonstrated to be extremely efficacious in determining second responses (82 % objective response rate). It is significant that persistent nephrotoxicity was moderate, as remarked also by other groups (Dome et al. 2002; Malogolowkin et al. 1994).

Malogolowkin et al. reported for the NWTS-5 Relapse protocol on 60 homogeneously treated children who relapsed after initial therapy with vincristine, actinomycin D, and doxorubicin plus radiotherapy (Abu-Ghosh et al. 2002). The 4-year EFS and OS were 42.3 and 48 %, respectively, for all patients and were 48.9 and 52.8 % for those with relapse to the lungs only. These results were obtained using alternate courses of the drug pairs cyclophosphamide/etoposide and carboplatin/etoposide; this regimen was 90 weeks long, and many children had discontinuation of therapy due to prolonged hematological toxicity. In a previous experience, Malogolowkin et al. treated 27 patients with alternating carboplatin/etoposide and ifosfamide/doxorubicin. The 3-year event-free survival and overall survival for these patients were 58 % (Malogolowkin et al. 1994).

7.7 High-Dose Chemotherapy and Autologous Stem Cell Rescue (ASCR)

The role of high-dose chemotherapy and ASCR in patients with *high-risk* recurrent WT is not fully defined. High-dose chemotherapy with ASCR has

Table 7.1 *High-risk* recurrent Wilms tumor – treatment results

Author	Group	Year	*N*	Induction chemotherapy	ASCR	Follow-up	EFS (%)	DFS (%)	OS (%)
Pein F[a]	France	1998	28	Various "conventional"	MEC	48 months		3 years 50	60
Abu-Ghosh AM	CCG	2002	11	ICE	No	4.2 years	3 years 63.6		63.6
				(1–12)	(2)				
Kremens B[b]	German	2002	20	Various	MEC	58 months	48.2		60.9
				± C, E	(15/20)				
Campbell AD	Chicago	2004	13	7/13	≠	30 month	4 years 60		73
				CPM/E/C	(1 or 2)				
Malogolowkin MH	NWTS-5	2007	60	CPM/E	No		4 years 42.3		48
				C/E					
Spreafico F	AIEOP	2008	20	ICE	MEC	36 months		4 years 56	55
				(15/20)	(8/15)				
Hale J	UK	2008	45	CPM/E	M		2 years		66
	CCLG			C/E					

Abbreviations: *M* melphalan, *E* etoposide, *C* carboplatin, *I* ifosfamide, *CPM* cyclophosphamide

[a]Exclusion of ten progressing patients before ASCR

[b]Inclusion of four patients in the 1st complete remission; exclusion of progressing patients before ASCR

been used worldwide and mostly outside controlled clinical trials. Since the first European Bone Marrow Transplant report (Garaventa et al. 1994), the number of WT patients registered in the EBMT registry has grown to more than 300 cases (Dallorso et al. 2008).

Overall, trials with high-dose chemotherapy and ASCR seemed to obtain a better outcome than historical controls, with 3- or 4-year overall survival (OS) rates ranging from 60 to 73 % (Pein et al. 1998; Kremens et al. 2002; Hale et al. 2008; Spreafico et al. 2008; Campbell et al. 2004). Pein et al. reported on 28 high-risk chemotherapy-responsive patients transplanted, and the 3-year OS and DFS were 60 and 50 %, respectively (Pein et al. 1998). Conditioning chemotherapy consisted of melphalan, etoposide, and carboplatin (MEC) in all the cases. Kremens et al. described 23 cases treated with high-dose chemotherapy and ASCR (18 children had the MEC conditioning course), after various reinduction regimens; the OS was 60.9 %, and the EFS 48.2 % (Kremens et al. 2002). Campbell et al. showed 4-year EFS and OS rates of 60 and 73 %, respectively, in 13 patients who underwent single or double ASCR after various conditioning regimens (Campbell et al. 2004). Spreafico et al. reported on 20 consecutive patients with high-risk features at recurrence: all patients received an intense-dose chemotherapy induction, most of them adopting ICE-based therapy and 15/20 receiving high-dose chemotherapy and ASCR as consolidation (Spreafico et al. 2008). This group electively reduced the drug dosage of the ICE and MEC associations vis-à-vis the doses used by others, in an attempt to reduce the expected toxicity without jeopardizing outcome; ICE consisted of ifosfamide 1,500 mg/m^2/day × 4 days, carboplatin 600 mg/m^2/day × 1 day, and etoposide 100 mg/m^2/day × 4 days. Three-year DFS and OS rates were 56 and 55 %, respectively.

The UK CCLG's strategy for patients with recurrent *high-risk* disease was based on reinduction dose-intense regimen and a consolidation with high-dose chemotherapy and ASCR (Hale et al. 2008). The reinduction chemotherapy alternated carboplatin and etoposide with cyclophosphamide and etoposide. After six chemotherapy courses, responding patients received high-dose single-agent melphalan with ASCR.

There are no randomized trials comparing conventional-dose to high-dose chemotherapy. However, the North American colleagues reported on a series of children who underwent one or the other strategy according to the quality of tumor response to induction chemotherapy. This Children's Cancer Group study of 66 patients with recurrent high-risk WT used cyclophosphamide (440 mg/m^2/day × 5 days) and etoposide (100 mg/m^2/day × 5 days) alternating with carboplatin (500 mg/m^2/day × 2 days) and etoposide (100 mg/m^2/day × 3 days) and gave a response rate of 78 % (42 % complete response and 36 % partial response after two courses) (Tannous et al. 2000). Patients who achieved complete tumor remission received maintenance therapy with a further five identical course pairs, while those with partial response or stable disease received ablative chemotherapy followed by ASCR. The 3-year EFS were 59 and 40 % for the maintenance and ASCR subgroups, while the 3-year OS were 64 and 42 %, respectively. Although the maintenance chemotherapy group had better outcomes than the ASCR group, there was a selection bias such that patients who were disease-free after induction therapy received standard-dose chemotherapy, whereas patients with residual disease received ASCR.

The abovementioned reports dealt with diverse inclusion criteria for patient selection (responding or not to miscellaneous reinduction chemotherapy, different disease status at the time of transplant, different histological types of renal tumors) and various conditioning regimens (single or tandem transplant, different agents). Direct comparisons are limited by these differences. It is not clear which preparative regimen is superior, but it does seem that there is a survival advantage in patients whose recurrent disease was chemosensitive and those without disease evidence prior to transplant.

Taken together, all these studies seem to suggest a role for dose-intensive strategies to treat children with relapsing *high-risk* WT, though there is no consensus on whether or not high-dose chemotherapy with ASCR accounts for the improvement in post-relapse outcome compared to historical published data.

In an effort to improve evidence on the role of high-dose chemotherapy and ASCR, an international analysis has attempted a synthesis of relevant published information, following a Bayesian framework, however remaining conscious of constraints that the underlined heterogeneity imposes on conclusions drawn (Ha et al. 2013). The authors have summarized EFS and OS experience of patients with relapsed or refractory WT with the objective of comparing patients who received high-dose therapy with those that did not. A total of 19 publications concerning 1,226 patients were identified (5 reporting on patients treated with high-dose chemotherapy, 6 reporting on patients treated without high-dose chemotherapy, and 8 including both categories of patients). The EFS and OS rates were combined in a weighted manner to derive hazard ratios. Pooling all studies suggested an advantage to high-dose therapy with a hazard ratio for EFS of 0.87 and 0.94 for OS. Further, analyses of those patients classified as high-risk suggested a hazard ratio of 0.90 (95 % CI 0.62 to 1.31), and for the very-high-risk patients 0.50 (CI 0.31 to 0.82). The authors concluded that the evidence was suggestive of the value of a high-dose option, particularly in the highest risk relapse group.

7.8 Topoisomerase Inhibitors

Topotecan, a camptothecin analogue that interacts with DNA topoisomerase I, demonstrated antitumor activity in different childhood cancers including WT (Nitschke et al. 1998). The schedule of administration was probably important in determining its activity, with the protracted schedule being more effective than an intermittent high-dose regimen. Investigators at St. Jude Children's Research Hospital studied its activity specifically on WT, both in preclinical models and in clinical phase I and II trials (Dome et al. 2005; Tubergen et al. 1996). In the WILTOP, a St. Jude-based phase II study, a response rate of 48 % was obtained in 25 evaluable heavily pretreated favorable histology WT patients (12 patients had partial remission, 6 patients had stable disease, and 7 patients had progression) (Metzger et al. 2007). Importantly, topotecan seemed to be less effective in anaplastic tumors. The encouraging results obtained in the WILTOP study differed from previous topotecan trials (Nitschke et al. 1998; Tubergen et al. 1996) and were ascribed to the protracted topotecan schedule (the action of poisons during S phase is optimized by longer exposure). Based on the St. Jude's experience, topotecan has been variably included into salvage strategies for high-risk recurrent WT patients in the past few years, but outside controlled clinical trials.

Prolonged and short schedules, as well as single infusions of irinotecan, a potent topoisomerase I inhibitor, alone or in combination with other agents, have been investigated in the traditional phase II setting in various pediatric tumors such as neuroblastoma, Ewing sarcoma, WT, and certain malignant brain tumors (Bomgaars et al. 2007; Vassal et al. 2008; Kushner et al. 2006; Turner et al. 2002; Wagner et al. 2007; Casey et al. 2009; Pappo et al. 2007). A recent Children's Oncology Group (COG) trial on rhabdomyosarcoma revealed no differences in response rates between two different schedules of irinotecan (prolonged versus short: daily for 5 days versus daily for 5 days, 2 days off, and then an additional 5 days, respectively), disproving the preclinical prediction of superior activity with a prolonged schedule (Mascarenhas et al. 2010).

Despite there were no response to single-agent irinotecan in previous early phase clinical trials, in a recent report four patients with multiply relapsing WT were treated with a combination of vincristine, irinotecan, temozolomide, and bevacizumab. Two had a complete response, and two had a partial response to treatment (Venkatramani et al. 2014). The respective dose-limiting toxicities were myelosuppression and diarrhea.

The Children's Oncology Group (COG) AREN0321 renal tumour study investigated the response to irinotecan in combination with vincristine (VI regimen) in patients with newly diagnosed stage IV diffuse anaplastic measurable WT in a upfront window (Perlman 2005; Daw et al. 2014). Preliminary data seem to support the use of the VI combination in diffuse anaplastic tumors at relapse, since 11/14 (79 %) patients treated with VI window displayed partial remission.

7.9 Very-High-Risk Relapsed Wilms Tumors

Patients with relapsed diffuse anaplastic tumors have dismal long-term survival rate regardless of the site of relapse (Dome et al. 2002, 2006; Green et al. 1994). Blastemal-type WT after primary chemotherapy has been identified by the SIOP colleagues as a poor prognosis group at diagnosis; patients bearing this histological type of WT who relapse displayed a dismal prognosis after recurrence, comparable to diffuse anaplastic tumors (Reinhard et al. 2008).

Overall, very poor responses to any drug or combination have been reported in these patients. In the analysis by Pinkerton et al., one out of seven patients with unfavorable histology responded to second-line chemotherapy (Pinkerton et al. 1991); in the WILTOP study two partial responses to topotecan were observed out of 11 diffuse anaplastic recurrent tumors (Metzger et al. 2007); no survivors were registered among nine anaplastic WT who relapsed, in the retrospective analysis of the S. Jude Hospital's survey (Dome et al. 2002).

Differently than for standard- or some high-risk patients with relapsed WT, the major cause of initial treatment failure was relative under treatment as opposed to the development of drug resistance, and we can speculate that for very-high-risk children, the intrinsic resistance to drugs is the main cause of failure, both at diagnosis and at relapse. Because very-high-risk patients will have received most conventional active agents in their initial therapy, inclusion into trials of novel agents is justified for these patients.

In general, these children should be referred to centers that are conducting research trials on novel agents in the treatment of children with solid tumors.

7.10 International Cooperative Trials

As a result of the success of the multidisciplinary approach for the therapy of these rare tumors, most of the reported trials on the treatment of relapsed WT are based on small cohorts of patients treated in a non-randomized fashion and compared to historical controls. Due to the small numbers of patients with relapsed WT investigators from the Children's Oncology Group, the International Society of Pediatric Oncology and the United Kingdom Children's Cancer and Leukemia Group have been working together to develop a cooperative trial to study important questions about the treatment of these patients. A trial for the treatment of high-risk relapsed WT patients was proposed to determine if treatment with conventional intensive chemotherapy or with high-dose chemotherapy followed by autologous stem cell transplantation (ASCT) would be associated with a better outcome. This study would also estimate the differences in resource utilization between these two therapeutic approaches by collecting data on the number of hospital days and the extent of transfusion support, as well as quality of life measurements associated with each therapeutic approach. Despite the international collaboration, this study would require a long period of patient accrual and follow-up and a large investment of time and effort to accomplish the study goals. With the decrease in financial support for pediatric cancer trials, this study was not opened and therefore the question of the role of ASCT will remain unanswered.

In spite of recognizing the importance of the development of an international cooperation, these groups decide to proceed with the development of studies to determine the feasibility and toxicity of a chemotherapy regimen including either ifosfamide or cyclophosphamide, carboplatin, etoposide, with or without topotecan for the treatment of high-risk favorable histology WT patients. This studies will potentially serve as the template for future studies that may explore the combination of chemotherapy with novel biologic agents.

7.11 New Agents, Novel Approaches

Since the number of relapsed WT cases is limited, there have been few WT children entered in phase I or II studies for relapsed pediatric solid tumors. Apart from isolated case reports on single promising agents, like taxane (Italiano et al. 2005; Ramanathan et al. 2000), scanty data come from controlled clinical trials.

Oxaliplatin has a broad antitumor activity including tumors resistant to carboplatin. However, since the data available is from two patients enrolled on two different phase I pediatric trials (oxaliplatin alone (Spunt et al. 2007) and oxaliplatin/etoposide (McGregor et al. 2009)), with no documented response, no conclusion can be made about the potential efficacy of this agent for the treatment of recurrent WT.

Antiangiogenic strategies have been investigated, concentrating on the activity of vascular endothelial growth factor (VEGF) as a potential target (Ghanem et al. 2003). However, what emerged was that the pathways regulating angiogenesis in WT are very complex, and single-drug therapy is likely to be unsuccessful due to the early onset of resistance. Bevacizumab, a monoclonal antibody directed against the VEGF, was administered in a phase I study conducted by the Children's Oncology Group (COG) that included two patients with WT. Neither patient had an objective response. Bevacizumab was also administered to two children with WT on a compassionate basis (no information on their histology is available) (Benesch et al. 2008). Temporary disease stabilization was achieved in both patients, the second case being treated in combination with topotecan. Instead of targeting the ligand, some of the newer agents inhibit the VEGF tyrosine kinase-signaling receptors, VEGFR-1 and VEGFR-2. As a group, the tyrosine-kinase inhibitors are less specific and may affect signaling at varying degrees through parallel angiogenic pathways platelet-derived growth factor receptor (PDGFR) and FGFR. In the more recent studies in adults, antiangiogenic agents have been tested in combination with cytotoxic chemotherapy, with a potential additive or even synergistic effect.

A phase II trial by the COG testing the differentiation effect of all-*trans*-retinoic acid and interferon-α2A enrolled 14 evaluable WT patients, and no responses were registered (Adamson et al. 2007). Despite this, a recent case report by Witt et al. of a patient with a chemotherapy-resistant refractory bilateral nephroblastomatosis showed an excellent response to 13-cis retinoic acid in combination with vincristine and dactinomycin (Witt et al. 2009).

7.12 Biology

Although there are increasing data on molecular genetic factors present in the tumor at diagnosis, there is little information regarding the molecular genetic events acquired between primary tumors and subsequent relapse, to gain insights into the molecular basis of tumor progression or relapse, or the mechanisms through which tumor cells home into different sites of relapse.

There are only scanty data on the specific cellular pathways involved in tumor progression or metastasis, mainly relating to presence of TP53 mutations (Bardeesy et al. 1995). Whether anaplasia and/or 17p/*TP53* acquired mutation also confers an additional higher attitude to disseminate is not clear. Natrajan et al. revealed that the most significant abnormality acquired between paired primary and recurrent tumors was loss of 17p, the locus of the TP53 gene (Natrajan et al. 2007).

There is an urgent clinical need to define the involvement of pathways for which targeted therapies already exist in the progression or relapse of WT. Natrajan et al. interestingly documented an acquired gain at 15q, to which the *IGF1R* gene maps. IGF1R copy number gain and overexpression may be seen as steps leading to relapse, opening to a possible role for anti-IGF1R in the therapy for recurrent Wilms tumor.

7.13 Future Directions

Advancements in the treatment of relapsed WT resulting in improvement in the outcomes of high-risk patients and in the decrease in the morbidity of relapse therapy for those who currently have a very good outcome with respect to disease control will only be feasible through the development of well-designed clinical trials and international cooperation.

These studies should include biologic evaluation of the recurrent tumors that may provide insights into the genetic mechanisms of drug resistance, tumor progression, and relapse. The identification of these molecular events may provide new targets for novel therapeutic approaches to be used in future trials for the treatment of these patients.

References

Abu-Ghosh AM, Krailo MD, Goldman SC et al (2002) Ifosfamide, carboplatin and etoposide in children with poor-risk relapsed Wilms' tumor: a Children's Cancer Group report. Ann Oncol 13:460–469

Adamson PC, Matthay KK, O'Brien M, Reaman GH, Sato JK, Balis FM (2007) A phase 2 trial of all-trans-retinoic acid in combination with interferon-alpha2a in children with recurrent neuroblastoma or Wilms tumor: a Pediatric Oncology Branch, NCI and Children's Oncology Group Study. Pediatr Blood Cancer 49:661–665

Bardeesy N, Beckwith JB, Pelletier J (1995) Clonal expansion and attenuated apoptosis in Wilms' tumors are associated with p53 gene mutations. Cancer Res 55:215–219

Benesch M, Windelberg M, Sauseng W et al (2008) Compassionate use of bevacizumab (Avastin) in children and young adults with refractory or recurrent solid tumors. Ann Oncol 19:807–813

Bomgaars LR, Bernstein M, Krailo M et al (2007) Phase II trial of irinotecan in children with refractory solid tumors: a Children's Oncology Group Study. J Clin Oncol 25:4622–4627

Campbell AD, Cohn SL, Reynolds M et al (2004) Treatment of relapsed Wilms' tumor with high-dose therapy and autologous hematopoietic stem-cell rescue: the experience at Children's Memorial Hospital. J Clin Oncol 22:2885–2890

Casey DA, Wexler LH, Merchant MS et al (2009) Irinotecan and temozolomide for Ewing sarcoma: the Memorial Sloan-Kettering experience. Pediatr Blood Cancer 53:1029–1034

D'Angio GJ, Evans AE, Breslow N et al (1976) The treatment of Wilms' tumor: results of the national Wilms' tumor study. Cancer 38:633–646

D'Angio GJ, Evans A, Breslow N et al (1981) The treatment of Wilms' tumor: results of the Second National Wilms' Tumor Study. Cancer 47:2302–2311

Dallorso S, Dini G, Faraci M, Spreafico F (2008) SCT for Wilms' tumour. Bone Marrow Transplant 41(Suppl 2):S128–S130

Daw NC, Anderson JR, Hoffer FA et al (2014) A phase 2 study of vincristine and irinotecan in mestastatic diffuse anaplastic Wilms tumor: results from Children's Oncology Group Study AREN0321. J Clin Oncol 32 (5s) suppl abstr 10032.

De Camargo B, Melarango R, Saba e Silva N et al (1994) Phase II study of carboplatin as a single drug for relapsed Wilms' tumor: experience of the Brazilian Wilms' Tumor Study Group. Med Pediatr Oncol 22:258–260

Dome JS, Liu T, Krasin M et al (2002) Improved survival for patients with recurrent Wilms tumor: the experience at St. Jude Children's Research Hospital. J Pediatr Hematol Oncol 24:192–198

Dome JS, Neale G, Hill DA et al (2005) Anti-tumor activity of topotecan against Wilms' tumor: translation of a xenograft model to phase II study. Pediatr Blood Cancer 45:432–433

Dome JS, Cotton CA, Perlman EJ et al (2006) Treatment of anaplastic histology Wilms' tumor: results from the fifth National Wilms' Tumor Study. J Clin Oncol 24:2352–2358

Fuchs J, Szavay P, Luithle T, Furtwangler R, Graf N (2008) Surgical implications for liver metastases in nephroblastoma–data from the SIOP/GPOH study. Surg Oncol 17:33–40

Garaventa A, Hartmann O, Bernard JL et al (1994) Autologous bone marrow transplantation for pediatric Wilms' tumor: the experience of the European Bone Marrow Transplantation Solid Tumor Registry. Med Pediatr Oncol 22:11–14

Ghanem MA, van Steenbrugge GJ, Sudaryo MK, Mathoera RB, Nijman JM, van der Kwast TH (2003) Expression and prognostic relevance of vascular endothelial growth factor (VEGF) and its receptor (FLT-1) in nephroblastoma. J Clin Pathol 56:107–113

Green DM, Breslow NE, Ii Y et al (1991) The role of surgical excision in the management of relapsed Wilms' tumor patients with pulmonary metastases: a report from the National Wilms' Tumor Study. J Pediatr Surg 26:728–733

Green DM, Beckwith JB, Breslow NE et al (1994) Treatment of children with stages II to IV anaplastic Wilms' tumor: a report from the National Wilms' Tumor Study Group. J Clin Oncol 12:2126–2131

Green DM, Cotton CA, Malogolowkin M et al (2007) Treatment of Wilms tumor relapsing after initial treatment with vincristine and actinomycin D: a report from the National Wilms Tumor Study Group. Pediatr Blood Cancer 48:493–499

Gross RE, Neuhauser EB (1950) Treatment of mixed tumors of the kidney in childhood. Pediatrics 6:843–852

Grundy P, Breslow N, Green DM, Sharples K, Evans A, D'Angio GJ (1989) Prognostic factors for children with recurrent Wilms' tumor: results from the Second and Third National Wilms' Tumor Study. J Clin Oncol 7:638–647

Ha TC, Spreafico F, Graf N, Dallorso S, Dome JS, Malogolowkin M, Furtwängler R, Hale JP, Moroz V, Machin D, Pritchard-Jones K (2013) An international strategy to determine the role of high dose therapy in recurrent Wilms' tumour. Eur J Cancer 49(1): 194–210. doi:10.1016/j.ejca.2012.07.010

Hale J, Hobson R, Moroz V, Satori P (2008) Results of UK Children's Cancer and Leukemia Group (CCLG) protocol for relapsed Wilms tumor (UKWR): unified relapse strategy improves outcome. In: 40th meeting of International Society of Paediatric Oncology, p 62

Italiano A, Sirvent N, Michiels JF, Peyrade F, Otto J, Thyss A (2005) Tumour response to paclitaxel in an adult with relapsed nephroblastoma. Lancet Oncol 6:252–253

Kremens B, Gruhn B, Klingebiel T et al (2002) High-dose chemotherapy with autologous stem cell rescue in children with nephroblastoma. Bone Marrow Transplant 30:893–898

Kung FH, Desai SJ, Dickerman JD et al (1995) Ifosfamide/carboplatin/etoposide (ICE) for recurrent malignant solid tumors of childhood: a Pediatric Oncology Group Phase I/II study. J Pediatr Hematol Oncol 17:265–269

Kushner BH, Kramer K, Modak S et al (2006) Irinotecan plus temozolomide for relapsed or refractory neuroblastoma. J Clin Oncol 24:5271–5276

Lemerle J, Voute PA, Tournade MF et al (1983) Effectiveness of preoperative chemotherapy in Wilms' tumor: results of an International Society of Paediatric Oncology (SIOP) clinical trial. J Clin Oncol 1:604–609

Malogolowkin MH, Casak SJ, Feusner J et al (1994) Carboplatin and etoposide alternating with ifosfamide and doxorubicin for the treatment of children with recurrent Wilms' tumors. Proc Am Soc Clin Oncol 13:424, (abstract no. 1453)

Malogolowkin M, Cotton CA, Green DM et al (2008) Treatment of Wilms tumor relapsing after initial treatment with vincristine, actinomycin D, and doxorubicin. A report from the National Wilms Tumor Study Group. Pediatr Blood Cancer 50:236–241

Mascarenhas L, Lyden ER, Breitfel PP et al (2010) Randomized phase II window trial of two schedules of irinotecan with vincristine in patients with first relapse or progression of rhabdomyosarcoma: a report from the Children's Oncology Group. J Clin Oncol 28:4658

McGregor LM, Spunt SL, Santana VM et al (2009) Phase 1 study of an oxaliplatin and etoposide regimen in pediatric patients with recurrent solid tumors. Cancer 115:655–664

Metzger ML, Stewart CF, Freeman BB 3rd et al (2007) Topotecan is active against Wilms' tumor: results of a multi-institutional phase II study. J Clin Oncol 25:3130–3136

Natrajan R, Little SE, Sodha N et al (2007) Analysis by array CGH of genomic changes associated with the progression or relapse of Wilms' tumour. J Pathol 211:52–59

Nitschke R, Parkhurst J, Sullivan J, Harris MB, Bernstein M, Pratt C (1998) Topotecan in pediatric patients with recurrent and progressive solid tumors: a Pediatric Oncology Group phase II study. J Pediatr Hematol Oncol 20:315–318

Pappo AS, Lyden E, Breitfeld P et al (2007) Two consecutive phase II window trials of irinotecan alone or in combination with vincristine for the treatment of metastatic rhabdomyosarcoma: the Children's Oncology Group. J Clin Oncol 25:362–9

Pein F, Pinkerton R, Tournade MF et al (1993) Etoposide in relapsed or refractory Wilms' tumor: a phase II study by the French Society of Pediatric Oncology and the United Kingdom Children's Cancer Study Group. J Clin Oncol 11:1478–1481

Pein F, Tournade MF, Zucker JM et al (1994) Etoposide and carboplatin: a highly effective combination in relapsed or refractory Wilms' tumor–a phase II study by the French Society of Pediatric Oncology. J Clin Oncol 12:931–936

Pein F, Michon J, Valteau-Couanet D et al (1998) High-dose melphalan, etoposide, and carboplatin followed by autologous stem-cell rescue in pediatric high-risk recurrent Wilms' tumor: a French Society of Pediatric Oncology study. J Clin Oncol 16:3295–3301

Pein F, Rey A, de Kraker J et al (1999) Multivariate analysis of adverse prognostic factors (APF) in children with recurrent (Rec) Wilms' tumor (WT) after initial treatment according to SIOP-6 or SIOP-9 strategies. Med Pediatr Oncol 33:170, (abstract no. 11)

Perlman EJ (2005) Pediatric renal tumors: practical updates for the pathologist. Pediatr Dev Pathol 8:320–338

Pinkerton CR, Groot-Loonen JJ, Morris-Jones PH, Pritchard J (1991) Response rates in relapsed Wilms' tumor. A need for new effective agents. Cancer 67:567–571

Ramanathan RK, Rubin JT, Ohori NP, Belani CP (2000) Dramatic response of adult wilms tumor to paclitaxel and cisplatin. Med Pediatr Oncol 34:296–298

Reinhard H, Schmidt A, Furtwangler R et al (2008) Outcome of relapses of nephroblastoma in patients registered in the SIOP/GPOH trials and studies. Oncol Rep 20:463–467

Spreafico F, Bisogno G, Collini P et al (2008) Treatment of high-risk relapsed Wilms tumor with dose-intensive chemotherapy, marrow-ablative chemotherapy, and autologous hematopoietic stem cell support: experience by the Italian Association of Pediatric Hematology and Oncology. Pediatr Blood Cancer 51:23–28

Spunt SL, Freeman BB 3rd, Billups CA et al (2007) Phase I clinical trial of oxaliplatin in children and adolescents with refractory solid tumors. J Clin Oncol 25:2274–2280

Tannous R, Giller R, Holmes E et al (2000) Intensive therapy for high risk (HR) relapsed Wilms' tumor (WT). A CCG-4921/POG-9445 study report. In: Proceeding of ASCO, p 588a, (abstract no. 2315)

Tournade MF, Lemerle J, Brunat-Mentigny M et al (1988) Ifosfamide is an active drug in Wilms' tumor: a phase II study conducted by the French Society of Pediatric Oncology. J Clin Oncol 6:793–796

Tubergen DG, Stewart CF, Pratt CB et al (1996) Phase I trial and pharmacokinetic (PK) and pharmacodynamics (PD) study of topotecan using a five-day course in children with refractory solid tumors: a pediatric oncology group study. J Pediatr Hematol Oncol 18:352–361

Turner CD, Gururangan S, Eastwood J et al (2002) Phase II study of irinotecan (CPT-11) in children with high-risk malignant brain tumors: the Duke experience. Neuro Oncol 4:102–108

Vassal G, Giammarile F, Brooks M et al (2008) A phase II study of irinotecan in children with relapsed or refractory neuroblastoma: a European cooperation of the Société Française d'Oncologie Pédiatrique (SFOP) and the United Kingdom Children Cancer Study Group (UKCCSG). Eur J Cancer 44:2453–2460

Venkatramani R, Malogolowkin MH, Mascarenhas L (2014) Treatment of multiply relapsed wilms tumor with vincristine, irinotecan, temozolomide and bevacizumab. Pediatr Blood Cancer 61:756–9

Vujanic GM, Sandstedt B, Harms D, Kelsey A, Leuschner I, de Kraker J (2002) Revised International Society of Paediatric Oncology (SIOP) working classification of renal tumors of childhood. Med Pediatr Oncol 38:79–82

Wagner LM, McAllister N, Goldsby RE et al (2007) Temozolomide and intravenous irinotecan for treatment of advanced Ewing sarcoma. Pediatr Blood Cancer 48:132–139

Witt O, Hammerling S, Stockklausner C et al (2009) 13-cis retinoic acid treatment of a patient with chemotherapy refractory nephroblastomatosis. J Pediatr Hematol Oncol 31:296–299

Imaging

8

Geetika Khanna and Øystein E. Olsen

Contents

G. Khanna (✉)
Mallinckrodt Institute of Radiology, Washington University School of Medicine,
510 S. Kingshighway, Campus, 8131-MIR,
St Louis, MO 63110, USA
e-mail: khannag@mir.wustl.edu

Ø.E. Olsen
Radiology Department, Great Ormond Street Hospital for Children NHS Trust,
Great Ormond Street, London WC1N 3JH, UK
e-mail: oystein.olsen@gosh.nhs.uk

Abstract

Ultrasound is the frontline imaging modality in any child with a clinically evident or suspected abdominal mass. Formal staging relies on computed tomography (CT) or magnetic resonance imaging (MRI), which both provide sufficiently accurate pretherapeutic staging in the abdomen. The major downside of MRI is the long acquisition time requiring sedation or anesthesia and of CT the poor tissue contrast and exposure to ionizing radiation. If CT is chosen, great care should be taken to keep the dose of ionizing radiation as low as possible, e.g., by only performing a single acquisition. For tissue characterization, MRI and positron emission tomography (PET) are more promising, but still largely unexplored in nephroblastoma. CT of the chest has a proven positive therapeutic efficacy when there are lung nodules that are not visible on plain radiographs. However, the main drawback is poor specificity, which may cause unjustified upstaging of some patients with "CT-only" lung nodules. In locoregional staging, emphasis should be on detecting (1) tumor rupture into the retroperitoneum or peritoneum;

K. Pritchard-Jones, J.S. Dome (eds.), *Renal Tumors of Childhood: Biology and Therapy*, Pediatric Oncology, DOI 10.1007/978-3-662-44003-2_8, © Springer-Verlag Berlin Heidelberg 2014

(2) invasion into the renal vein, inferior vena cava, and right heart; (3) invasion of the upper urinary tract; and (4) lymph node metastases, where there is currently low specificity vis-à-vis reactive lymph nodes. In bilateral disease it is of particular importance to distinguish active tumor from nephrogenic rests, scars, and normal variants, since it is important to preserve as much renal tissue as deemed safe oncologically. This remains challenging with ultrasound and CT; however, new techniques (e.g., MRI) are promising. For this group of children, observation over time is particularly important. There is now general agreement that children with genetic predispositions for nephroblastoma should undergo ultrasound screening every 3–4 months up to the age of 7 years, whereas screening of children with isolated hemihypertrophy remains controversial.

8.1 Introduction

The imaging disciplines are developing so rapidly that it becomes challenging to assess the efficacy of the modalities. Further, the accuracy of imaging is fundamentally depending on how standardized the image acquisition and interpretation are performed. Keeping this in mind, one can see how difficult it is to specify absolute imaging guidelines for any clinical context, and not least in pediatric oncology where there is such variation in presentation, and in patient size, age, and compliance. This chapter will give a brief overview of the most commonly used imaging modalities, ultrasound, computed tomography (CT), magnetic resonance imaging (MRI), and positron emission tomography (PET), and discuss the preference of CT or MRI for abdominal imaging. We will then focus on local and distant staging, with particular emphasis on the challenges encountered in bilateral disease, small lung nodules, and tumors that show paradoxical change in size during chemotherapy. We will further discuss some imaging-related issues related to undesirable effects of treatment and finally discuss long-term follow-up after treatment, as well as screening for nephroblastoma in children with predisposing conditions.

8.2 Imaging Modalities

8.2.1 Ultrasound

Ultrasound is the first-line modality for any child with a suspected abdominal mass. It has high availability, is very cost-effective, allows real-time observation, does not require sedation, and does not use ionizing radiation. However, being highly operator dependent, it is very important that the person(s) carrying out the scan is/are sufficiently experienced with pediatric abdominal ultrasound, since even the fundamental interpretation, such as distinguishing a suprarenal from an intrarenal mass, may be challenging.

Due to continuous technical advancement, the lifetime of ultrasound equipment should be no more than 10 years. Pediatric scanning requires a good selection of probes with a combination of high-frequency range curvilinear and linear probes. Capability of tissue harmonic imaging (important for definition of interface normal-abnormal) and duplex Doppler (for definition of vascular involvement and relations) is mandatory.

The environment is of importance, and effort should be made to facilitate a relaxed and inviting atmosphere for child and family and should offer some form of distraction (toys, entertainment system, etc).

8.2.2 Computed Tomography

CT made a significant technological leap with the introduction of multidetector CT (MDCT) in 1992 (Cody 2002). The newer MDCT machines have rows of detectors aligned along the patient as well as in the transverse plane. Their advantages include high-speed acquisition, increased anatomic coverage, and improved three-dimensional post-processing, all of which expand the scope of imaging. Increased speed has reduced scanning time to a few seconds, reducing motion blur and also diminishing the need for sedation in children.

Improved image resolution along the length of the patient (providing isotropic volume elements for image construction) allows post-processing of high-quality images in any arbitrary plane and high-quality three-dimensional images. Sagittal and coronal reconstructions, now performed routinely, aid the delineation of the organ of origin of a mass and helps define relationships to surrounding structures. Though multiphase images should not be acquired routinely due to ionizing radiation, CT may be used to obtain angiographic images when planning partial nephrectomy. Similarly, delayed phase images can be used to obtain a CT urogram to delineate the relationship between the mass and the renal collection system. For further discussion, see Sect. 8.3.4 for issues related to ionizing radiation and Sect. 8.3.5 for contrast media.

8.2.3 Magnetic Resonance Imaging

For its superior soft tissue contrast alone, MRI would be the first modality of choice following ultrasound. While CT forms images based exclusively on electron density, MRI depends on a range of physical-chemical tissue characteristics (energy exchange, magnetic heterogeneity, diffusion barriers, fat/water distribution, etc). Its nonionizing radiation nature allows acquisition of multiple image weightings and allows repeat imaging following intravenous contrast media administration so that dynamic properties may be captured. Scan planes are arbitrary, and MRI is also capable of true three-dimensional image acquisition. Although not yet established in clinical use, several quantitative techniques are now commonly available, e.g., calculation of apparent diffusion coefficients and tissue perfusion parameters. These add to the tissue characterization capabilities of MRI. Although some evidence exists on the accuracy of MRI in detection of lung nodules (Frericks et al. 2008), lung staging with MRI is currently not recommended.

The operator dependence in MRI is mainly down to local experience in adaptation of scan settings across different age groups and body sizes and adaptation of image weighting to pediatric malignancies (whose tissue characteristics differ from adult tumors; Fig. 8.1). A suggested scan protocol for upper abdominal tumors is given in Table 8.1. Particular attention should be paid to the three-dimensional fast T1-weighted acquisitions in early phase following contrast medium bolus injection, which is useful for demarcating tumor and normal renal parenchyma and for assessment of the renal vein(s) and the inferior vena cava. T2-weighted images without fat suppression are excellent for relating tumor to adjacent anatomic planes, which is important with tumor rupture. Inversion recovery images and, when acquired, diffusion-weighted images are sensitive for metastatic deposits both in the liver and in regional lymph nodes.

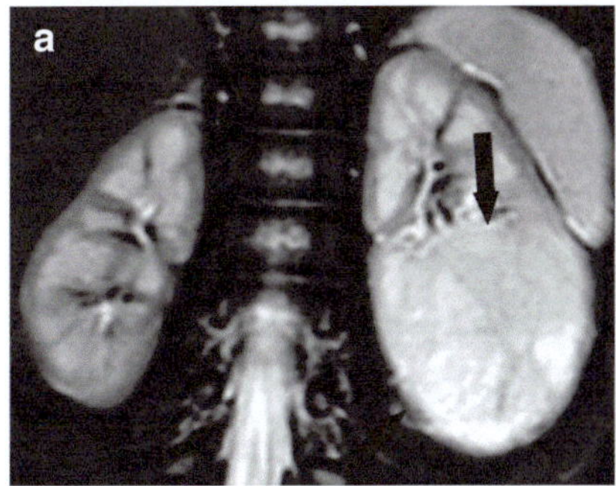

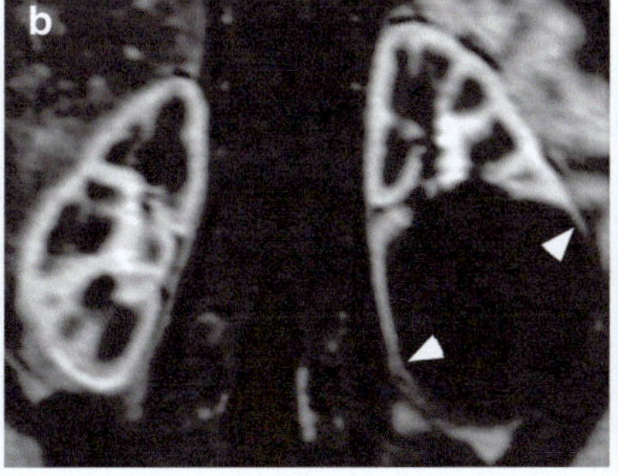

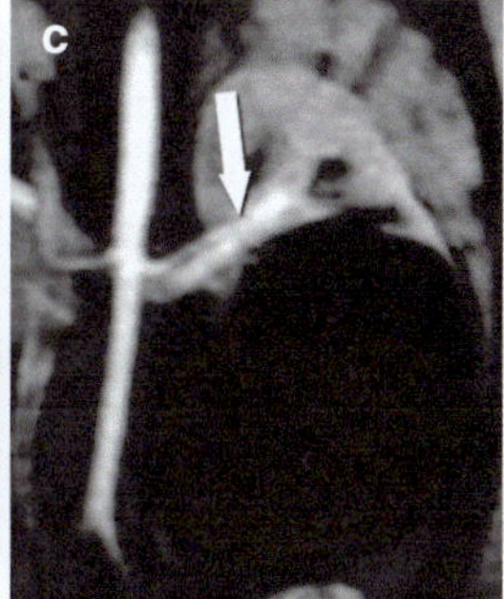

Fig. 8.1 Left lower pole nephroblastoma imaged with coronal sections on MRI. (**a**) Fat-suppressed T2-weighted technique, the often preferred pulse sequence in adult tumor imaging, provides poor contrast between the renal tissue and the mass (*black arrows*). (**b**) Fast T1-weighted gradient echo sequence acquired in arterial phase following intravenous gadolinium contrast administration provides an excellent contrast between the low-enhancing tumor and the avidly enhancing renal parenchyma. The "claw sign" (*arrowheads*) is now evident. (**c**) Thick slab maximum intensity projection-reconstruction demonstrates the renal vessels (*white arrow*)

Table 8.1 Suggested MRI pulse sequence protocol for upper abdominal mass lesions

Pulse sequence	Plane	Gating/breath control	Contrast medium	Technical detail
Short-tau inversion recovery turbo spin echo	Coronal[a] Transaxial	Prospective diaphragmatic gating	–	Preferable relatively long echo-time
T2-weighted fast spin-echo	Transaxial	Prospective diaphragmatic gating		Phase encoding left to right may further reduce motion artifact from the anterior abdominal wall
Diffusion-weighted imaging	Transaxial	–		b values of 0 and >800
Fat-suppressed T1-weighted fast spin-echo	Transaxial	–	Pre-contrast for comparison	–
3D fast low-angle shot spoiled gradient echo	Axial or coronal[a]	Breath-hold (about 30 s acquisition)	Pre-contrast for comparison and optional subtraction In arterial/renal venous phase following contrast medium administration[b]	Voxels should be close to isotropic to allow reformatting
Fat-suppressed T1-weighted fast spin-echo	Transaxial	–	Delayed following contrast administration	–

Notes
Unless contraindicated, peristaltic suppression (e.g., intravenous hyoscine) will reduce imaging artifact
[a]In an established renal lesion, a tilted coronal plane along the long axis of the kidneys may be preferable
[b]Peripheral injection using a power injector, with a chaser bolus of saline. Use of a monitoring slice allows better timing

8.2.4 Positron Emission Tomography

^{18}F-fluorodeoxyglucose (FDG)-PET has revolutionized oncologic imaging. PET/CT-scanners allow a combination of functional assessment along with anatomic detail that has never before been available in a single diagnostic modality. Though FDG remains the workhorse, several new radionuclides, such as ^{18}F-3′-fluoro-3′-deoxy-L-thymidine, have been developed, aiming at higher specificity. Few studies have evaluated FDG-PET in Wilms tumor. Despite avid FDG uptake in normal renal parenchyma, FDG-PET has been shown able to detect Wilms tumor, detect metastatic disease, differentiate malignant and benign lesions, and demonstrate therapy response (Moinul Hossain et al. 2010; Murphy et al. 2008; Shulkin et al. 1997). An important role for PET may be in guiding biopsy to viable and biologically aggressive parts of tumor and possibly in early assessment of therapy response. It has been suggested that PET may be useful for differentiating high-risk from intermediate-risk histology tumors, as the former are more FDG avid; however, this needs confirmation in larger series (Misch et al. 2008; Begent et al. 2011). There is no proof that PET offers diagnostic improvement within the current staging systems, particularly because it has limited sensitivity for detection of small lung metastases.

8.3 CT or MRI for Staging?

8.3.1 Can We Scientifically Judge?

Stringent evidence is hard to find. Structured search of the two major knowledge databases EMBASE and MEDLINE yields thousands of MRI studies published over the last 10 years; however, of the fewer than 70 papers on non-CNS pediatric oncologic MRI, under a third utilized any statistical analysis for objective assessment of results and even fewer studies tried to assess outcome beyond diagnostic impact. It is exceedingly rare in pediatric oncologic imaging to find published data from efficacy studies that reach beyond comparison between modalities.

The lack of traditional evidence should, however, not discourage a scientific approach to the issue, and we should definitely not base our decision on personal preferences, such as surgeons, oncologists, or radiologists being more comfortable with one particular modality (Olsen 2008). Although local limitations in availability and infrastructure are unavoidable decision-making factors, it is also important to stress that children with cancer deserve the best available imaging if it has a potential impact on their treatment and outcome.

8.3.2 CT: Pros and Cons

CT is readily available. Recent technological development has lead to very short scan times and consequently less movement artifact, improved multiplanar and three-dimensional capability, and reduced need for sedation. CT also allows very high spatial resolution, which is attractive for lung and bone imaging where inherent contrast is high. However, CT image formation is fundamentally only based on electron density and is therefore extremely limited, although contrast administration partly compensates by allowing information on large vessels, perfusion, and vascular permeability. These parameters cannot be quantified with CT. Also, some reader dependence is likely in the accuracy of lung nodule, liver lesion, and lymph node detection and interpretation. Although new detector technology and intensive work on radiation dose awareness have had huge impacts on dose reduction in CT, there is inevitably a risk related to ionizing radiation, in particular when scanning younger individuals, larger areas, and when doing multiple follow-up scans (see Sect. 8.3.4).

8.3.3 MRI: Pros and Cons

MRI is capable of true three-dimensional imaging, and of time-resolved imaging, e.g., following contrast medium administration. The main clinical advantage is excellent soft tissue contrast. MRI is therefore much more flexible in terms of tailoring the image acquisition in order to achieve the desired contrast, and this will improve accuracy of lesion detection and delineation. A potential, still not well explored, advantage is in quantitative imaging, such as the study of cellular packing with diffusion-weighted imaging and study of perfusion and leakage with dynamic contrast-enhanced MRI. MRI allows coverage of large anatomic areas without a radiation risk penalty.

The main drawback with MRI is the long scan time, which often requires sedation/deep sedation/general anesthesia, and whereas this is generally well accepted and safe (Sury and Smith 2008), it carries costs in terms of staff, equipment, and increased logistic complexity. Since MRI is currently not recommended for lung imaging, a CT scan of the thorax becomes an additional requirement and an extra logistic complication. MRI also requires rather large investments (time and knowledge) by the radiologist, which may sometimes be difficult to justify.

8.3.4 How Much Ionizing Radiation Is Acceptable?

Cohort studies, mostly in atomic bomb survivors, estimate an excess of 50 deaths from cancer per one million individuals exposed to 1 mSv medical radiation, that is to say, one death per 20 Sv exposure (International Commission on Radiological Protection 1991). Although the translational value of these studies may be questioned, no alternative empirical risk assessment tool is available, and it is currently believed that there is a linear, non-threshold relation between radiation dose and risk (Little et al. 2009). One multidetector CT scan of the abdomen delivers the equivalent radiation dose of 150–250 chest radiographs. In a pediatric

Table 8.2 Radiation dose and risk estimates for CT of the chest and CT of the abdomen/pelvis in neonates and young children

Patient age	Scan region	Dose estimate, mSv[a]	Equivalent number of AP chest radiographs[b]	Attributable deaths per 1,000,000 scans[c]	
				Male	Female
Neonate	Chest	1.6	80	2.4	4.8
	Abdomen/pelvis	4.0	200	6	12
8 years	Chest	1.6	80	1.6	3.2
	Abdomen/pelvis	4.4	220	4.4	8.8

Notes

[a]Estimate for Siemens (Siemens, Erlangen, Germany) Somatom® 64-slice scanner with collimation 0.6 mm, tube voltage 80–100 kV, and reference tube current 30–70 mAs; calculated using CT Expo ver 1.6 (Stamm and Nagel 2002)

[b]Assuming a constant dose of 0.01 mSv for a chest radiograph in one plane

[c]Based on the 1993 revision of atomic bomb survivors data (United Nations Scientific Committee on the Effects of Atomic Radiation 1993)

context, the traditional estimates of radiation risk are probably too low since it is thought that the lifetime risk equivalent is about three times as high in male and six times in female infants due to longer life expectancy and more radiation-sensitive tissues (Thomsen et al. 2007; Mayo et al. 2003). Some dose and risk comparisons are shown in Table 8.2.

Several steps should be taken to reduce the radiation dose: (1) *avoid multiphase* scanning (da Costa e Silva and da Silva 2007); (2) scan only the relevant anatomy; (3) use weight-based tube voltage and automated tube current modulation (Paterson and Frush 2007); and, of course, (4) use alternative imaging modalities if feasible. However, since alternatives are not always available, and since we are discussing children with a life-threatening condition, certain pragmatism must be allowed.

8.3.5 CT and MRI Contrast Media and Safety

Contrast media used in CT (iodinated compounds) and MRI (chelated gadolinium ions) are generally safe and well tolerated. Patients with renal neoplasm may have reduced renal function due to local effects of the primary tumor, reduced nephron population following resection, or toxic effects of therapy. Particular considerations are therefore required.

Contrast delivery is mandatory for abdominal CT, and the main concern is the associated nephrotoxicity. CT with contrast may therefore be contraindicated in a renally compromised patient (Frush 2008). If the patient is already on dialysis, this is not a contraindication per se.

MRI contrast is not nephrotoxic; however, impaired clearance is a caveat since slow elimination may lead to more dissociated gadolinium being deposited in the tissues. Free gadolinium is toxic, and this is thought to be the etiology of nephrogenic systemic fibrosis (Thomsen et al. 2007; Sadowski et al. 2007). Low (estimated) GFR (<30 ml/min/1.73 m^2) whether physiological (infants) or pathological, dialysis, and end-stage liver disease are contraindications for gadolinium (Mendichovszky et al. 2008). MRI without gadolinium is still possible and is definitely preferable to a non-contrast CT, but there will be limited depiction of small vascular branches, and perfusion studies will be virtually impossible.

Both for CT and MRI contrast, local guidelines, complying with national and international recommendations, should be followed.

8.4 Current Clinical Imaging

8.4.1 Unilateral Disease

Imaging in a child with a clinically suspected abdominal mass should begin with ultrasound.

If a mass is confirmed, the next step is to determine its origin. Renal masses typically distort the normal renal parenchyma by expansion, whereas extrarenal masses displace and compress the kidney. The “claw” or “beak” sign of normal renal tissue surrounding the mass is useful as verification of its renal origin (Figs. 8.1 and 8.2). Renal masses typically move with the kidney during breathing, contrary to hepatic or adrenal masses. Ventilation synchronous motion may however be absent in renal masses that breach the capsule and infiltrate adjacent organs. Appearance on ultrasound can vary from uniform echogenicity, typical of entirely viable tumors, to the rather heterogeneous echotexture seen with tissue necrosis and hemorrhage. If a biopsy is planned, ultrasound is invaluable for defining the solid elements of a heterogeneous mass. As tumor can rupture and spill into the peritoneum or retroperitoneum (Figs. 8.3 and 8.4), evaluation

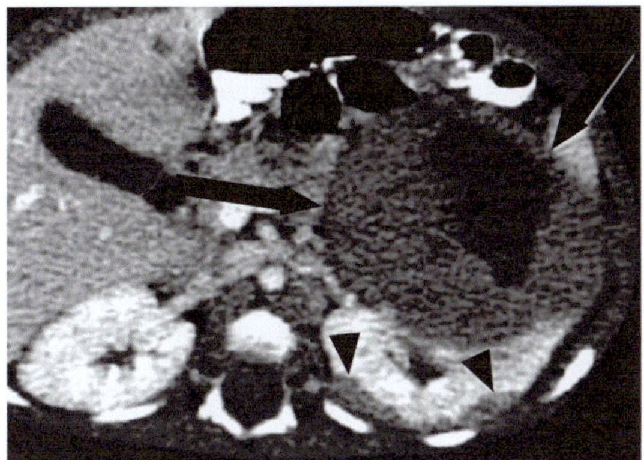

Fig. 8.2 Left-sided Wilms tumor (*arrows*) and perilobar nephrogenic rests (*arrowheads*) on a transaxial section from a contrast-enhanced CT in a 6-month-old

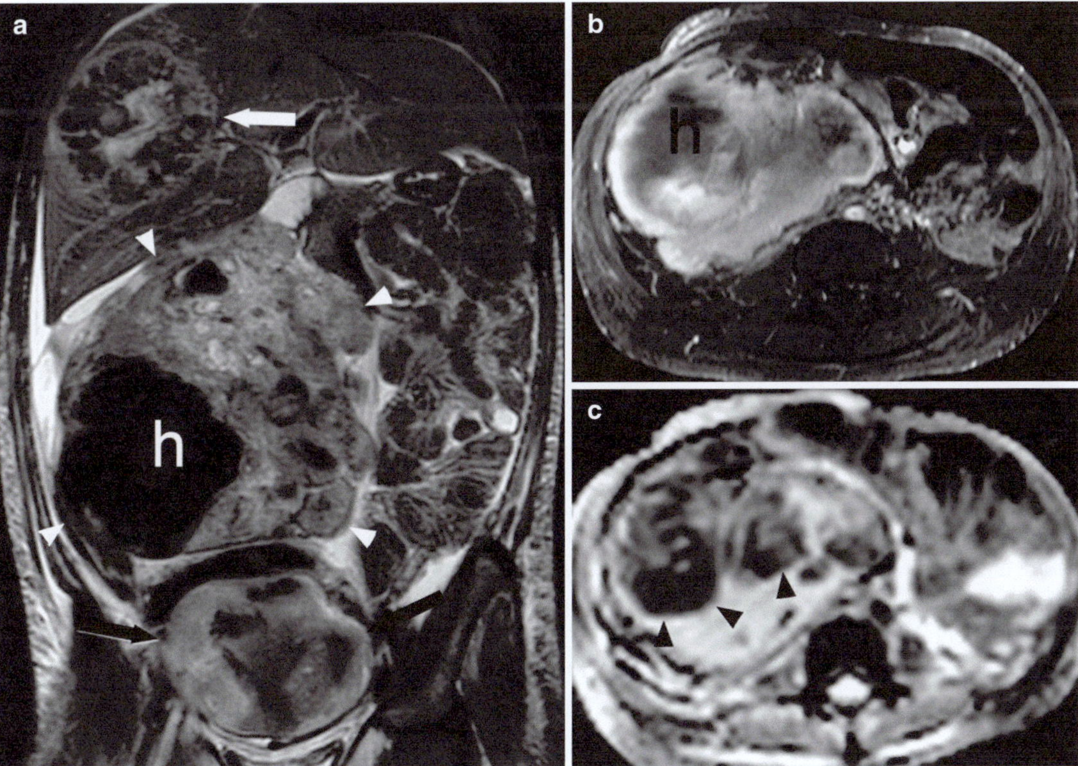

Fig. 8.3 A 6-year-old with Wilms tumor. (**a**) Coronal fat-suppressed T2-weighted MR image demonstrates the large mass (*white arrowheads*) with central hemorrhage (h). A large metastatic deposit is seen in the right lobe of the liver (*white arrow*) and in the pelvis (*black arrows*). (**b**) Post-contrast fat-suppressed T1-weighted image confirms the nonviable area (h) centrally in the primary lesion. (**c**) In this extensively necrotic tumor, diffusion-weighted imaging helped guide the diagnostic biopsy. Dark areas (*black arrowheads*) on this ADC map correspond to moderately enhancing areas on the post-contrast image (**b**) and are therefore assumed to represent viable tumor

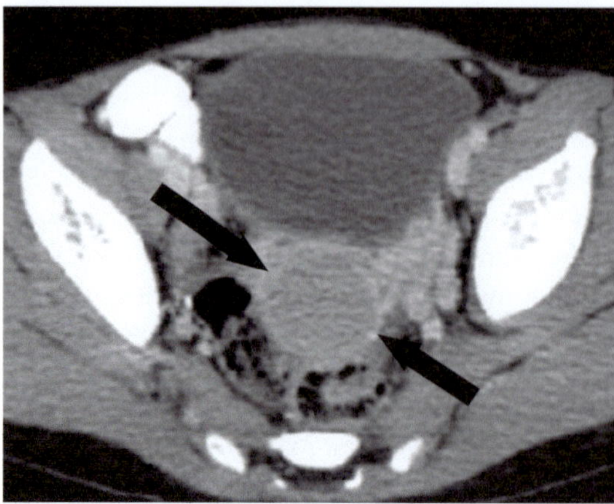

Fig. 8.4 Transaxial section from a contrast-enhanced CT scan in a 6-year-old with Wilms tumor demonstrates a pelvis drop metastasis (*arrows*)

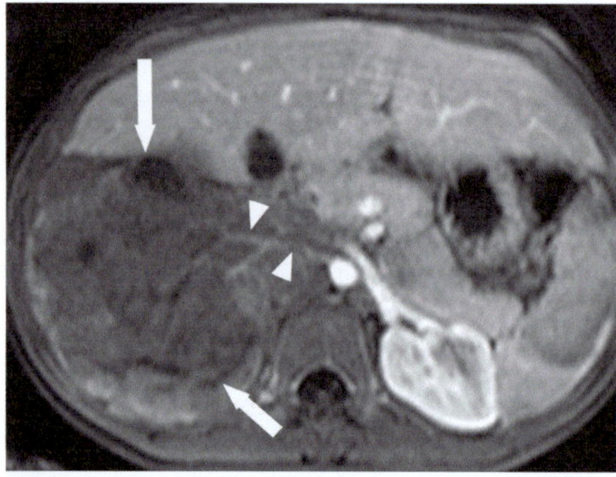

Fig. 8.5 Atypical right-sided Wilms tumor (*arrows*) on MRI (fat-suppressed T1-weighted sequence in arterial phase following intravenous contrast administration): there is encasement of the renal vessels (*arrowheads*). This is a sign of either rupture and retroperitoneal infiltration or of extensive regional lymphadenopathy

of the entire abdominal cavity is important; however, detection of small deposits is highly operator dependent.

Ultrasound should be used for evaluating the renal vessels. While renal tumors tend to invade or displace vessels, neuroblastoma tends to encase vessels. This feature is useful for differentiating renal tumors and neuroblastoma, although there are exceptions to this rule (Fig. 8.5). Combined grayscale and color Doppler evaluation of the renal veins is essential also for diagnosing tumor thrombus (Fig. 8.6). Color Doppler alone may give false-negative results, as tumor thrombus is vascular. Benign masses such as pyelonephritis, specifically xanthogranulomatous pyelonephritis, should be considered so as to avoid unnecessary interventions. Once a renal mass is diagnosed with ultrasound, further evaluation with formal cross-sectional imaging (CT or MRI) is recommended for confirmation and for staging.

If CT is chosen, it should include the chest, abdomen, and pelvis. There is *no place for a precontrast run* (da Costa e Silva and da Silva 2007). Portal venous phase images alone are sufficient. Delayed phase images may however be helpful for evaluating the collecting system before nephron-sparing surgery (Fig. 8.7). Multiplanar reconstructions are helpful in confirming the organ of origin and delineating the extent of disease. As on ultrasound, Wilms tumor is often heterogeneous in appearance due to focal necrosis and hemorrhage, seen as areas of low density (i.e., with little or no contrast uptake). Calcification is unusual in Wilms tumor.

On MRI, Wilms tumor shows intermediate signal intensity on T1-weighted images, hyperintensity on T2-weighted images, and heterogeneous contrast enhancement. A heterogeneous appearance has been proved useful in differentiating Wilms tumor from nephrogenic rests (Gylys-Morin et al. 1993). Even with MRI, distinction between stage I and II is inaccurate, as capsular invasion is often microscopic. This is especially true in young children where the lack of significant perinephric fat makes detection of capsular infiltration more difficult (Schenk et al. 2005). Lymph node metastases have prognostic significance. However, the anatomic criterion for detection of lymph node involvement, i.e., short axis diameter of 1 cm or greater, has limited accuracy. Hence, lymph node sampling at the time of surgery remains crucial for accurate staging (Gow et al. 2000).

Intravascular tumor extension (Fig. 8.6) has been reported in up to 11.3 % of children with Wilms tumor and with tumor thrombus extending into the inferior vena cava or heart in up to 8.1 % (Ritchey et al. 1990, 1988; Shamberger et al. 2001; Lall et al. 2006). Tumor thrombus

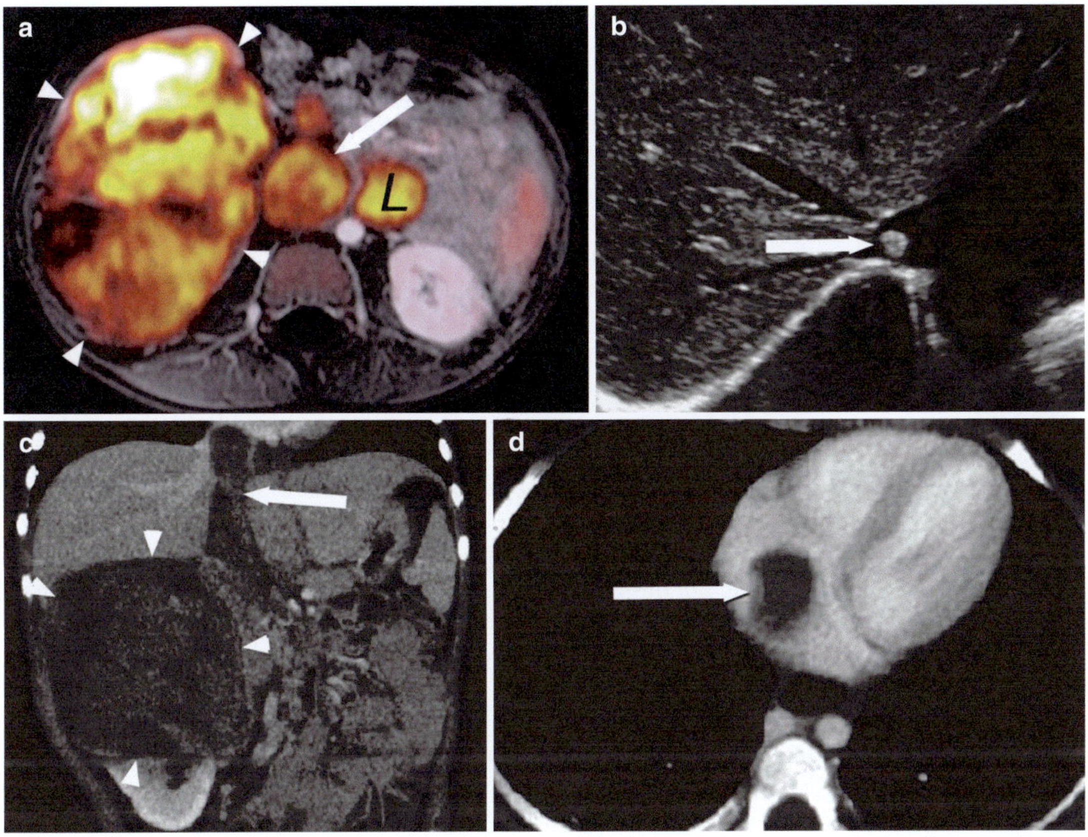

Fig. 8.6 Venous invasion in three different patients with three different modalities. (**a**) MRI with diffusion-weighted (*red scale*) overlay on T1-weighted post-contrast (*grayscale*) sequence demonstrates a large right-sided renal tumor (*arrowheads*), large lymph node mass (L), and tumor thrombus in the inferior vena cava (*arrow*). (**b**) Ultrasound is very sensitive for small thrombi; a fine thrombus is here seen (*arrow*) in the upper IVC at the confluence of the hepatic veins. (**c**, **d**) Contrast-enhanced CT in one patient with a right-sided Wilms tumor (*arrowheads*) demonstrating tumor thrombus in the IVC on coronal reformats (**c**) and in the right atrium on axial slice through the lower thorax (**d**)

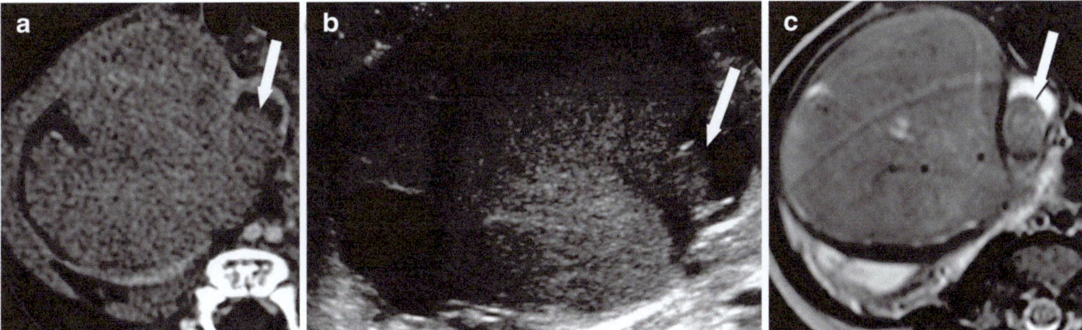

Fig. 8.7 A large right renal mass invades the renal collection system and proximal ureter. Images with three different modalities: CT (**a**), ultrasound (**b**), and T2-weighted MRI (**c**) all demonstrate the tumor-urine interface (*arrows*)

does not affect survival (Ritchey et al. 1990). However, it increases the risk of perioperative complications. In NWTS-4, the rate of perioperative complications in patients with extension of tumor thrombus into the IVC and heart was estimated at 17 and 37 %, respectively (Shamberger et al. 2001). Presence of cavoatrial thrombus may influence the decision about preoperative chemotherapy and may change the surgical approach. Preoperative knowledge of tumor thrombus has been shown to decrease the rate of perioperative complications (Nakayama et al. 1986).

There is limited information regarding the diagnostic performance of individual imaging modalities for detection of tumor thrombus. In NWTS-3, ultrasound was shown to have a sensitivity of 59 % in detection of all tumor thrombus, as compared to 42 % for CT (Ritchey et al. 1990). In the same study, a correct preoperative diagnosis of renal vein thrombosis was made in only 2 % of cases. Diagnostic performance of individual imaging modalities was not evaluated in NWTS-4 (Shamberger et al. 2001). In the adult population with renal cell carcinoma, CT has a concordance rate of 84 % with pathology findings for vascular invasion into the renal hilum or beyond (Guzzo et al. 2009). The same study also showed that CT accurately predicted the level of tumor thrombus in 96 %.

CT has high sensitivity for detection of tumor rupture. In a study of 250 Wilms tumor patients enrolled by the International Society for Pediatric Oncology (SIOP), CT demonstrated signs of tumor rupture (intraperitoneal or retroperitoneal) in 25 % of patients, and a third of whom had no clinical signs of rupture (Brisse et al. 2008a). Intraperitoneal rupture upstages the patient to stage IIIc (COG) or III (SIOP) and has been shown to increase the risk of abdominal recurrence. The findings in intraperitoneal rupture include peritoneal fluid (hyperdense on CT, suggesting it is hemorrhagic) and/or nodules in the peritoneal cavity. A small amount of peritoneal fluid should however not be regarded as a sign of rupture as it may be reactive or secondary to venous stasis. Intratumoral hemorrhage or a subcapsular bleed is not regarded as a sign of rupture.

8.4.2 Bilateral Disease

Bilateral disease is seen in 4–13 % of children with Wilms tumor and can be synchronous or metachronous (Breslow et al. 1993; Coppes et al. 1989). Bilateral synchronous disease is seen in 5 % and is usually associated with nephrogenic rests (Figs. 8.2 and 8.8), genetic abnormalities, or predisposing syndromes. Contrast-enhanced CT or MRI is more sensitive than ultrasound at detecting small contralateral lesions, as nephrogenic rests can be isoechoic relative to normal renal parenchyma (Gylys-Morin et al. 1993; Rohrschneider et al. 1998). Ninety percent of patients with synchronous and 94 % of patients with metachronous bilateral Wilms have nephrogenic rests (Merchant and Badhe 1995). Though intraoperative exploration of the contralateral kidney for detection of bilateral disease was recommended in the past, studies have shown CT and MRI to have sufficient sensitivity for detection of bilateral disease. In a review of NWTS-4, there were 188 patients with bilateral disease noted intraoperatively. In all but 11 of these, bilateral involvement was seen on preoperative imaging. So, 5.9 % (11/188) of all bilateral lesions were missed, which was only 0.3 % (11/3,335) of all enrolled children. Six of the missed lesions were less than 1 cm in diameter, and three measured 1–2 cm (Ritchey et al. 2005). Based on this data, routine intraoperative exploration of the contralateral kidney is no longer recommended; however, preoperative contrast-enhanced CT or MRI is essential for detecting small lesions.

Distinguishing nephrogenic rests from Wilms tumor is difficult. While nephrogenic rests tend to have a more homogeneous appearance on both pre- and post-contrast CT and MRI, heterogeneity favors Wilms tumor. Both tumor and rests tend to be bright on T2-weighted images, while sclerotic rests will be dark. Nephrogenic rests usually are ovoid or lenticular, while tumor tends to be spherical. The size of the lesion per se is not reliable for differentiation, as nephrogenic rests up to 5 cm in diameter have been reported (Rohrschneider et al. 1998).

When faced with bilateral lesions, the possibility of renal involvement in a lymphoproliferative disorder must also be considered. This is

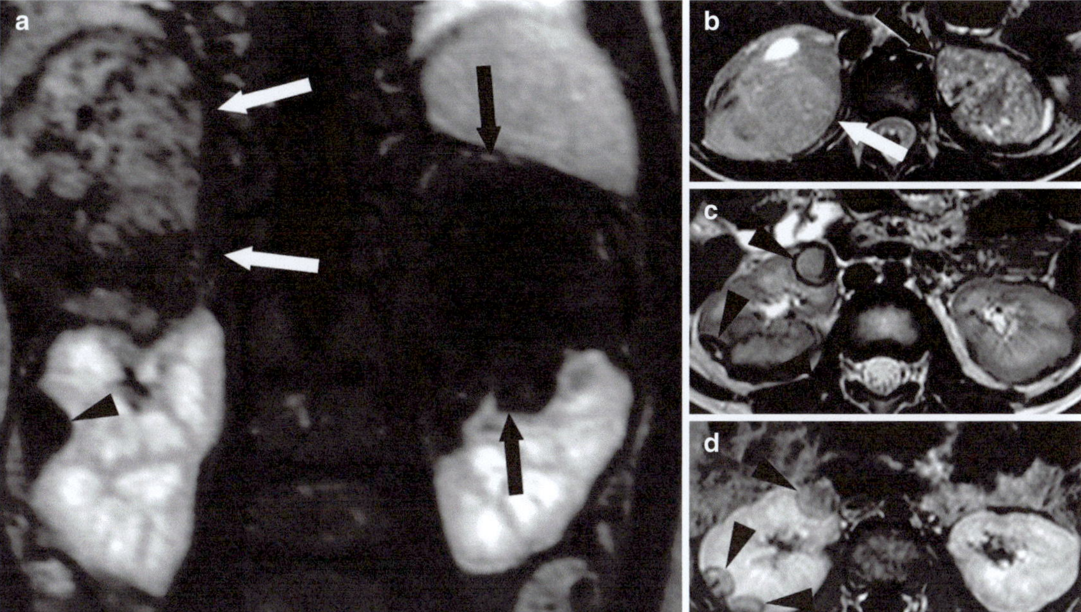

Fig. 8.8 Bilateral nephrogenic rests (*arrowheads*) and bilateral exophytic nephroblastomas (*left upper* pole mass, *black arrows*; *right upper* pole mass, *white arrows*). The rests show very little enhancement in the arterial phase following contrast administration (**a**), more enhancement in a delayed phase (**d**). The overall contrast between the tumor and kidney is poor on the T2-weighted image (**b**), whereas the nephrogenic rests are clearly demarcated (**c**)

generally accompanied by extensive lymphadenopathy and more diffuse renal involvement, unusual for Wilms tumor.

The major challenge in bilateral disease is to achieve cure and at the same time to preserve functional renal tissue. Imaging with CT using multiplanar reconstructions or multiplanar MRI can play an important role by identifying candidates for nephron-sparing surgery. Contraindications to nephron-sparing surgery include tumor rupture, extrarenal infiltration of tumor, intra-abdominal spread of tumor, tumor thrombus in the renal vein or IVC, more than 1/3 of the kidney involved by tumor is not the threshold for BWT. This applies only for non-syndromic unilateral WT. The radiologist therefore needs to assess all these features.

8.4.3 Staging

Advances in multidetector CT have increased the sensitivity for lung nodules, CT scans now being performed with a typical collimation of 0.6–1.5 mm and image reconstruction at slice thickness less than 5 mm (Fischbach et al. 2003). However, the clinical significance of detection of tiny lung nodules remains questionable. There are still no diagnostic criteria that reliably differentiate metastases from benign pulmonary nodules, such as granulomatous disease or intrapulmonary lymph nodes (Silva et al. 2010). NWTS-5 data showed that in children with "CT-only" (i.e., not visible on chest radiographs) nodules, 26 % (11/42) of biopsied nodules were benign (Ehrlich et al. 2006). The accuracy of pediatric radiologists with expertise in oncology in differentiating benign and malignant CT-only nodules has been shown to be 67 % at best. In a retrospective review of lung nodules in children with solid tumors, the most reliable predictors of malignancy were distinct nodule margins and the development of new nodules during follow-up (Fig. 8.9). Size did not differentiate benign and malignant nodules (McCarville et al. 2006).

The significance of CT-only nodules remains unclear. Owens et al. retrospectively studied 141

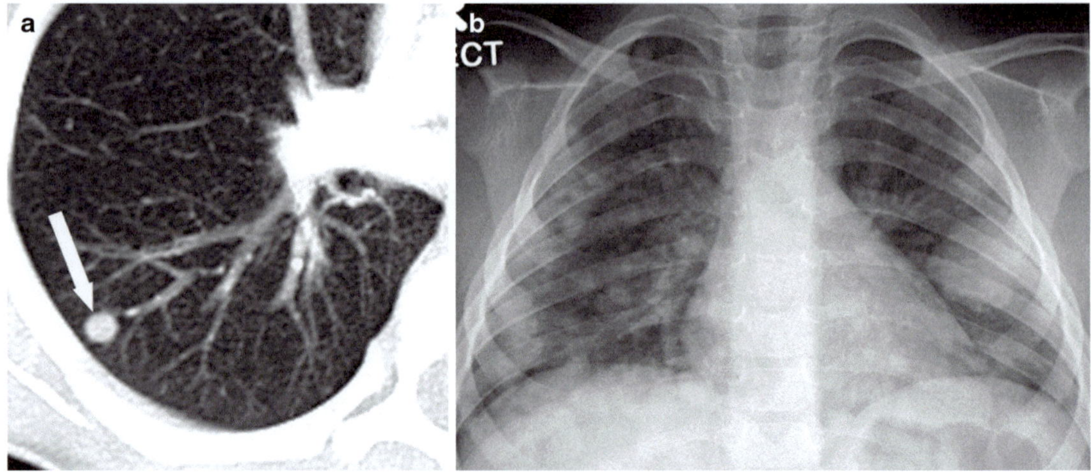

Fig. 8.9 Large (cannonball) lung metastases seen on chest radiograph (**a**), small metastasis seen on CT (**b**). A round, well-demarcated lesion raises the suspicion of metastatic lung disease even with a small number of low-volume lesions

children, who had a normal two-view chest radiograph at diagnosis and had undergone a pretreatment chest CT. They found a significant difference in the relapse rate in stage I patients treated with single agent chemotherapy who were CT positive (43 % relapse) versus those who were CT negative (10 % relapse) (Owens et al. 2002). Conversely, data from NWTS-3 and NWTS-4 did not show a statistically significant difference in event-free and overall survival between children who were treated as stage IV based on chest CT nodules (n=53, 89 and 91 %, respectively) and those with CT nodules who were treated based on their locoregional disease only (n=37, 80 and 85 %), respectively (Meisel et al. 1999).

In the current COG Wilms tumor study, biopsy proof of lung metastasis is recommended if small (<1 cm) lesions are identified on chest CT in stage I or II patients. These patients and all patients with stage III and IV disease receive 6 weeks of chemotherapy. If lung lesions are still present at the end of these 6 weeks, biopsy confirmation of residual disease is recommended prior to whole lung irradiation and intensification of chemotherapy.

8.4.4 Assessment of Treatment Response

Patients enrolled in the SIOP studies receiving presurgical chemotherapy should have formal cross-sectional imaging (MRI or CT) both at diagnosis and preoperatively. This group therefore provides a unique opportunity to study possible relations between histopathological findings and clinical outcome on one side and therapy-associated changes in imaging features on the other. Unfortunately, the previous imaging guidelines have not been sufficiently stringent to allow large-scale comparisons, and only a limited number of spin-off publications exist (Ng et al. 1991; Olsen et al. 2004). Observed change in imaging features over the course of chemotherapy therefore has no proven significance and no formal role in the current management of children with Wilms tumor.

Some kind of estimate or surrogate measurement for physical size of tumor is often the only reported expression for radiological change. Whereas increased size (WHO criteria) during chemotherapy is an independent prognosticator of poor outcome (Ora et al. 2007), it is clear that size alone is a crude parameter, as tumors that end up differentiated or almost completely necrotic may actually increase in size, and those that shrink may still be predominantly blastematous (Olsen et al. 2004).

Improved availability of high-quality imaging along with development of new quantitative (MRI) and "functional imaging" (molecular labeling; PET) techniques will allow more sophisticated staging and thereby more individually tailored treatment in future. Currently, two modalities seem to stand out: MRI being able to quantify several tissue properties, e.g., water diffusion, perfusion, and vascular leakage, none of which has been adequately explored in pediatric tumor imaging and positron emission tomography, which is very sensitive in pediatrics (Moinul Hossain et al. 2010; Murphy et al. 2008). Very low specificity is a major problem with FDG-PET, but the specificity of PET is presumed to improve with development of new tracers more specifically targeting malignant cells.

8.4.5 Imaging of Complications

The radiologically most relevant complications to surgery are, in the early stage, different types of collections (hemorrhagic, urine containing, pyogenic), which can usually be assessed with ultrasound, even bedside if required. Tumor spillage is usually microscopic and can only be assessed at a later stage.

Acute complications to chemotherapy with relevance to imaging include toxic pneumonitis, opportunistic infections, and neutropenic colitis. Rational imaging should be guided by clinical and laboratory findings. Pulmonary toxicity is a late diagnosis on chest radiographs. Specific clinical suspicion therefore justifies the use of computed tomography with a "high-resolution" algorithm, i.e., imaging in thin sections with relatively wide intersection gaps through the lungs. Typical findings in pneumonitis include diffuse bilateral ground glass opacification and variable interstitial thickening (Silva and Müller 2006). These findings may per se be nonspecific, but would strengthen a clinical suspicion of pneumonitis and help target lung biopsy if necessary. Suspicion of opportunistic airway infection requires volumetric imaging of the entire lungs and sometimes of the paranasal sinuses. Since clinically significant lesions can be small, it is important that the volumetric CT data is reviewed directly as lesions may be difficult to detect on reconstructed slices (Thomas et al. 2003).

Opportunistic infection in the abdomen (hematogenous, urinary) is best investigated with ultrasound or MRI; ultrasound is for practical reasons and the first choice. As in the chest, clinically significant lesions may be small and are easily missed when using a standard (curvilinear) ultrasound transducer. It is therefore mandatory to use a high-definition linear transducer, particularly for the spleen, liver, and kidneys. With suspicion of digestive tract complications, there should be a low threshold for obtaining an abdominal radiograph, which should be used to exclude hollow viscus perforation (seen as free gas), obstruction (dilated loops, paucity of distal bowel content), and paralytic bowel (featureless dilated bowel loops with gas-fluid levels). Bowel wall thickening and intramural gas suggest neutropenic colitis and can be seen throughout the colon, but most frequently in the cecum and ascending colon. Ultrasound with a high-definition linear transducer is more sensitive than radiographs for detecting bowel wall thickening and should be used liberally. A relevant differential diagnosis for intramural gas is pneumatosis intestinalis, which can be very pronounced, but usually asymptomatic. The distinction is therefore usually easy clinically.

Above-baseline incidence of focal nodular hyperplasia (FNH) of the liver has been reported in survivors of pediatric malignancies. These benign lesions have been reported from 2 to 26 years after completion of therapy (Marabelle et al. 2008). They are usually incidental findings and could be mistaken for metastatic or new malignant disease. FNH is made of hyperplastic, polyclonal hepatocytes divided by septa that may radiate from a central stellate fibrous scar. The mass is usually supplied by a central hepatic artery, resulting in intense enhancement on the arterial phase imaging. The pathogenesis of FNH is poorly understood. One hypothesis is hepatic reperfusion post-thrombosis of hepatic vessels, such as can be caused by cytotoxic chemotherapy and radiation therapy. If the lesion shows characteristic imaging findings on MRI, it can be followed conservatively without the need for biopsy or resection.

8.5 Screening and Follow-Up

8.5.1 Children with Predisposing Conditions

Though the vast majority of Wilms tumors occur sporadically, several predisposition syndromes for Wilms tumor have been described. Patients with Beckwith-Wiedemann syndrome (BWS) are at increased risk for a variety of embryonal tumors, most commonly Wilms tumor. In a survey from the BWS registry, 13 children with tumors before the fourth year of life were reported in a cohort of 183 children (DeBaun and Tucker 1998). The overall tumor risk in BWS is in the range 5–10 % (Lapunzina 2005; Sotelo-Avila et al. 1980; Weng et al. 1995). The peak incidence of Wilms tumor associated with BWS is between the first and second birthdays (DeBaun et al. 1996). Hemihypertrophy in association with BWS increases the risk of tumor fourfold (RR=4.6, 95 % CI=1.5–14.2), as compared to BWS alone (DeBaun and Tucker 1998). Other conditions associated with increased risk of Wilms tumor include Perlman syndrome, Sotos syndrome, WAGR (Wilms tumor, aniridia, genitourinary malformation, and mental retardation) syndrome, isolated aniridia, and Denys-Drash syndrome (Clericuzio and Johnson 1995).

An increased risk of Wilms tumor has also been reported in children with isolated hemihypertrophy. Isolated hemihypertrophy was reported in 2.5 % of Wilms tumor patients in the National Wilms Tumor Study and in 3.2 % enrolled by SIOP (Pastore et al. 1988). A tumor risk of about 6 % has been reported in children with isolated hemihypertrophy, with the average age of 3 years at presentation (Hoyme et al. 1998). There is some controversy surrounding this group of children since hemihypertrophy is a poorly defined entity and because some studies suggest the risk of Wilms tumor in this group is as low as 3.5 % (Hoyme et al. 1998). Whereas active surveillance is advocated by COG, the United Kingdom surveillance guidelines do not include children with isolated hemihypertrophy (Scott et al. 2006).

The recommended screening protocol for the predisposition syndromes is ultrasound every 3–4 months, up to the age of 7 years (Scott et al. 2006) (Fig. 8.10). These recommendations are based on the detection of early-stage Wilms tumor by 3 monthly sonography in BWS (Andrews and Amparo 1993; Azouz et al. 1990). Screening of children with BWS or idiopathic hemihypertrophy at least three times a year has been shown to significantly decrease the proportion of late-stage (stages III–IV) Wilms tumors (Choyke et al. 1999). Though another study of 41 children with predisposition syndromes showed no statistically significant difference in stage of tumor at diagnosis between the screened and unscreened populations, however, in this study no standardized imaging protocols were used for screening (Craft et al. 1995).

8.5.2 Children with Nephrogenic Rests/Nephroblastomatosis

As discussed in Sect. 8.4.2, synchronous tumors are seen in 5 %, and of these 90 % have nephrogenic rests. Among patients with metachronous tumors, 94 % have nephrogenic rests (Merchant and Badhe 1995). Balancing the need for oncologic disease control against the need for conserving nephrons, distinguishing neoplastic tissue from nephrogenic rests is a huge challenge for the imaging disciplines. The required accuracy cannot be achieved with current technology, although certain features suggest a diagnosis of nephrogenic rests: wedge-shaped, ovoid, or lentiform lesions; little or no mass effect on surrounding tissue; and low signal on T2-weighted MRI (Rohrschneider et al. 1998; Gylys-Morin et al. 1993). Hyperplastic rest may however be mistaken for tumor (Subhas et al. 2004); conversely, early neoplastic degeneration of rests may not be detectable (Owens et al. 2008). While there is a need for more accurate techniques, current technology should be optimized in the follow-up of these patients. Change over time is invaluable in these cases, and it is therefore important to ensure a consistent imaging strategy, i.e., a preference

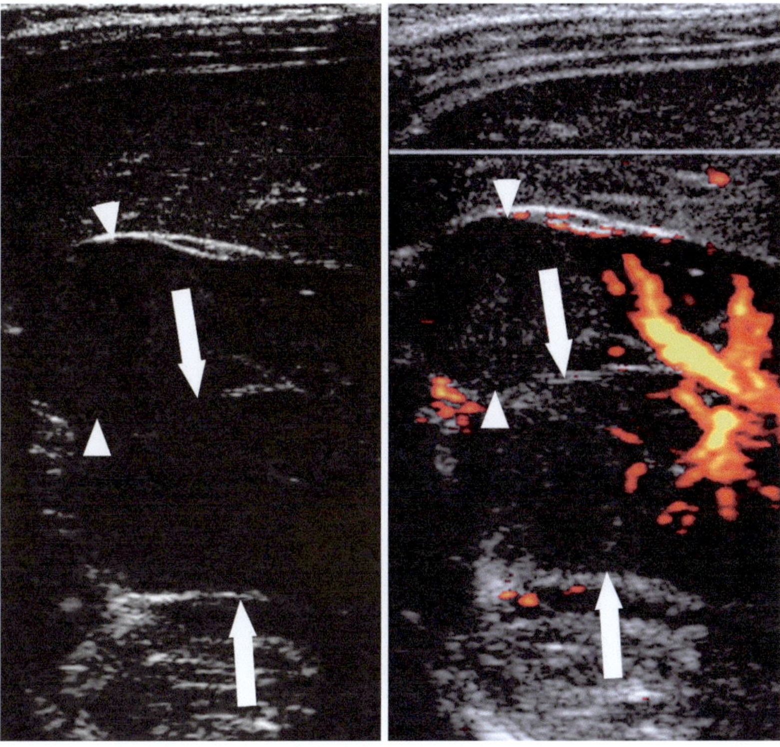

Fig. 8.10 A 17-month-old recently noted to have hemihypertrophy was referred for a screening ultrasound. Ultrasound with grayscale (*left*) and color Doppler (*right*) demonstrates two very similar hypovascular renal masses. Despite imaging similarities, the anterior one (*arrowheads*) was a Wilms tumor, and the posterior (*arrows*) represented a hyperplastic nephrogenic rest

for formal cross-sectional imaging (CT or MRI), use of standardized scan protocols, and interpretation by one or a limited number of radiologists (Fig. 8.11). In the right hands, MRI is the modality of choice because it offers numerous tissue contrasts, however, with the limitations discussed in Sect. 8.3.3.

8.5.3 Long-Term Follow-Up

As the overall prognosis of children with Wilms tumor is good, follow-up imaging should be tailored keeping cost-effectiveness, radiation risk, and inconvenience to the child and family in mind. Most relapses occur within the first 4 years of diagnosis with the most common sites of recurrence being the lung (58 %) and abdomen (29 %) (3, 4). The risk of local recurrence is highest in patients with lymph node involvement, tumor spillage during surgery, and those with unfavorable histology (5). Recommendations from SIOP include the use of chest radiographs and abdominal ultrasound for detection of recurrence. The COG recommendations are currently more stratified and prescriptive with chest CT for the first 2–3 years, depending on disease stage and histology, before switching to chest radiographs. Abdominal evaluation is recommended with CT or MRI during the first 2 years after treatment. Details about recommended imaging surveillance are given in Table 8.3.

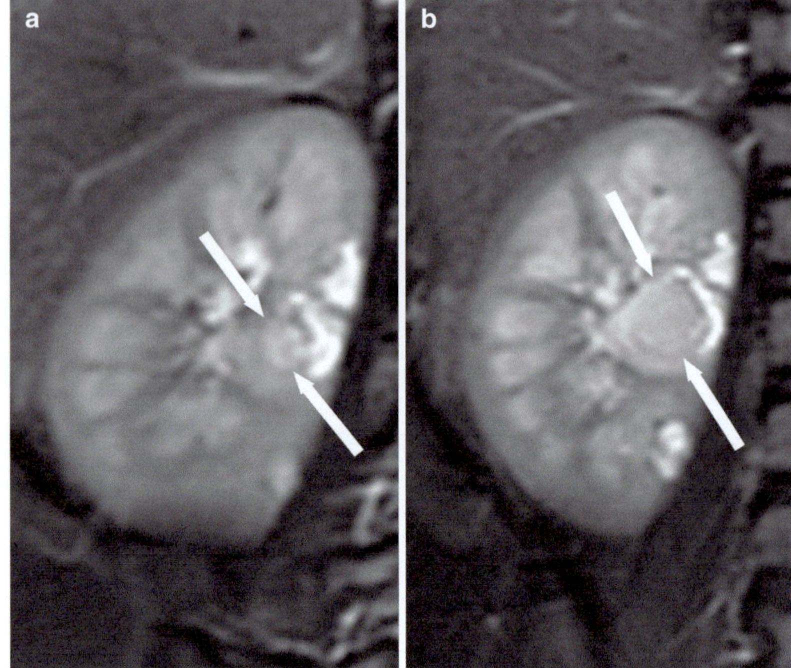

Fig. 8.11 A child with Denys-Drash syndrome had undergone left nephrectomy for Wilms tumor and was followed up with MRI. (**a**) A very ill-defined abnormality was seen centrally in the right kidney (*arrows*), which prompted closer follow-up. (**b**) After 3 months, the mass (metachronous Wilms) was unequivocal

Table 8.3 Recommended surveillance imaging during the first 6 years after end of treatment for nephroblastoma

Months from end of treatment		2	3	4	6	9	12	15	18	21	24	27	30	33	36	42	48	54	60	72
SIOP 2001 as adapted by (Brisse et al. 2008b)																				
Initial stage IV with lung mets	Chest	–	CXR	–	CXR	CXR	CXR	CXR	CXR	CXR	CXR	–	CXR	–	CXR	CXR	CXR	–	CXR	–
Nephrogenic rests, local stage III and/or high-risk histopathology	Abdomen/ pelvis	–	US	–	US	US	US	US	US	US	US	–	US	–	US	US	US	US	US	US
Else	Chest	–	CXR	–	CXR	CXR	CXR	–	CXR	–	CXR	–		–	CXR	–	CXR	–	CXR	–
	Abdomen/ pelvis	–	–	–	US		US	–	US	–	US	–		–	US	–	US	–	US	–
Current COG recommendations																				
Very low risk, stage I	Chest	CT	–	CT	CT	CT	CT	CT	CT	CXR	CXR	CXR	CXR	–	CXR	CXR	CXR	CXR	CXR	–
	Abdomen/ pelvis	CT/ MRI	–	CT/ MRI	CT/ MRI	CT/ MRI	CT/ MRI	CT/ MRI	CT/ MRI	US	US	US	US	–	US	US	US	US	US	–
Low and standard risk, stage I-III	Chest	–	CXR	–	CT	CXR	CT	CXR	CT	CXR	CT	CXR	CT	CXR	CT	CXR	CXR	CXR	CXR	–
	Abdomen/ pelvis	–	US	–	CT/ MRI	US	CT/ MRI	US	CT/ MRI	US	CT/ MRI	US	CT/ MRI	US	CT/ MRI	US	US	US	US	–
Higher risk, favorable histology	Chest	–	CT	–	CT	CT	CT	CT	CT	CT	CT	–	CXR	–	CXR	–	CXR	–	CXR	CXR
	Abdomen/ pelvis	–	CT/ MRI	–	CT/ MRI	CT/ MRI	CT/ MRI	CT/ MRI	CT/ MRI	CT/ MRI	CT/ MRI	–	US	–	US	–	US	–	US	US

Notes

CXR chest radiograph, *US* ultrasound, *SIOP* International Society for Pediatric Oncology, *COG* Children's Oncology Group

CT/MRI: It is recommended to aim at using the same modality for all follow-up scans

Conclusion

Imaging in Wilms tumor should follow best practice guidelines as per the relevant treatment protocols in order to ensure consistent and correct oncologic staging. Current deficiencies in imaging include the accurate diagnosis of small lung nodules seen on CT only, dealing with non-size-related treatment response and differentiation between nephrogenic rests and neoplastic tissue. These challenges are mostly linked to the current lack of specificity of all imaging modalities. However, the technological development is fast, and new techniques to be seen over the coming years include quantitative MRI and PET with more specific tracers. Technical development combined with a better understanding of the biological implications of imaging findings will hopefully result in both improved survival and reduced side effects as imaging will increasingly help tailoring more stratified treatment strategies.

References

Andrews MW, Amparo EG (1993) Wilms' tumor in a patient with Beckwith-Wiedemann syndrome: onset detected with 3-month serial sonography. AJR Am J Roentgenol 160:139–140

Azouz EM, Larson EJ, Patel J et al (1990) Beckwith-Wiedemann syndrome: development of nephroblastoma during the surveillance period. Pediatr Radiol 20:550–552

Begent J, Sebire NJ, Levitt G et al (2011) Pilot study of F(18)-Fluorodeoxyglucose Positron Emission Tomography/computerised tomography in Wilms' tumour: correlation with conventional imaging, pathology and immunohistochemistry. Eur J Cancer 47:389–396

Breslow N, Olshan A, Beckwith JB et al (1993) Epidemiology of Wilms tumor. Med Pediatr Oncol 21:172–181

Brisse HJ, Schleiermacher G, Sarnacki S et al (2008a) Preoperative Wilms tumor rupture: a retrospective study of 57 patients. Cancer 113:202–213

Brisse HJ, Smets AM, Kaste SC et al (2008b) Imaging in unilateral Wilms tumour. Pediatr Radiol 38:18–29

Choyke PL, Siegel MJ, Craft AW et al (1999) Screening for Wilms tumor in children with Beckwith-Wiedemann syndrome or idiopathic hemihypertrophy. Med Pediatr Oncol 32:196–200

Clericuzio CL, Johnson C (1995) Screening for Wilms tumor in high-risk individuals. Hematol Oncol Clin North Am 9:1253–1265

Cody DD (2002) AAPM/RSNA physics tutorial for residents: topics in CT. Image processing in CT. Radiographics 22:1255–1268

Coppes MJ, de Kraker J, van Dijken PJ et al (1989) Bilateral Wilms' tumor: long-term survival and some epidemiological features. J Clin Oncol 7:310–315

Craft AW, Parker L, Stiller C et al (1995) Screening for Wilms' tumour in patients with aniridia, Beckwith syndrome, or hemihypertrophy. Med Pediatr Oncol 24:231–234

da Costa e Silva EJ, da Silva GA (2007) Eliminating unenhanced CT when evaluating abdominal neoplasms in children. AJR Am J Roentgenol 189:1211–1214

DeBaun MR, Brown M, Kessler L (1996) Screening for Wilms' tumor in children with high-risk congenital syndromes: considerations for an intervention trial. Med Pediatr Oncol 27:415–421

DeBaun MR, Tucker MA (1998) Risk of cancer during the first four years of life in children from The Beckwith-Wiedemann Syndrome Registry. J Pediatr 132:398–400

Ehrlich PF, Hamilton TE, Grundy P et al (2006) The value of surgery in directing therapy for patients with Wilms' tumor with pulmonary disease. A report from the National Wilms' Tumor Study Group (National Wilms' Tumor Study 5). J Pediatr Surg 41:162–167, discussion 162–167

Fischbach F, Knollmann F, Griesshaber V et al (2003) Detection of pulmonary nodules by multislice computed tomography: improved detection rate with reduced slice thickness. Eur Radiol 13:2378–2383

Frericks BB, Meyer BC, Martus P et al (2008) MRI of the thorax during whole-body MRI: evaluation of different MR sequences and comparison to thoracic multidetector computed tomography (MDCT). J Magn Reson Imaging 27:538–545

Frush DP (2008) MDCT in children: scan techniques and contrast issues. In: Kalra MK, Sanjay S, Rubin GD (eds) Multidetector CT: from protocols to practice. Springer, Heidelberg

Gow KW, Roberts IF, Jamieson DH et al (2000) Local staging of Wilms' tumor–computerized tomography correlation with histological findings. J Pediatr Surg 35:677–679

Guzzo TJ, Pierorazio PM, Schaeffer EM et al (2009) The accuracy of multidetector computerized tomography for evaluating tumor thrombus in patients with renal cell carcinoma. J Urol 181:486–490

Gylys-Morin V, Hoffer FA, Kozakewich H et al (1993) Wilms tumor and nephroblastomatosis: imaging characteristics at gadolinium-enhanced MR imaging. Radiology 188:517–521

Hoyme HE, Seaver LH, Jones KL et al (1998) Isolated hemihyperplasia (hemihypertrophy): report of a prospective multicenter study of the incidence of neoplasia and review. Am J Med Genet 79:274–278

International Commission on Radiological Protection (1991) ICRP publication 60: 1990 recommendations of The International Commission on Radiological Protection. Elsevier, New York

Lall A, Pritchard-Jones K, Walker J et al (2006) Wilms' tumor with intracaval thrombus in the UK Children's Cancer Study Group UKW3 trial. J Pediatr Surg 41: 382–387

Lapunzina P (2005) Risk of tumorigenesis in overgrowth syndromes: a comprehensive review. Am J Med Genet C Semin Med Genet 137C:53–71

Little MP, Wakeford R, Tawn EJ et al (2009) Risks associated with low doses and low dose rates of ionizing radiation: why linearity may be (almost) the best we can do. Radiology 251:6–12

Marabelle A, Campagne D, Dechelotte P et al (2008) Focal nodular hyperplasia of the liver in patients previously treated for pediatric neoplastic diseases. J Pediatr Hematol Oncol 30:546–549

Mayo JR, Aldrich J, Muller NL et al (2003) Radiation exposure at chest CT: a statement of the Fleischner Society. Radiology 228:15–21

McCarville MB, Lederman HM, Santana VM et al (2006) Distinguishing benign from malignant pulmonary nodules with helical chest CT in children with malignant solid tumors. Radiology 239:514–520

Meisel JA, Guthrie KA, Breslow NE et al (1999) Significance and management of computed tomography detected pulmonary nodules: a report from the National Wilms Tumor Study Group. Int J Radiat Oncol Biol Phys 44:579–585

Mendichovszky IA, Marks SD, Simcock CM et al (2008) Gadolinium and nephrogenic systemic fibrosis: time to tighten practice. Pediatr Radiol 38:489–496

Merchant SA, Badhe PB (1995) Nephroblastomatosis–pathologic and imaging characteristics. J Postgrad Med 41:72–80

Misch D, Steffen IG, Schonberger S et al (2008) Use of positron emission tomography for staging, preoperative response assessment and posttherapeutic evaluation in children with Wilms tumour. Eur J Nucl Med Mol Imaging 35:1642–1650

Moinul Hossain AK, Shulkin BL, Gelfand MJ et al (2010) FDG positron emission tomography/computed tomography studies of Wilms' tumor. Eur J Nucl Med Mol Imaging. doi:10.1007/s00259-010-1396-2

Murphy JJ, Tawfeeq M, Chang B et al (2008) Early experience with PET/CT scan in the evaluation of pediatric abdominal neoplasms. J Pediatr Surg 43:2186–2192

Nakayama DK, Norkool P, deLorimier AA et al (1986) Intracardiac extension of Wilms' tumor. A report of the National Wilms' Tumor Study. Ann Surg 204:693–697

Ng YY, Hall-Craggs MA, Dicks-Mireaux C et al (1991) Wilms' tumour: pre- and post-chemotherapy CT appearances. Clin Radiol 43:255–259

Olsen ØE (2008) Imaging of abdominal tumours: CT or MRI? Pediatr Radiol 38(Suppl 3):S452–S458

Olsen ØE, Jeanes AC, Sebire NJ et al (2004) Changes in computed tomography features following preoperative chemotherapy for nephroblastoma: relation to histopathological classification. Eur Radiol 14:990–994

Ora I, van Tinteren H, Bergeron C et al (2007) Progression of localised Wilms' tumour during preoperative chemotherapy is an independent prognostic factor: a report from the SIOP 93–01 nephroblastoma trial and study. Eur J Cancer 43:131–136

Owens CM, Brisse HJ, Olsen ØE et al (2008) Bilateral disease and new trends in Wilms tumour. Pediatr Radiol 38:30–39

Owens CM, Veys PA, Pritchard J et al (2002) Role of chest computed tomography at diagnosis in the management of Wilms' tumor: a study by the United Kingdom Children's Cancer Study Group. J Clin Oncol 20:2768–2773

Pastore G, Carli M, Lemerle J et al (1988) Epidemiological features of Wilms' tumor: results of studies by the International Society of Paediatric Oncology (SIOP). Med Pediatr Oncol 16:7–11

Paterson A, Frush DP (2007) Dose reduction in paediatric MDCT: general principles. Clin Radiol 62: 507–517

Ritchey ML, Kelalis PP, Breslow N et al (1988) Intracaval and atrial involvement with nephroblastoma: review of National Wilms Tumor Study-3. J Urol 140: 1113–1118

Ritchey ML, Othersen HBJ, de Lorimier AA et al (1990) Renal vein involvement with nephroblastoma: a report of the National Wilms' Tumor Study-3. Eur Urol 17:139–144

Ritchey ML, Shamberger RC, Hamilton T et al (2005) Fate of bilateral renal lesions missed on preoperative imaging: a report from the National Wilms Tumor Study Group. J Urol 174:1519–1521

Rohrschneider WK, Weirich A, Rieden K et al (1998) US, CT and MR imaging characteristics of nephroblastomatosis. Pediatr Radiol 28:435–443

Sadowski EA, Bennett LK, Chan MR et al (2007) Nephrogenic systemic fibrosis: risk factors and incidence estimation. Radiology 243:148–157

Schenk JP, Schrader C, Furtwangler R et al (2005) MRI-morphology and staging of congenital mesoblastic nephroma: evaluation of a collection with 20 patients. Rofo 177:1373–1379

Scott RH, Walker L, Olsen ØE et al (2006) Surveillance for Wilms tumour in at-risk children: pragmatic recommendations for best practice. Arch Dis Child 91:995–999

Shamberger RC, Ritchey ML, Haase GM et al (2001) Intravascular extension of Wilms tumor. Ann Surg 234:116–121

Shulkin BL, Chang E, Strouse PJ et al (1997) PET FDG studies of Wilms tumors. J Pediatr Hematol Oncol 19:334–338

Silva CI, Müller NL (2006) Drug-induced lung diseases: most common reaction patterns and corresponding high-resolution CT manifestations. Semin Ultrasound CT MR 27:111–116

Silva CT, Amaral JG, Moineddin R et al (2010) CT characteristics of lung nodules present at diagnosis of extrapulmonary malignancy in children. AJR Am J Roentgenol 194:772–778

Sotelo-Avila C, Gonzalez-Crussi F, Fowler JW (1980) Complete and incomplete forms of Beckwith-Wiedemann syndrome: their oncogenic potential. J Pediatr 96:47–50

Stamm G, Nagel HD (2002) CT-expo–a novel program for dose evaluation in CT. Rofo 174:1570–1576

Subhas N, Argani P, Gearhart JP et al (2004) Nephrogenic rests mimicking Wilms' tumor on CT. Pediatr Radiol 34:152–155

Sury MR, Smith JH (2008) Deep sedation and minimal anesthesia. Paediatr Anaesth 18:18–24

Thomas KE, Owens CM, Veys PA et al (2003) The radiological spectrum of invasive aspergillosis in children: a 10-year review. Pediatr Radiol 33:453–460

Thomsen HS, Marckmann P, Logager VB (2007) Nephrogenic systemic fibrosis (NSF): a late adverse reaction to some of the gadolinium based contrast agents. Cancer Imaging 7:130–137

United Nations Scientific Committee on the Effects of Atomic Radiation (1993) Sources and effects of ionizing radiation: UNSCEAR 1993 report to the General Assembly, with scientific annexes, New York

Weng EY, Moeschler JB, Graham JMJ (1995) Longitudinal observations on 15 children with Wiedemann-Beckwith syndrome. Am J Med Genet 56:366–373

Biological Prognostic Factors in Wilms Tumors

9

Kathy Pritchard-Jones, Mariana Maschietto, and Paul Grundy

Contents

K. Pritchard-Jones (✉)
Department of Developmental Biology and Cancer, Institute of Child Health, University College London, 30 Guilford Street, London, WC1N 1EH, UK
e-mail: k.pritchard-jones@ucl.ac.uk

M. Maschietto
Post-doctoral research scientist, Institute of Child Health, Cancer Section University College London (UCL), 30 Guilford Street, London, WC1N 1EH, UK
e-mail: m.maschietto@ucl.ac.uk

P. Grundy
Cancer Control Alberta, Alberta Health Services, Calgary, Alberta, Canada
e-mail: paul.grundy@albertahealthservices.ca

Abstract

The outcome is now good for most patients with Wilms tumor of the kidney. Over and above the gains in survival, the ability to progressively regulate the amount of chemotherapy and radiation so that groups of patients are receiving dosing adequate to achieve cure, but not more, has been made possible by the use of prognostic factors. We often now think of prognostic factors as molecular or biological findings, but factors used to predict outcome in patients with Wilms tumor – to thereby stratify therapy – include histology (favorable vs anaplastic), stage (using criteria such as lymph node involvement, local or intravascular tumor extension, and presence of metastatic disease), age at diagnosis, response to therapy, and now molecular or genetic changes (loss of heterozygosity (LOH) for chromosomes 1p and 16q).

Prognostic factors are determined retrospectively and must always be validated in a second population of patients. Furthermore, prognostic factors are dependent on the treatment used in the population in which they are identified. Thus, as therapy changes from study to study, so too can prognostic factors change, so they must be constantly reassessed. Examples of these principles are discussed and information on current prognostic factors being utilized is presented.

K. Pritchard-Jones, J.S. Dome (eds.), *Renal Tumors of Childhood: Biology and Therapy*, Pediatric Oncology, DOI 10.1007/978-3-662-44003-2_9,

9.1 Introduction

Almost all patients with renal tumors in the Western world are treated according to protocols developed through the prospective, multicentre trials conducted by the SIOP-RTSG (International Society of Paediatric Oncology (SIOP) Renal Tumours Study Group, Europe) or the COG (Children's Oncology Group, formerly NWTSG, North America). The main objectives of these trials and studies have been to treat patients according to well-defined risk groups to achieve the highest cure rates, to decrease the frequency and intensity of acute and late toxicity, and to minimize the cost of therapy. Until the 2000s, the approach to risk stratification relied solely on clinical factors of patient age and tumor stage and histological subtype. Impressive improvements in outcome have been achieved while actually using shorter duration and lower total doses of chemotherapy and radiation (Green et al. 1998a, b). Current trials are examining the benefit of intensified chemotherapy for specific subsets of patients, while maintaining overall reduced doses for most, and attempting to eliminate adjuvant therapy for one small subset of patients in COG. It is likely that we have almost exhausted the generation of clinical indicators of outcome, except perhaps for refinements of tumor response – by imaging or histology – and that the way to continue to improve the accuracy of relapse prediction and selection of higher risk patients for novel therapies is through better insights into the many faces of Wilms tumor biology.

Even though the genetic basis of a subgroup of Wilms tumors was characterized during the 1990s, as involving the *WT1* gene or imprinting abnormalities of the *IGF2/H19* locus on chromosome 11p15.5, neither of these molecular changes was clearly associated with clinical outcome, when treatment was applied according to the classical clinical risk groups. However, analysis of loss of heterozygosity (LOH) as a strategy to identify the chromosomal locations of the so-called tumor suppressor genes highlighted regions on chromosome 1p and 16q as being of potential prognostic significance. Subsequently, extensive studies of genomic copy number, gene expression profiles, and most recently whole exome sequencing have been applied to determine the genetic landscape of Wilms tumor. While these analyses have started to give insights into the genetic complexity of the various molecular pathways involved in Wilms tumor, their results are not yet at a stage where they are ready for routine clinical application. Advances in the field will be discussed in the context of the evolving clinical and pathological prognostic factors identified by the two main clinical trial groups.

9.2 Stage

The first prognostic factor used in NWTS-1 was tumor stage (stage was called group in NWTS-1) which was assigned according to the extent of disease prior to the administration of chemotherapy (Table 9.1) (D'Angio et al. 1972). In fact, the very first staging system was developed somewhat empirically (although logically) since there was no prior large series of cases to analyze, to establish, or to validate the importance of the various staging criteria. The outcomes in NWTS-1, however, did validate the staging criteria in general. Patients in group I had a significantly better outcome compared with similarly treated group II/III patients. There was no apparent difference in outcomes between group II and III though.

This study, which utilized a single chemotherapeutic agent, actinomycin D, for group I patients and for a randomized subset of group II/III patients, demonstrated two principles of the use of prognostic factors. There may be interactions between factors, and these interactions are dependent on the treatment utilized. In group I patients, treated only with actinomycin D, there was a clear effect of age with those less than age 2 years having a significantly better outcome than those greater than age 2 (D'Angio et al. 1976). Interestingly, this same phenomenon has been reported by the United Kingdom Children's Cancer Study Group (UKCCSG) who observed better outcomes for children with stage I tumors treated with vincristine only if under age two at

Table 9.1 Clinical grouping used in NWTS-1 trial

The patient's group is decided by the surgeon in the operating room and is confirmed by the pathologist. If the histological diagnosis and grouping will take more than 48 hours, the surgical grouping stands, the patient is registered and started on treatment
Group I – tumor limited to kidney and completely resected
The surface of the renal capsule is intact. The tumor was not ruptured before or during removal. There is no residual tumor apparent beyond the margins of resection
Group II – tumor extends beyond the kidney but is completely resected
There is local extension of the tumor, i.e., penetration beyond the pseudocapsule into the perirenal soft tissues or periaortic lymph node involvement. The renal vessels outside the kidney substance are infiltrated or contain tumor thrombus. There is no residual tumor apparent beyond the margins of resection
Group III – residual nonhematogenous tumor confined to the abdomen
Any one or more of the following occur: (1) the tumor has been biopsied or ruptured before or during surgery; (2) there are implants on peritoneal surfaces; (3) there are involved lymph nodes beyond the abdominal periaortic chains; (4) the tumor is not completely resectable because of local infiltration into vital structures
Group IV – hematogenous metastases
Deposits beyond group III, e.g., lung, liver, bone, and brain
Group V – bilateral renal involvement either initially or subsequently

diagnosis (Pritchard-Jones et al. 2003). This effect of age was not observed in group II/III children nor has it been found to be an independent prognostic factor in subsequent NWTSG studies (unpublished data), all of which have used combination chemotherapy. This demonstrates the principle that the prognostic power of any given factor is dependent on the treatment context. In this example, age at diagnosis is predictive of outcome, but only in the context of minimal therapy. With more effective therapy, this predictive effect is lost.

We also see in NWTS-1 that patients with group II/III tumors treated with the combination of actinomycin D and vincristine actually fared better than the subset of patients who were older than age two with group I disease treated with actinomycin D only and without radiation. These data do not invalidate the staging/grouping system but demonstrate the interactions of multiple prognostic factors and the therapeutic context. These conclusions may seem self-evident, but particularly when complex, state-of-the-art molecular genetic assays are proposed as predictors; these simple tenets are often forgotten.

Since prognostic factors are identified retrospectively, their significance may change when more effective treatment regimens are developed. This in fact has occurred with the sequential evaluation of prognostic factors among children treated on the National Wilms Tumor Studies. The current definitions are listed in Table 9.2. The most significant recent change has been in the distinction between stages I and II (Beckwith 1998). Prior to NWTS-5, one of the criteria for stage II included extension of the tumor past the hilar plane, an imaginary boundary marked by the medial border of the renal sinus. The renal sinus is biologically quite important because it contains the major renal vessels, a potential route for hematogenous and lymphatic spread. However, this "hilar plane" has proven difficult to reliably and objectively assess and so the hilar plane criterion for staging was removed from NWTS-5 and replaced by the criterion of renal sinus vascular invasion which is assessed microscopically. Applying the new criteria, the difference in survival between stage I and II Wilms tumors continues to be statistically significant.

Another major change in the staging criteria for the current Children's Oncology Group (COG) studies is the categorization of tumor spill. In prior NWTS studies, tumor spill was classified as "local," a criterion for stage II, or "diffuse," a criterion for stage III. The difficulty was that although one could provide examples which everyone would agree represented either a local or diffuse spill, there was no objective definition of the difference between the two. Furthermore, a study of NWTS-4 patients led by John Kalapurakal showed that patients with stage II disease with local spill had lower 8-year relapse-free survival, 79 % vs 87 % ($p=0.07$), and overall survival, 90 % vs 95 % ($p=0.04$),

Table 9.2 Current staging criteria used by the Children's Oncology Group

Staging	Description
Stage I	Tumor limited to kidney, completely resected. The renal capsule is intact. The tumor was not ruptured or biopsied prior to removal. The vessels of the renal sinus are not involved. There is no evidence of tumor at or beyond the margins of resection. Note: for a tumor to qualify for certain therapeutic protocols as stage I, regional lymph nodes must be examined microscopically
Stage II	The tumor is completely resected and there is no evidence of tumor at or beyond the margins of resection. The tumor extends beyond kidney, as is evidenced by any one of the following criteria:
	There is regional extension of the tumor (i.e., penetration of the renal capsule or extensive invasion of the soft tissue of the renal sinus, as discussed below)
	Blood vessels within the nephrectomy specimen outside the renal parenchyma, including those of the renal sinus, contain tumor
	Note: rupture or spillage confined to the flank, including biopsy of the tumor, is no longer included in stage II and is now included in stage III
Stage III	Residual nonhematogenous tumor present following surgery and confined to the abdomen. Any one of the following may occur:
	Lymph nodes within the abdomen or pelvis are involved by tumor (Lymph node involvement in the thorax or other extra-abdominal sites is a criterion for stage IV)
	The tumor has penetrated through the peritoneal surface
	Tumor implants are found on the peritoneal surface
	Gross or microscopic tumor remains postoperatively (e.g., tumor cells are found at the margin of surgical resection on microscopic examination)
	The tumor is not completely resectable because of local infiltration into vital structures
	Tumor spillage occurring either before or during surgery
	The tumor is treated with preoperative chemotherapy (with or without a biopsy regardless of type – tru-cut, open, or fine-needle aspiration) before removal
	Tumor is removed in greater than one piece (e.g., tumor cells are found in a separately excised adrenal gland; a tumor thrombus within the renal vein is removed separately from the nephrectomy specimen). Extension of the primary tumor within vena cava into thoracic vena cava and heart is considered stage III, rather than stage IV even though outside the abdomen
Stage IV	Hematogenous metastases (lung, liver, bone, brain, etc.) or lymph node metastases outside the abdominopelvic region are present (The presence of tumor within the adrenal gland is not interpreted as metastasis and staging depends on all other staging parameters present)
Stage V	Bilateral renal involvement by tumor is present at diagnosis. An attempt should be made to stage each side according to the above criteria on the basis of the extent of disease

compared with stage II patients without spill when treated without abdominal radiation therapy (Kalapurakal et al. 2010). It was thus concluded that the group of patients with any form of intraoperative spill would have a better outcome if treated with irradiation (as stage III) and spill was then changed to a criterion for stage III. It will be difficult to prove that this change is beneficial. Certainly, we can monitor the outcomes of patients on the current trials who are stage III for spill alone – but not only is this a small group, and a single arm study, but the distribution of children whose spill might have been classified as diffuse vs local will be impossible to know.

According to SIOP protocols, the primary staging allocates patients to one of three pretreatment groups: localized unilateral Wilms tumors (regardless of regional lymph node status on imaging), metastatic Wilms tumors, or bilateral Wilms tumors/disease. Precise local-regional staging is performed after preoperative chemotherapy and takes into account the extent of the disease at that time only (de Kraker et al. 2004).

Staging criteria for Wilms tumor are based exclusively on the anatomic extent of the tumor, without consideration of genetic, biological, or molecular markers. Adequate exploration of the abdominal cavity and biopsy or excision of all suspicious structures is essential, including biopsy of lymph nodes at the level of renal vessels which is obligatory even if they seem not to be invaded.

Even with centralized pathological review, staging may still represent a problem, partly because renal tumors are usually large at nephrectomy and often it is very difficult to assess their relationship with normal renal anatomical structures such as the renal capsule and the renal sinus. Preoperative chemotherapy may result in tumor necrosis/regression outside of the kidney making staging even more difficult. SIOP studies have shown that the presence of necrotic tumor or chemotherapy-induced changes in the renal sinus or perirenal fat is of no adverse prognostic significance and it should be ignored for staging purposes. However, the presence of the same features at resection margins and lymph nodes should be regarded as stage III since a possibility of having viable tumor tissue in non-resected tumor or lymph nodes could not be excluded (Vujanic et al. 2002).

Approximately 5 % of children with Wilms tumor have disease affecting both kidneys; this may be either bilateral Wilms tumor, bilateral rests, or unilateral Wilms tumor with contralateral nephrogenic rests (Coppes et al. 1989; Stiller and Parkin 1990). Bilateral tumors were associated with somatic H19 epimutation (Scott et al. 2012). These children have stage V tumors with treatment adapted to their disease.

9.3 Histology

The histological finding of anaplasia was first identified as an important determinant of prognosis by Beckwith and Palmer in 1978 (Beckwith and Palmer 1978). The criteria for the diagnosis of anaplasia include: (1) the identification of nuclei with a diameter at least three times those of adjacent cells, (2) hyperchromasia of the enlarged cells providing evidence for increased chromatin content, and (3) the presence of multipolar or otherwise recognizably polyploid mitotic figures (Zuppan et al. 1988). Anaplasia is not common, approximately 5 % of all Wilms tumors, and correlates with patient age. It is rare in the first 2 years of life and then increases to a relatively stable rate of about 13 % in patients older than 5 years.

Table 9.3 Outcomes for stages II–IV diffuse anaplastic Wilms tumor on NWTS-3, -4, and -5

	4 years relapse-free survival % (*n*)		
	Reg DD4A RT	Reg J	Reg I
Stage	VDA	VDA + cyclo	VDC/CE
II	40 (12)	72 (11)	82 (23)
III	33 (9)	59 (13)	64 (43)
IV	0 (8)	17 (6)	33 (15)

Anaplasia has remained the most adverse prognostic factor since being defined. The results in Table 9.3 show the value of identifying this small subset (Dome et al. 2006). While overall treatment intensity has been reduced for patients with favorable histology Wilms tumor, these data have allowed the sequential intensification of therapy – adding doxorubicin, cyclophosphamide, and now etoposide – with modest but definite improvements in outcome. Without this factor these children would still be included in the larger group and would not have benefited from improvements in therapy.

Other more limited correlations between outcome and histology have been reported. In the setting of chemotherapy-naïve tumors, blastemal-rich tumors tend to be extremely invasive but often respond well to chemotherapy. In contrast, predominantly epithelial and rhabdomyomatous Wilms tumors more frequently present at a low stage, reflecting less aggressiveness, yet are often resistant to chemotherapy. While these prognostic trends have been observed and attempts made to exploit them, it has not been possible to define them in such a way as to show reproducible significant differences in outcome and so they have not been incorporated into staging or risk-based schemas by the COG or SIOP-RTSG.

Histology is also the most important prognostic factor for Wilms tumor in the SIOP trials, where it is a direct indicator of the individual tumor's in vivo response to chemotherapy. Wilms tumors can be classified as low, intermediate, or high risk (HR) according to the overall necrosis percentage and the cell type predominance in the residual viable tumor (Delemarre et al. 1996).

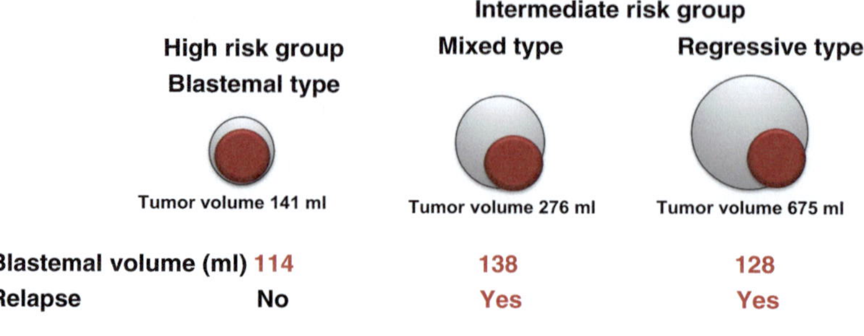

Fig. 9.1 Three tumors from the SIOP WT 2001 trial that have similar total volume of residual blastema after pre-operative chemotherapy but different histological risk groups according to the current SIOP classification scheme. The dark circle represents the size of the viable tumor component.

In this context, tumors with blastemal predominance as defined by the SIOP classification (see pathology Chap. 4) are high risk (Graf et al. 2000; Green et al. 1994). The unanswered question at present is whether it is the total residual volume of viable blastemal component that remains after pre-op chemotherapy that is the more important for prognosis, rather than its relative proportion. Figure 9.1 shows three tumors from the SIOP WT 2001 trial to illustrate the challenge.

Diffuse anaplasia is also placed in the high-risk category whether identified in a chemotherapy-naïve tumor or one that has been exposed to pre-nephrectomy chemotherapy. Special consideration is required for the anaplastic and blastemal subtypes that are metastatic at diagnosis – these should be considered as a very-high-risk group because they currently have an event-free survival of only ~30 % even with intensive treatment. These children are in need of new biological insights into their disease in order to introduce novel therapies.

After preoperative chemotherapy, the total residual volume of blastema is a potential new biomarker that could be used to further refine the current definition of "high-risk" histology. This is defined as less than 2/3 of the tumor being necrotic and more than 2/3 of the viable tumor comprising blastemal cells. However, this definition is somewhat subjective and it should be noted that detailed quantification of residual blastema was only defined on central pathology review (Vujanic et al. 2009), not by local pathologists in the SIOP 93–01 trial. A preliminary analysis of the SIOP 2001 trial data has shown that there is a threshold of between 20 and 50 ml residual blastemal volume in localized Wilms tumors that confers adverse event-free survival (~75 %) (Graf et al. 2011). However, it would be premature to introduce this into clinical risk stratification, especially as overall survival remains excellent (>90 %) for these children if they do not have "blastemal-type" WT. Rather, efforts should be made to understand the biology of blastemal cells that are resistant to chemotherapy treatment and to translate this into a robust gene alteration or protein expression test for routine use by pathologists.

9.4 Response of Metastatic Disease

SIOP investigators have long based the need for whole-lung irradiation for pulmonary metastases on whether there is a complete response to the first 6 weeks of chemotherapy. Seventy-five percent of patients with stage IV FH WT treated on SIOP trials have thus been spared whole-lung irradiation with apparently comparable outcomes to the NWTSG (de Kraker et al. 1990). These results cannot be immediately utilized in North America because the chemotherapy regimen used by the SIOP is more intensive, particularly with regard to anthracycline dosage. It is therefore possible that withholding radiation in the context of the lesser chemotherapy regimen used by COG might result in more recurrences. This question is being currently examined in the COG trial, with the further differences that complete response is being defined by CT scan at week 6, rather than by chest X-ray and that the response must be attained following chemotherapy only, not surgery. These criteria are therefore more conservative than the SIOP approach. Finally, the COG is using the failure to attain a complete response as a predictor of adverse outcome and is testing intensification of chemotherapy for this subset of patients.

9.5 Tumor Volume After Preoperative Chemotherapy

The use of preoperative chemotherapy provides the opportunity to assess tumor response – whether by volume reduction (imaging) or by histological response, as discussed above. Tumor volume reduction, although clearly associated with outcome, must be correlated with predominant histology. For example, rhabdomyomatous or stromal predominant tumors may not shrink at all in response to chemotherapy yet have a favorable outcome if resected completely (Verschuur et al. 2010). Although this correlation exists, a clear criterion has not yet been defined to allow the incorporation of volume reduction into treatment-determining risk strata. The COG takes tumor volume into account for treatment stratification purposes by defining the very-low-risk group as primarily operated young patients with a tumor volume below 550 ml.

It is expected that increase in tumor volume during preoperative chemotherapy is a reflection of the proliferative property and biological aggressiveness (Ora et al. 2007). Following this, the GPOH (Germany) is looking to answer the question if a more intense treatment is beneficial for patients with poor response according to tumor volume. These patients comprise around 14 % of the stage II and III tumors and are defined by tumor volume greater than 500 ml after chemotherapy. Excluding those with stromal- or epithelial-type Wilms tumor, they receive more intensive post-nephrectomy chemotherapy in Germany (Graf et al. 2012).

9.6 Patient Age

In patients with favorable histology Wilms tumors, age is a prognostic factor but not an independent one. Usually, patients with stage I favorable histology Wilms tumor are significantly younger than those with higher stages. Age older than 4 years at diagnosis is clearly an adverse prognostic factor but, probably related to tumors with more adverse biological features (Pritchard-Jones et al. 2003). The incidence of anaplasia (unfavorable histology) in children less than 2 years old is about 2 %, increasing significantly to 13 % in children diagnosed at ages greater than 5 years. Interestingly, age at diagnosis is lower in sporadic tumors with somatic WT1 mutations (Scott et al. 2012).

However, contrary to previous reports that showed that age below 2 year was a positive prognostic factor (Pession et al. 2008), a more recent study that evaluated only tumors with stage II and III did not found a correlation between age and the risk of relapse or death (Graf et al. 2012).

9.7 Molecular Markers

In 1994, Pediatric Oncology Group investigators showed that, among 232 children with Wilms tumor registered on NWTS-3 and -4, loss of heterozygosity (LOH) for polymorphic DNA markers on chromosome 16q, present in tumor tissue from 17.2 % of those with favorable or anaplastic histology tumors, was associated with statistically significantly poorer 2-year relapse-free and overall survival percentages even when adjusted for stage or histology (17). LOH for chromosome 1p, present in tumor tissue from 11 % of children, was also associated with poorer relapse-free and overall survival although these results were not statistically significant. By contrast, LOH for 11p, a region thought to contain at least two Wilms tumor-related genes, found in 33 % of cases, was not associated with any difference in outcome (Grundy et al. 1994).

NWTS-5 was designed to prospectively test this proposed association between LOH for chromosome 16q or chromosome 1p and outcome

Table 9.4 RFS and OS by joint LOH at chromosomes 1p and 16q for clinical stage I/II favorable histology Wilms tumor patients

LOH status	# pts	Relapse-free survival			Overall survival		
		# relapses	4 years RFS %	RR (95 % CI) *p*-value[a]	# deaths	4 years OS %	RR (95 % CI) *p*-value[a]
Neither	750	60	91.2	–	14	98.4	–
1p only	60	11	80.4	2.19 (1.15–4.17) $p=0.02$	4	91.2	4.03 (1.20–12.43) $p=0.02$
16q only	114	19	82.5	1.91 (1.14–3.21) $p=0.01$	3	98.1	1.40 (0.40–4.95) $p=0.60$
Both	46	11	74.9	2.88 (1.51–5.49) $p=0.001$	4	90.5	4.25 (1.37–13.19) $p=0.01$

[a]RRs are calculated with stratification on stage I/age <24 months/Wt <550 g, stage I/age ≥24 months or Wt ≥550 g, and stage II

Table 9.5 RFS and OS by joint LOH at chromosomes 1p and 16q for stage III/IV favorable histology Wilms tumor patients

LOH status	# pts	Relapse-free survival			Overall survival		
		# relapses	4 years RFS %	RR (95 % CI) *p*-value[a]	# deaths	4 years OS %	RR (95 % CI) *p*-value[a]
Neither	500	82	83.0	–	38	91.9	–
1p only	56	6	89.0	0.69 (0.30–1.57) $p=0.37$	2	97.6	0.52 (0.12–2.14) $p=0.36$
16q only	100	15	85.3	0.89 (0.51–1.54) $p=0.67$	7	92.0	0.88 (0.39–1.97) $p=0.76$
Both	30	9	65.9	2.41 (1.20–4.82) $p=0.01$	5	77.5	2.66 (1.04–6.82) $p=0.04$

[a]RRs are calculated with stratification on stage III and IV

in favorable histology Wilms tumor, all of whom were treated with common, stage-specific treatment regimens. The study was designed to detect clinically significant associations within stages of disease, namely, stages I/II and III/IV, and to provide more accurate estimates of the outcomes. As shown in Tables 9.4 and 9.5, patients with stage I/II tumors had worse outcomes with either LOH chromosome 1p or 16q but it was the subset with LOH of both which had a threefold risk of relapse, which equated to a 75 % relapse-free survival, a clinically significant difference relative to those with LOH for neither chromosome who had a 90 % RFS. Similarly, for stage III/IV patients, those with LOH for 1p and 16q had a 2.5 increased risk of relapse and death – a 65 % RFS compared with 83 % for those without LOH. This has now been added to stage and histology to generate "risk" groups (Table 9.6). It is important to note that although combined LOH 1p/16q is now proven to be associated with an adverse outcome, intensified therapy has not yet been shown to improve relapse-free or overall survival. That is one of the questions of the current COG trials.

Messahel has reported on the prognostic significance of loss of heterozygosity (LOH) on 1p and 16q in 426 favorable histology Wilms tumors treated with either immediate nephrectomy (63 %) or preoperative chemotherapy (37 %) in the United Kingdom. Intriguingly, although they found the same incidence of LOH 1p and 16q as in the NWTS series, only LOH 16q was associated with an increased risk of relapse (hazard ratio (HR) 2.69, 95 % CI: 1.47–4.92) and death (HR 2.67, 95 % CI: 1.17–6.06) while LOH 1p showed no significant associations (Messahel

Table 9.6 Favorable histology Wilms tumor

Patient age	Tumor weight	Stage	LOH*	Rapid response	Risk group
<2 years	<550 g	I	Any	N/A	Very low
Any	≥550 g	I	None	N/A	Low
>2 years	Any	I	None	N/A	Low
Any	Any	II	None	N/A	Low
>2 years	Any	I	LOH	N/A	Standard
Any	≥550 g	I	LOH	N/A	Standard
Any	Any	II	LOH	N/A	Standard
Any	Any	III	None	Any	Standard
Any	Any	III	LOH	Any	Higher
Any	Any	IV	LOH	Any	Higher
Any	Any	IV	None	Yes	Standard
Any	Any	IV	None	No	Higher
Any	Any	V	Any	Any	Bilateral

*Combined LOH 1p/16q

et al. 2009). Whether this difference between the North American and UK results reflects the inability of the smaller UK series to detect a significant association with 1p LOH (the first NWTS study which was also smaller also showed 16q but not 1p to be associated with adverse outcome) or a difference in the biology of Wilms tumors in different populations is not known.

Use of loss of heterozygosity assays (LOH) to determine areas of allele loss has shown that the majority of Wilms tumors have few or no changes and these tend to be restricted to a few loci, mainly at 11p, 1p, 16q, 11q, and 22q (Ruteshouser et al. 2005; Williams et al. 2010, 2011; Wittmann et al. 2007). The better characterized finding regarding LOH with clinical prognostic value is the combined LOH 1p and 16q for tumors treated by immediate surgical removal (Grundy et al. 2005). However, these prognostic markers have not yet been shown to confer additional prognostic information in the setting of the histological risk groups defined after preoperative chemotherapy, as used in the SIOP-RTSG trials.

Although utilized clinically as a biomarker, the mechanisms by which LOH 1p or 16q might be directly responsible for tumor resistance remain unknown. Mutational screening of candidate genes selected on the basis of their putative role in nephrogenesis or location within rare regions of homozygous loss has so far failed to pinpoint the critical genes involved in either 1p36 or 16q21-24 (Safford et al. 2003; Tamimi et al. 2007). It is possible that LOH at these loci is not always the driving factor but a marker of change elsewhere in the genome. For example, cytogenetic analyses of Wilms tumors have shown an association of 16q loss with 1q gain due to unbalanced translocation (Bown et al. 2002; Segers et al. 2013).

A well-designed case-cohort analysis in a COG trial showed a correlation of increased expression of telomerase components with adverse relapse-free but not overall survival. However, the ultimate test of telomerase activity, the TRAP assay, could not confirm this correlation, perhaps due to the higher failure rate and the inherent variability in an in vitro test of enzymatic activity (Dome et al. 2005).

Subsequently, several groups have taken a whole-genome approach to the identification of prognostic biomarkers in Wilms tumor (Huang et al. 2009; Li et al. 2005; Williams et al. 2004). To date, it has been difficult to define a reproducible molecular signature predictive of relapse. Genomic copy number appears a better classifier than expression profiling (Williams et al. 2004, 2011). This may be due to the complexity of cellular composition of Wilms tumor, with retention of expression patterns reflecting embryonic counterparts (Maschietto et al. 2008).

Table 9.7 Molecular markers studied in Wilms tumors

Molecular marker	Type of association	Size of studied population	Found by independent studies	Reference
Gain of 1q	Adverse outcome	>1,000 patients	Yes	Hing et al. (2001), Natrajan et al. (2006a, c)
				Gratias et al. (2013) and unpublished results
Mutation in *TP53*	Unfavorable histology	3–40 patients	Yes	Bardeesy et al. (1994, 1995), El Bahtimi et al. (1996) Maschietto et al. (2014)
Overexpression of *NTRK2*	Relapse	39 patients	No	Eggert et al. (2001)
Gain/overexpression of *IGF1R*	Relapse	68 patients	No	Natrajan et al. (2006b)
Gain of *MYCN*	Unfavorable histology	More than 400 patients	Yes	Williams et al. (2010, 2011)
Reduced retinoic pathway activity	High-risk tumor	200 patients	Yes	Wegert et al. (2011), Zirn et al. (2006)

Several studies have shown a strong association between gain of the whole or part of chromosome 1q and adverse outcome (Bown et al. 2002; Hing et al. 2001; Natrajan et al. 2006a, c; Segers et al. 2013). Such copy number abnormalities of 1q are a frequent finding (~30 % of cases), but the region of gain is generally very large.

Other analyses have highlighted alterations of insulin-like growth factor II signaling and retinoic acid pathways as of potential prognostic significance (Huang et al. 2009; Wegert et al. 2011; Zirn et al. 2005). For instance, *IGF1R* overexpression (transcript and protein) in the blastemal cells and 15q26.3 amplification, where *IGF1R* is located, were associated with relapse in patients with Wilms tumors presenting favorable histology (Natrajan et al. 2006b). In primary culture of high-risk Wilms tumors, a reduced retinoic acid pathway activity was described compared to low- and intermediate-risk Wilms tumors suggesting a beneficial impact of RA on advanced Wilms tumors cases (Wegert et al. 2011).

These findings are of particular interest as relevant therapies are already in clinical use. Genomic amplification of 2p24.3, where *MYCN* is located, is associated with unfavorable histology. Initially this finding was described in patients treated in the SIOP trials, but a later study showed that amplification of *MYCN* is also present in the diffuse anaplastic tumors from COG trials (Williams et al. 2010, 2011). The observed levels of copy number gain are generally modest, though occasional cases show high-level gain comparable with that seen in neuroblastoma. However, much further research remains to be done before any of these potential biomarkers could be used for treatment decision making.

Other genomic loci were associated with unfavorable histology including gain on 13q31 and losses at 12q24, 18q21, 1q32.1, and 2q36.3–2q37.1 (Natrajan et al. 2006c; Williams et al. 2011), but their role in tumor outcome, is not clear.

Somatic defects at several loci where the so-called Wilms tumor genes are located, including mutations in *WT1*, *CTNNB1*, *WTX*, *TP53,* and *FBXW7,* and the disruption of the imprinted 11p15 region, have been implicated in Wilms tumor. However, the clinical association of these alterations is not always clear. Overexpression of genes such as *NTRK2* (Eggert et al. 2001) and *KIT* (Jones et al. 2007) was also associated with poor prognosis in patients with favorable Wilms tumor treated in the SIOP trials (Table 9.7).

However, for the patients treated in the SIOP trials, it is still necessary to clarify if these prognostic factors are associated with tumor biology itself or if they arise as a consequence of the chemotherapy treatment.

9.8 The Search for Additional Biomarkers in Wilms Tumor

Neither the SIOP nor COG treatment approaches have yet succeeded in defining a prognostic biomarker that is sufficiently sensitive or specific to identify the majority of patients with poor outcome: "high-risk" histology (blastemal type or diffuse anaplasia) is found in only ~25 % of all relapses with the SIOP approach, and combined LOH 1p/16q occurs in only ~10 % of all relapses with the COG approach. It is likely that multiple prognostic factors will be required to accurately define the highest risk group. Conversely, there is a need to more reliably identify patients whose current treatment can be safely reduced, e.g., by omission of doxorubicin, as in the current SIOP WT 2001 trial.

In the past, many studies of individual genes were underpowered and hence could not take account of established prognostic factors such as age, stage, and histology. The large size of the NWTSG-5 trial sample collection permitted a well-designed case-cohort analysis of the prognostic impact of telomerase activity (Dome et al. 2005). This showed a correlation of increased expression of telomerase components with adverse relapse-free but not overall survival. However, the ultimate test of telomerase activity, the TRAP assay, could not confirm this correlation.

Based on the results of their prospective biomarker trial (NWTSG-5), COG renal tumor trials now apply the molecular marker of combined loss of heterozygosity (LOH) covering fairly large genomic regions of chromosomes 1p (8 Mb) and 16q (25 Mb), to allocate tumors to more intensive regimens (Grundy et al. 2005). A more recent study evaluated 1q gain, 1p loss, and 16q loss in 212 patients with favorable histology WT enrolled in the NWTSG-5 and concluded that gain of 1q is associated with inferior event-free survival in all stages and might be used to stratify therapy in the next studies of this group (Gratias et al. 2013).

Blastemal-type tumor is a prognostic factor exclusively used by SIOP. LOH of 1p with LOH of 16q are used as a prognostic factor only by COG. Both clinical trials groups recognize diffuse anaplasia as high risk and intensify treatment accordingly. However, recent analysis of the prevalence of *TP53* mutations and/or 17p loss (where *TP53* is located) in diffuse anaplastic Wilms tumor found that only 55% of cases have detectable mutation and this is associated with increased risk of relapse and death compared to cases without *TP53* mutation or loss (Maschietto et al. 2014). This suggests that molecular analysis may help to optimise treatment planning for these intensively treated patients, but also emphasises the importance of meticulous selection of tumor tissue for molecular testing.

There are many ongoing translational research studies that aim to discover new Wilms tumor genes through whole exome mutational analyses and to define the molecular pathways involved. Such approaches are already bearing fruit. Recently, *DROSHA* was found to be mutated in 12% of a cohort of 222 mixed histology tumors, with a recurrent mutation (E1147K) affecting a metal-binding residue of the RNase IIIb domain in 81% of the *DROSHA*-mutated tumors. As a key component of the microRNA biogenesis pathway, these mutations found in *DROSHA* and at much lower frequency in some other genes in the pathway, suggest that microRNAs play an important role for Wilms tumor development (Torrezan et al. 2014). Epigenetic changes may also be important, particularly in those Wilms tumors that lack identifiable somatic mutations, and may provide a biomarker that is detectable in circulating cell free DNA (Charlton et al. 2014). Molecular characterization of large numbers of tumors with linked clinical demographic, treatment and outcome data, will be essential to determine the place of these in potentially guiding current treatment. Such studies are a focus for ongoing work to optimize current treatment approaches and to prioritise new agents for testing in early phase trials in very high risk Wilms tumor.

References

Bardeesy N, Falkoff D, Petruzzi MJ, Nowak N, Zabel B et al (1994) Anaplastic Wilms' tumour, a subtype displaying poor prognosis, harbours p53 gene mutations. Nat Genet 7:91–97

Bardeesy N, Beckwith JB, Pelletier J (1995) Clonal expansion and attenuated apoptosis in Wilms' tumors are associated with p53 gene mutations. Cancer Res 55:215–219

Beckwith JB (1998) National Wilms Tumor Study: an update for pathologists. Pediatr Dev Pathol 1(1):79–84

Beckwith JB, Palmer NF (1978) Histopathology and prognosis of Wilms tumors: results from the First National Wilms' Tumor Study. Cancer 41(5):1937–1948

Bown N, Cotterill SJ, Roberts P, Griffiths M, Larkins S, Hibbert S et al (2002) Cytogenetic abnormalities and clinical outcome in Wilms tumor: a study by the U.K. cancer cytogenetics group and the U.K. Children's Cancer Study Group. Med Pediatr Oncol 38(1):11–21

Charlton J, Williams RD, Weeks M, Sebire NJ, Popov S, Vujanic G, Mifsud W, Alcaide-German M, Butcher LM, Beck S, Pritchard-Jones K (2014) Methylome analysis identifies a Wilms tumor epigenetic biomarker detectable in blood. Genome Biol 15(8):434

Coppes MJ, de Kraker J, van Dijken PJ, Perry HJ, Delemarre JF, Tournade MF et al (1989) Bilateral Wilms' tumor: long-term survival and some epidemiological features. J Clin Oncol 7(3):310–315

D'Angio GJ, Beckwith JB, Bishop HC, Breslow N, Evans AE, Goodwin WE et al (1972) Proceedings: the national Wilms' tumor study: a progress report. Proc Natl Cancer Conf 7:627–636

D'Angio GJ, Evans AE, Breslow N, Beckwith B, Bishop H, Feigl P et al (1976) Treatment of Wilms tumor – results of national Wilms tumor study. Cancer 38(2):633–646

de Kraker J, Lemerle J, Voute PA, Zucker JM, Tournade MF, Carli M (1990) Wilms' tumor with pulmonary metastases at diagnosis: the significance of primary chemotherapy. International Society of Pediatric Oncology Nephroblastoma Trial and Study Committee. J Clin Oncol 8(7):1187–1190

de Kraker J, Graf N, van Tinteren H, Pein F, Sandstedt B, Godzinski J et al (2004) Reduction of postoperative chemotherapy in children with stage I intermediate-risk and anaplastic Wilms' tumour (SIOP 93–01 trial): a randomised controlled trial. Lancet 364(9441):1229–1235

Delemarre JFM, Sandstedt B, Harms D, Boccon-Gibod L, Vujanić GM (1996) The new SIOP (Stockholm) working classification of renal tumours of childhood. Med Pediatr Oncol 26(2):145–146

Dome JS, Bockhold CA, Li SM, Baker SD, Green DM, Perlman EJ et al (2005) High telomerase RNA expression level Is an adverse prognostic factor for favorable-histology Wilms' tumor. J Clin Oncol 23(36):9138–9145

Dome JS, Cotton CA, Perlman EJ, Breslow NE, Kalapurakal JA, Ritchey ML et al (2006) Treatment of anaplastic histology Wilms' tumor: results from the fifth National Wilms' Tumor Study. J Clin Oncol 24(15):2352–2358

el Bahtimi R, Hazen-Martin DJ, Re GG, Willingham MC, Garvin AJ (1996) Immunophenotype, mRNA expression, and gene structure of p53 in Wilms' tumors. Mod Pathol 9:238–244

Eggert A, Grotzer MA, Ikegaki N, Zhao H, Cnaan A, Brodeur GM et al (2001) Expression of the neurotrophin receptor TrkB is associated With unfavorable outcome in Wilms' tumor. J Clin Oncol 19(3):689–696

Graf N, Tournade MF, de Kraker J (2000) The role of preoperative chemotherapy in the management of Wilms' tumor. The SIOP studies International Society of Pediatric Oncology. Urol Clin North Am 27(3):443–454

Graf N, van Tinteren H, Pritchard-Jones K, Bergeron C, Sandstedt B, Leuschner I et al (2011) Is the absolute blastemal volume after pre-operative chemotherapy relevant for prognosis? Pediatr Blood Cancer 57(5):741(O138)

Graf N, van Tinteren H, Bergeron C, Pein F, van den Heuvel-Eibrink MM, Sandstedt B et al (2012) Characteristics and outcome of stage II and III non-anaplastic Wilms' tumour treated according to the SIOP trial and study 93–01. Eur J Cancer 48(17):3240–3248

Gratias EJ, Jennings LJ, Anderson JR, Dome JS, Grundy P, Perlman EJ (2013) Gain of 1q is associated with inferior event-free and overall survival in patients with favorable fistology Wilms tumor: a report from the Children's Oncology Group. Cancer 119:3887–3894

Green DM, Breslow NE, Beckwith JB, Moksness J, Finklestein JZ, D'Angio GJ (1994) Treatment of children with clear-cell sarcoma of the kidney: a report from the National Wilms' Tumor Study Group. J Clin Oncol 12(10):2132–2137

Green DM, Breslow NE, Beckwith JB, Finklestein JZ, Grundy P, Thomas PR et al (1998a) Effect of duration of treatment on treatment outcome and cost of treatment for Wilms' tumor: a report from the National Wilms' Tumor Study Group. J Clin Oncol 16(12):3744–3751

Green DM, Breslow NE, Beckwith JB, Finklestein JZ, Grundy PE, Thomas PR et al (1998b) Comparison between single-dose and divided-dose administration of dactinomycin and doxorubicin for patients with Wilms' tumor: a report from the National Wilms' Tumor Study Group. J Clin Oncol 16(1):237–245

Grundy PE, Telzerow PE, Breslow N, Moksness J, Huff V, Paterson MC (1994) Loss of heterozygosity for chromosomes 16q and 1p in Wilms' tumors predicts an adverse outcome. Cancer Res 54(9):2331–2333

Grundy PE, Breslow N, Li S, Perlman E, Beckwith JB, Ritchey ML, Shamberger RC, Haase GM, D'Angio GJ, Donaldson M, Coppes MJ, Malogolowkin M, Shearer P, Thomas PR, Macklis R, Tomlinson G, Huff V, Green DM, National Wilms Tumor Study Group (2005) Loss of heterozygosity for chromosomes 1p and 16q is an adverse prognostic factor in favorable-histology Wilms tumor: a report from the National Wilms Tumor Study Group. J Clin Oncol 23(29):7312–7321

Hing S, Lu Y-J, Summersgill B, King-Underwood L, Nicholson J, Grundy P, Grundy R, Gessler M, Shipley J, Pritchard-Jones K (2001) Gain of 1q is associated with adverse outcome in favorable histology Wilms' tumors. Am J Pathol 158(2):393–398

Huang CC, Gadd S, Breslow N, Cutcliffe C, Sredni ST, Helenowski IB et al (2009) Predicting relapse in favorable histology Wilms tumor using gene expression analysis: a report from the Renal Tumor Committee of the Children's Oncology Group. Clin Cancer Res 15(5):1770–1778

Jones C, Rodriguez-Pinilla M, Lambros M, Bax D, Messahel B, Vujanic GM et al (2007) c-KIT overexpression, without gene amplification and mutation, in paediatric renal tumours. J Clin Pathol 60(11):1226–1231

Kalapurakal JA, Li SM, Breslow NE, Beckwith JB, Ritchey ML, Shamberger RC et al (2010) Intraoperative spillage of favorable histology Wilms tumor cells: influence of irradiation and chemotherapy regimens on abdominal recurrence. A report from the National Wilms Tumor Study Group. Int J Radiat Oncol Biol Phys 76(1):201–206

Li W, Kessler P, Yeger H, Alami J, Reeve AE, Heathcott R et al (2005) A gene expression signature for relapse of primary Wilms tumors. Cancer Res 65(7): 2592–2601

Maschietto M, de Camargo B, Brentani H, Grundy P, Sredni ST, Torres C, Mota LD, Cunha IW, Patrão DF, Costa CM, Soares FA, Brentani RR, Carraro DM (2008) Molecular profiling of isolated histological components of Wilms tumor implicates a common role for the Wnt signaling pathway in kidney and tumor development. Oncology 75:81–91

Maschietto M, Williams RD, Chagtai T, Popov SD, Sebire NJ, Vujanic G, Perlman E, Anderson JA, Grundy P, Dome JS, Pritchard-Jones K (2014) TP53 mutational status is a potential marker for risk stratification in Wilms tumour with diffuse anaplasia. Plos One (in press)

Messahel B, Williams R, Ridolfi A, A'Hern R, Warren W, Tinworth L et al (2009) Allele loss at 16q defines poorer prognosis Wilms tumour irrespective of treatment approach in the UKW1-3 clinical trials: a Children's Cancer and Leukaemia Group (CCLG) Study. Eur J Cancer 45(5):819–826

Natrajan R, Little SE, Reis-Filho JS, Hing L, Messahel B, Grundy PE et al (2006a) Amplification and overexpression of CACNA1E correlates with relapse in favorable histology Wilms' tumors. Clin Cancer Res 12(24):7284–7293

Natrajan R, Reis-Filho JS, Little SE, Messahel B, Brundler MA, Dome JS et al (2006b) Blastemal expression of type I insulin-like growth factor receptor in Wilms' tumors is driven by increased copy number and correlates with relapse. Cancer Res 66(23):11148–11155

Natrajan R, Williams RD, Hing SN, Mackay A, Reis-Filho JS, Fenwick K et al (2006c) Array CGH profiling of favourable histology Wilms tumours reveals novel gains and losses associated with relapse. J Pathol 210(1):49–58

Ora I, van Tinteren H, Bergeron C, de Kraker J (2007) Progression of localised Wilms' tumour during preoperative chemotherapy is an independent prognostic factor: a report from the SIOP 93–01 nephroblastoma trial and study. Eur J Cancer 43(1):131–136

Pession A, Dama E, Rondelli R, Magnani C, De Rosa M, Locatelli F et al (2008) Survival of children with cancer in Italy, 1989–98. A report from the hospital based registry of the Italian Association of Paediatric Haematology and Oncology (AIEOP). Eur J Cancer 44(9):1282–1289

Pritchard-Jones K, Kelsey A, Vujanic G, Imeson J, Hutton C, Mitchell C (2003) Older age is an adverse prognostic factor in stage I, favorable histology Wilms' tumor treated with vincristine monochemotherapy: a study by the United Kingdom Children's Cancer Study Group, Wilms' Tumor Working Group. J Clin Oncol 21(17):3269–3275

Ruteshouser EC, Hendrickson BW, Colella S, Krahe R, Pinto L, Huff V (2005) Genome-wide loss of heterozygosity analysis of WT1-wild-type and WT1-mutant Wilms tumors. Genes Chromosomes Cancer 43(2):172–180

Safford SD, Goyeau D, Freemerman AJ, Bentley R, Everett ML, Grundy PE et al (2003) Fine mapping of Wilms' tumors with 16q loss of heterozygosity localizes the putative tumor suppressor gene to a region of 6.7 megabases. Ann Surg Oncol 10(2):136–143

Scott RH, Murray A, Baskcomb L, Turnbull C, Loveday C, Al-Saadi R et al (2012) Stratification of Wilms tumor by genetic and epigenetic analysis. Oncotarget 3(3):327–335

Segers H, van den Heuvel-Eibrink MM, Williams RD, van Tinteren H, Vujanic G, Pieters R, Pritchard-Jones K, Bown N; on behalf of the Children's Cancer and Leukaemia Group and the UK Cancer Cytogenetics Group (2013) Gain of 1q is a marker of poor prognosis in Wilms' tumors. Genes Chromosomes Cancer 52(11):1065–1074

Stiller CA, Parkin DM (1990) International variations in the incidence of childhood renal tumours. Br J Cancer 62(6):1026–1030

Tamimi Y, Ziebart K, Desaulniers N, Dietrich K, Grundy P (2007) Identification of a minimal region of loss on the short arm of chromosome 1 in Wilms tumor. Genes Chromosomes Cancer 46(4):327–335

Torrezan GT, Ferreira EN, Nakahata AM, Barros BD, Castro MT, Correa BR, Krepischi AC, Olivieri EH, Cunha IW, Tabori U, Grundy PE, Costa CM, de Camargo B, Galante PA, Carraro DM (2014) Recurrent somatic mutation in DROSHA induces microRNA profile changes in Wilms tumour. Nat Commun 5:4039. doi:10.1038/ncomms5039

Verschuur A, Vujanic G, van Tinteren H, Pritchard-Jones K, de Kraker J, Sandstedt B (2010) Stromal and epithelial predominant Wilms tumours have an excellent outcome: the SIOP 93 01 experience. Pediatr Blood Cancer 55:233–238

Vujanic GM, Sandstedt B, Harms D, Kelsey A, Leuschner I, de Kraker J (2002) Revised International Society of Paediatric Oncology (SIOP) working classification of renal tumors of childhood. Med Pediatr Oncol 38(2):79–82

Vujanic GM, Sandstedt B, Kelsey A, Sebire NJ (2009) Central pathology review in multicenter trials and studies: lessons from the nephroblastoma trials. Cancer 115(9):1977–1983

Wegert J, Bausenwein S, Kneitz S, Roth S, Graf N, Geissinger E et al (2011) Retinoic acid pathway activity in Wilms tumors and characterization of biological responses in vitro. Mol Cancer 10:136

Williams RD, Hing SN, Greer BT, Whiteford CC, Wei JS, Natrajan R et al (2004) Prognostic classification of relapsing favorable histology Wilms tumor using cDNA microarray expression profiling and support vector machines. Genes Chromosomes Cancer 41(1):65–79

Williams RD, Al-Saadi R, Chagtai T, Popov S, Messahel B, Sebire N et al (2010) Subtype-specific FBXW7 mutation and MYCN copy number gain in Wilms tumour. Clin Cancer Res 16(7):2036–2045

Williams RD, Al-Saadi R, Natrajan R, Mackay A, Chagtai T, Little S et al (2011) Molecular profiling reveals frequent gain of MYCN and anaplasia-specific loss of 4q and 14q in Wilms tumor. Genes Chromosomes Cancer 50(12):982–995

Wittmann S, Zirn B, Alkassar M, Ambros P, Graf N, Gessler M (2007) Loss of 11q and 16q in Wilms tumors is associated with anaplasia, tumor recurrence, and poor prognosis. Genes Chromosomes Cancer 46(2):163–170

Zirn B, Samans B, Spangenberg C, Graf N, Eilers M, Gessler M (2005) All-trans retinoic acid treatment of Wilms tumor cells reverses expression of genes associated with high risk and relapse in vivo. Oncogene 24(33):5246–5251

Zirn B, Hartmann O, Samans B, Krause M, Wittmann S, Mertens F et al (2006) Expression profiling of Wilms tumors reveals new candidate genes for different clinical parameters. Int J Cancer 118(8):1954–1962

Zuppan CW, Beckwith JB, Luckey DW (1988) Anaplasia in unilateral Wilms' tumor: a report from the National Wilms' Tumor Study Pathology Center. Hum Pathol 19(10):1199–1209

10 Molecular-Targeted Therapy for Pediatric Renal Tumors

James I. Geller and Peter Hohenstein

Contents

J.I. Geller (✉)
Division of Oncology, Cincinnati Children's Hospital Medical Center, University of Cincinnati, Cincinnati, OH, USA
e-mail: James.Geller@cchmc.org

P. Hohenstein
The Roslin Institute, University of Edinburgh, Easter Bush Campus, Midlothian EH25 9RG, UK
e-mail: peter.hohenstein@roslin.ed.ac.uk

Abstract

Advances in Wilms' tumor therapy have undeniably enabled cure of the majority of infants and children with favorable histology of Wilms' tumor in developed countries, and as such, treatment of Wilms' tumor is regarded as one of the great successes in pediatric oncology. Without diminishing the import of such progress, it should be noted, however, that universal cure is not a reality and cure rates remain poor in developing countries where the delivery of current toxic therapies is not easily accomplished and for those that do survive, "cure" is often associated with both acute and chronic morbidity. Even "minimal two-drug" vincristine and dactinomycin chemotherapy, forming the basis for Wilms' tumor therapy used worldwide for more than four decades presents significant risk for acute hepatic toxicity in the form of venoocclusive disease, among other acute toxicities not limited to peripheral neuropathy and bone marrow suppression. Similarly, nephrectomy with or without chemotherapy, a second widely used therapy for Wilms' tumor, automatically implies a stage I

K. Pritchard-Jones, J.S. Dome (eds.), *Renal Tumors of Childhood: Biology and Therapy*, Pediatric Oncology, DOI 10.1007/978-3-662-44003-2_10, © Springer-Verlag Berlin Heidelberg 2014

chronic kidney disease (CKD) status. It is becoming increasingly clear that Wilms' tumor survivors demonstrate "abnormal" renal function early on post-therapy, with an uncertain prognosis for long-term renal function beyond 20 years. Late effects resulting from surgery, radiotherapy, and chemotherapy for Wilms' tumor can also include musculoskeletal effects, cardiac toxicity, reproductive problems, and the development of second malignant neoplasms.

10.1 Introduction

Advances in Wilms' tumor therapy have undeniably enabled cure of the majority of infants and children with favorable histology of Wilms' tumor in developed countries, and as such, treatment of Wilms' tumor is regarded as one of the great successes in pediatric oncology. Without diminishing the import of such progress, it should be noted, however, that universal cure is not a reality and cure rates remain poor in developing countries where the delivery of current toxic therapies is not easily accomplished and for those that do survive, "cure" is often associated with both acute and chronic morbidity. Even "minimal two-drug" vincristine and dactinomycin chemotherapy, forming the basis for Wilms' tumor therapy used worldwide for more than four decades presents significant risk for acute hepatic toxicity in the form of venoocclusive disease, among other acute toxicities not limited to peripheral neuropathy and bone marrow suppression (Jagt et al. 2009). Similarly, nephrectomy with or without chemotherapy, a second widely used therapy for Wilms' tumor, automatically implies a stage I chronic kidney disease (CKD) status. It is becoming increasingly clear that Wilms' tumor survivors demonstrate "abnormal" renal function early on post-therapy, with an uncertain prognosis for long-term renal function beyond 20 years (Stefanowicz et al. 2010; Daw et al. 2009). Late effects resulting from surgery, radiotherapy, and chemotherapy for Wilms' tumor can also include musculoskeletal effects, cardiac toxicity, reproductive problems, and the development of second malignant neoplasms (Wright et al. 2009).

Unfortunately, an additional reality is that despite optimized currently available medical care, approximately 10–15 % of all children affected with favorable histology of Wilms' tumor, the most common kidney cancer in childhood, relapse and an additional 8 and 9 % demonstrate bilateral disease or unfavorable histology (anaplastic histology), respectively, each associated with a poorer prognosis (Ehrlich 2009; Dome et al. 2006). The prognosis for children with rhabdoid tumor of the kidney and advanced renal cell carcinoma remains dismal. Thus, "high-risk" renal tumors of childhood, including relapsed favorable histology of Wilms' tumor, bilateral Wilms' tumor, anaplastic Wilms' tumor, rhabdoid tumor of the kidney, advanced clear cell sarcoma of the kidney, and renal cell carcinoma, as a group, account for approximately one in four infants and children affected by Wilms' tumor and one in three infants and children affected by any type of pediatric kidney cancer. To improve cure rates and to decrease short- and long-term morbidity, continued expansion of our understanding of the molecular biology of pediatric renal tumors and the development of novel more tolerable biologically targeted therapies for all infants and children affected by pediatric kidney cancer is necessary.

This chapter will address Wilms' tumorigenesis and ongoing efforts to identify new drug targets for pediatric renal tumors, with specific focus on Wilms' tumor and their progress in reaching the clinic. The kidney developmental background of Wilms' tumors provides extra challenges but maybe also new possibilities for directed design of new or improved therapies.

10.2 Kidney Development and Wilms' Tumorigenesis

The development of Wilms' tumors (WTs) can be considered an archetypical example of normal development going awry, eventually leading to a metastasizing tumor. Rightfully and emphasizing this fact, WTs have been described as a "malignant developing kidney" (Nicholson 1950). Histological and microarray data has further established the close resemblance of Wilms' tumor (WT) to the developing kidney (Rivera and Haber 2005). This has several implications for drug development and treatment of WT patients, as a detailed understanding of the developmental processes that give rise to

WTs when disturbed could identify genes and pathways that need to be targeted for correction. When we consider WTs the result of blocked and/or uncontrolled differentiation, (re)activation of the pathways and signals downstream of or parallel to the affected step might force the early tumor cells to continue their normal differentiation and go out of cycle. A developmental cancer like WTs might be specifically well suited to such an approach, if the details of normal kidney development and how these are affected in the tumors would be sufficiently known.

Development of the mammalian metanephric kidney starts when several thousand cells in the caudal part of the intermediate mesoderm lying adjacent to the Wolffian duct condense to form the blastema, also referred to as the metanephric mesenchyme. The cascade of events that follows is a classic example of how reciprocal signals between epithelial and mesenchymal components can give rise to a complex organ. Excellent and detailed overviews of kidney development are available (Vize et al. 2003), and for our purpose here a brief overview is provided.

The starting event is the induction of formation of the ureteric bud. The blastemal cells produce GDNF, while the Wolffian duct expresses the c-RET receptor and GFRA-1 co-receptor (Dressler 2006). This signal induces the outgrowth of the ureteric bud from the Wolffian duct. The growing ureteric bud invades the metanephric mesenchyme and the mesenchyme response by inducing the first branching event of the bud. In its turn, the mesenchyme responds to this by forming a condensate of three to four cells thick around the newly formed bud tip called the cap mesenchyme. Gene-targeting studies identified Wnt9b expressed in tips of the ureteric bud as a strong candidate for this inductive signal (Basson 2005). In the cap mesenchyme an autocrine Wnt4 loop is the result, which is essential for the subsequent mesenchymal-to-epithelial transition (MET) (Stark et al. 1994). *Six2*-positive cells in the cap mesenchyme have been identified as a renewing progenitor population that gives rise to the complete nephron (Kobayashi 2008). Initially, a pre-tubular aggregate is formed by mesenchymal cells being left behind by the growing ureteric bud, which subsequently forms the polarized renal vesicle. Patterning processes lead to a clearly recognizable (initially via marker gene expression, later on morphologically) proximal and distal half, and via intermediate comma and S-shaped body stages, the distal and proximal tubules and the glomerulus are formed. At the same time, the distal end of the renal vesicle fuses to the ureteric bud, and the basic architecture of the nephron and collecting duct system is a fact.

The genetics of WTs have been studied for a long time and identify the important steps in kidney development from a WT objective. The first gene to be implicated in WTs was the *WT1* tumor suppressor gene (Lee 1999). It encodes a four Zn-finger multifunctional protein that can function in transcriptional regulation and RNA metabolism (Hohenstein and Hastie 2006). Its expression during kidney development starts in the intermediate mesoderm, stays expressed in the metanephric mesenchyme, and starts to increase in the cap mesenchyme. After the MET, WT1 expression becomes restricted to the proximal half of the developing nephron, until eventually only podocytes express WT1 in the postnatal kidney. *WT1* is essential for early kidney development as *WT1* knockout mice show massive apoptosis in the uninduced mesenchyme, even before the invasion of the ureteric bud, leading to complete absence of the kidneys (Kreidberg 1993). Additionally, heterozygous knockout mice and isoform-specific knockouts of *WT1* have shown that WT1 is indispensible for podocyte integrity (Menke 2003; Hammes 2001).

A second gene deregulated in WT is *β-catenin*. The protein functions as an intracellular signaling transducer for WNT signals and is mutated in many types of cancer. Oncogenic mutations in *β-catenin* result in stabilization of the protein leading to increased and constitutive signaling and can be detected via nuclear accumulation of the protein. *WT1* loss in WTs is frequently combined with oncogenic activation of the *β-catenin* proto-oncogene (Maiti et al. 2000; Koesters 1999). As different WNT signals are essential for normal development of the kidney, β-catenin has been widely implicated in normal kidney development as well. Wnt9b is expressed in the stalk of the ureteric bud and is believed to be the inducer of mesenchyme condensation via a β-catenin-mediated process (Carroll et al. 2005). β-catenin is essential for nephron induction and constitutively active β-catenin can compensate for the loss of *Wnt9b* or

Wnt4 (Burn et al. 2011; Tanigawa et al. 2011) in this process; however, its signaling needs to be inhibited at a later stage to complete nephron formation (Birney 2007). Interestingly, in the developing testis, β-catenin signaling was shown to be downregulated by WT1 (Chang 2008).

A third gene implicated in the development of Wilms' tumors is *WTX*. The gene was identified on the X chromosome, and, as one would expect, in female patients, the mutations are specifically found on the active copy of the chromosome, confirming it acts as a tumor suppressor gene (Rivera 2007). It was suggested to account for up to 30 % of WT cases. WTX function has been directly implicated in controlling the stability of the β-catenin protein (Major 2007). Accordingly, the initial publication suggested that *WTX* and *WT1*/β-catenin mutations are mutually exclusive (Rivera 2007); however, later data on additional WT samples showed this is not the case, and much reduced frequencies of *WTX* mutations have since then been reported (Ruteshouser et al. 2008; Perotti 2008). Interestingly, germline *WTX* mutations where identified in families with sclerosing skeletal dysplasia without any signs of increased tumorigenesis (WT or other) (Jenkins 2009). At present no specific functions for *WTX* in the developing kidney have been described, nor have *Wtx* mouse models been reported that could further enlighten these contradictions.

Another important genetic aberration linked to WT formation is increased expression of *IGF2*. The gene is maternally imprinted (so paternally expressed) in the kidney, and early work suggested increased expression through loss of imprinting or duplication of the paternal alleles in WT (Ogawa 1993) and BWS (Beckwith-Wiedemann syndrome, an overgrowth syndrome associated with increased incidence of WTs) (Weksberg et al. 1993). Imprinting of this locus at 11p15 is controlled by expression of the *H19* gene, and methylation of its promoter is now one of the best studied examples of epigenetic aberrations in cancer (Steenman 1994; Moulton 1994). Despite the clear importance of IGF2 activation in a large subset of WTs, it has so far been difficult to couple this to specific functions during kidney development. Mice that receive a mutated paternal allele of *H19* or are homozygous mutants are severely growth retarded (60 % of wild-type littermates) but viable (Dechiara et al. 1990; Dechiara et al. 1991). Maternal loss of *H19* results in increased *IGF2* expression and a 28 % increase in body weight but no other phenotypes (Leighton et al. 1995). Further increase in IGF2 levels through loss of its IGF2r receptor (leading to decreased IGF2 turnover) results in further overgrowth symptoms resembling BWS but no WTs (Eggenschwiler 1997). Combination of the *IGF2* imprinting mutant with loss of $p57^{Kip2}$ (also found mutated in BWS) gives additional BWS phenotypes but still no WTs (Caspary 1999). The kidney dysplasia observed in these mice is believed to be an augmentation of the $p57^{Kip2}$ knockout phenotype. Comparable overgrowth symptoms were found in transgenic lines with additional copies of the complete *IGF2* locus in a dose-dependent manner (Sun et al. 1997). Combined these models demonstrate a subtle dependence of normal embryonic growth in general of IGF2 activity, but a clear mechanistic role for IGF2 in kidney development or Wilms' tumor development has not been demonstrated yet.

An important factor in the understanding of WTs from a developmental point of view is the need for proper classification of subsets of Wilms' tumors. Different subtypes are likely to develop through different mechanisms with potentially different cells of origin and different genetics. Two clear subtypes can been distinguished based on the type of nephrogenic rests they associate with and potentially originate from. Intralobar nephrogenic rests (ILNR) are found within the renal lobe and are usually found with *WT1* mutant WTs, whereas perilobar nephrogenic rests (PLNR) are found in the periphery of the lobe and is usually found in conjunction with overgrowth syndromes like BWS (Beckwith 1998). Genome-wide expression analysis can clearly distinguish the *WT1*-mutant from *WT1* wild-type subgroups and confirms the importance of β-catenin activation in the former (Li 2004). *IGF2* loss-of-imprinting tumors (the PLNR type) have been suggested to arise from a later stage of renal development than *WT1*-mutant (ILNR) tumors (Ravenel et al. 2001). Myogenesis has mainly been found in the *WT1* mutant subset (Miyagawa 1998). Combined the data suggests that ILNR-associated WTs arise through loss of

WT1 function, with subsequent oncogenic activation of β-catenin from an early cell type that still has maximal plasticity to form different cell and tissue types (even transdifferentiation of the target cell into a cell type with increased plasticity can at present not be excluded). A recent publication describing five new *WT1*-mutant WT cell lines even suggested a mesenchymal stem cells/paraxial mesodermal origin of these tumors, which would, if correct, take this possibility even further (Royer-Pokora 2010). The PLNR-associated subset arises from a (slightly) later developmental stage due to deregulation of the IGF2 pathway. This later developmental origin could be the reason why these *WT1* wild-type tumors appear to show an even increased expression level of the WT1 protein; it might simply reflect the higher normal expression of endogenous *WT1* in these later stages. The same could be argued to increased β-catenin levels in the absence of activating mutation.

Does the present knowledge of normal kidney development and how disturbance of this results in WT formation provides sufficient leads for hypothesis-driven therapy design? The answer so far is maybe. Key players in kidney development and WT formation, such as IGFR, RET, and HGF/c-MET, are current clinical targets being tested in WT patients, and agents targeting the Wnt-beta-catenin pathway are the subject of vigorous pharmaceutical industry attention. Further understanding of Wilms' tumorigenesis is necessary, however, not just for new target identification, but also to increase the possibility of introducing rationale differentiation therapy. To that end, the biggest remaining question is the exact cell of origin of different subtypes of WTs. Microarray analysis has previously suggested that the blastemal cells in WT appear arrested in the earliest committed stage after the mesenchymal to epithelial transition (Li 2002), but it is not clear how far this dataset represents different subtypes of tumors. In vitro RNAi in kidney organ culture has shown that *WT1* is responsible for induction of this MET (Davies 2004) providing some rationale for its role in WT development. Much larger tumor expression datasets combined with a thorough histological and genetic analysis will be needed to provide more clarity, but even then this is not guaranteed to identify the tumor-initiating cell type(s). In rapidly developing tissues like the kidney, it is not unreasonable to suggest that between the moment of the tumor-initiating genetic event(s) and the disruption leading to tumor formation, one or more developmental steps (with present knowledge recognizable or not) have been taken. This will never be elucidated in patient material representing the final tumor, and for obvious reason the earliest events in WT formation will never be accessible in patients. Therefore well-defined animal models for WTs will be essential to fully understand the origin and development of WTs. An ENU mutagenesis rat model for WT is available (Sharma et al. 1994), but it is not clear in how far the genetics of this provide an accurate enough model to understand WT formation from a renal developmental perspective (Ehrlich 2010). For the purpose of testing therapies, any model might be better than no model, but this is a different question and purpose. Genetically modified mouse models for WTs will likely be the only way of obtaining a defined, reproducible, and predictable model that will allow the study of the earliest steps of different subsets of WTs and provide the basis for rational drug candidates. With the exception of a single mouse chimeric for a *WT1* Denys-Drash mutation (Patek 1999), no such model has been reported. It is clear that the lack of WTs (Hu et al. 2011) in the existing models for *WT1*, *β-catenin*, and *IGF2* means it will not be easy to develop these models. It is hoped that the development of conditional mouse models for *Wt1* (Martinez-Estrada 2010), *β-catenin* (Harada 1999), and other genes implicated in WT development, separate or combined, will help in the development of these models. Obviously, not knowing the identity of the WT initiating cell(s) will still complicate the use of these mice, but at least these conditional models might provide an experimental tool to identify these cells. Once proper mouse models for the different subsets of WTs are established, they will allow the analysis of the earliest steps of WT development from a normal developing kidney. Alternatively, nonmammalian animal models like the zebra fish might provide additional in vivo models to study the role of known genetic players in WT development in the context of the developing kidney (Perner et al. 2007; White et al. 2009) and provide new clues for rational drug design.

10.3 Wilms' Tumor Cell Line and Primary Tumor Tissue Study

A major limiting factor in the study of WT biology is the fact that established primary WT cell lines have largely been unstable, monophasic (representative of only one part of the original heterogeneous cancer), or incorrectly characterized. The T3/73 and WTCL-1–WTCL-4 cell lines, as well as additional cell lines established from human WTs, demonstrate limited life-span or the requirement for specialized media for successful passage (Kumar et al. 1987; Zumkeller et al. 1993; Qing et al. 1996; Schmitt et al. 1997; Brown et al. 1989). Purported WT cell lines including HFWT, WitP3, and a group of cell lines recently established from *WT1* mutated WTs each appear to represent stromal components of WT only (Ishiwata et al. 1991; Hueber et al. 2009; Royer-Pokora et al. 2010). The SKNEP1 cell line, initially purported to be a derivative anaplastic WT cell line, has now been confirmed to represent a Ewing sarcoma (Smith et al. 2008). Similarly, the G401 cell line represents a rhabdoid tumor (Garvin et al. 1993). The WCC-1 cell line is reportedly derived from a "sarcomatoid" WT model (Talts et al. 1993).

The WiT49 anaplastic WT cell line, established at The Hospital for Sick Children in Toronto, has been recently used by laboratories and thus far has proven to be a useful sustainable line (Alami et al. 2003a). Using WiT49, it has been shown that (1) WT demonstrates and may depend upon autocrine c-Met/HGF signaling as a proliferative signal (Stanhope-Baker et al. 2004), (2) activated beta-catenin signaling with evidence of high levels of beta-catenin co-localized to membranous c-Met, constitutive activation of MMP9 and latent MMP2, and only weak expression of Wnt5A (Alami et al. 2003b), (3) opposing regulation of podocalyxin (an antagonist of cellular adhesion) by WT1 and p53, via interaction with ezrin Stanhope-Baker et al. 2004), (4) apoptosis induced by downregulation of C/EBPB via siRNA (Piva et al. 2006; Li et al. 2005), (5) a pro-survival role for STAT1 in WT (Timofeeva et al. 2006), and (6) a role for sphingosine-1-phosphate in Wilms' tumor cell migration and invasion, as well as proliferation via induction of connective tissue growth factor (Li et al. 2008, 2009). An orthotopic model derived from theWiT49 cell line has been characterized demonstrating biphasic expression of stromal and epithelial components (Li et al. 2010).

Despite limitations inherent with a historic lack of primary WT cell lines, studies of primary WT tissues have provided many insights. Specifically, published data suggest the importance of IGFR signaling, Wnt-beta-catenin-driven transcription, the VEGFR and EGFR pathways, c-Met/HGF signaling, the apoptotic pathway, sphingosine metabolism, telomerase function, epigenetic control, and cell cycle machinery in WT pathophysiology.

10.3.1 IGFR Signaling

IGF2, the current target of numerous current molecular therapeutic agents in early phase clinical cancer trials is a well characterized fetal mitogen implicated in the pathogenesis of WT. IGF signaling can provide an antiapoptotic signal, promote tumorigenesis, and mediate proliferation (Werner et al. 1993; Kurmasheva and Houghton 2006; Reidemann and Macaulay 2006). The precise role of IGF2 in Wilms' tumorigenesis, as previously discussed, has not been absolutely clearly identified. Nonetheless, IGF2 LOI and IGF2 LOH are reported to occur in 25–40 % and 35 % of sporadic WT, respectively (Ravenel et al. 2001; Pritchard-Jones and Vujanic 2006; Grundy et al. 1994). IGF2 dosage can also increase via aberrant imprinting of the *IGFR2* receptor (Xu et al. 1997). Both *IGF2* and *IGFR1* are subject to WT1-mediated transcriptional repression, and similar to IGF2, IGFR1 is increased in WT at the RNA and protein levels (Drummond et al. 1992; Gansler et al. 1988; Werner et al. 1993). Gain in IGFR1 gene copy number has been found in WT associated with 15q gain and with relapse (Natrajan et al. 2006, 2007a). Lastly, autocrine IGF2/IGFR1 signaling has been demonstrated in WT (Qing et al. 1996; Schmitt et al. 1997). Thus, in part due to the purported although incompletely understood role of IGF2/IGFR1 signaling in the kidney and WT development and in part due to genetic and epigenetic dysregulation and autocrine signaling leading to increased IGF2 function in WT, IGF2/IGFR1 has emerged as an important pathway for molecular targeting in WT, either alone or in various combinations of additional targeted agents. The downstream dependence on mTOR and the interplay between IGF signaling and both beta-catenin signaling and EGFR pathway function, as well as the Ras/Raf cascade, present opportunities for combination therapy strategies (Desbois-Mouthon et al. 2001).

As of May 2010, the Children's Oncology Group has completed a Phase I study of IMCA12, a monoclonal antibody targeting IGFR, in pediatric patients with relapsed/refractory solid tumors. Additionally, the initial WT strata (ten WT patients) has completed enrollment on the COG IMCA12 Phase II study, but efficacy results are not yet available. A Phase I study of IMCA12 plus the mTOR inhibitor temsirolimus is currently being completed, with preliminary plans for formal Phase II testing of this combination in pediatric solid tumor patients, with a planned WT strata. Several other IGFR monoclonal antibodies as well as small molecule inhibitors of IGFR are in preclinical and clinical development.

10.3.2 Wnt-Beta-Catenin Signaling

Similar to IGF2, the Wnt-Beta-catenin signaling pathway plays an important role in the kidney and likely WT development; it is activated in WT via various mechanisms, and it is the subject of broader anticancer therapy developmental interest. Transcription driven by activated beta-catenin regulates survival/apoptosis, differentiation, proliferation, and motility, all key elements of the malignant phenotype. The role of Wnt-4 in the mesenchymal to epithelial transition and finding of *beta-catenin* or *WTX* mutations in WT has been previously discussed. In sum, between the two mutations, at least 45 % of sporadic WT have overactive beta-catenin signaling. In addition, the gene encoding the APC protein, a known binding partner that targets beta-catenin for proteosomal degradation, has been found to demonstrate either microsatellite instability or LOH in 16 % and 30 % of WT tested, respectively [86]. It is not surprising then that an overwhelming majority of WT demonstrated beta-catenin expression in various subcellular localizations and in various Wilms' tumor histological compartments. Such wide expression prohibits the easy use of such expression as a prognostic marker; however, nuclear beta-catenin expression has been found to be specifically increased in metastatic WT and in WT associated with *beta-catenin* mutations (Alami et al. 2003b; Koesters et al. 2003).

Recently, using a cDNA microarray platform comparing *beta-catenin* mutated WT vs. non-mutated WT, genes *PITX2*, *APCDD1*, and the endothelin proteins *EDN3* and *EDNRA* were shown to be activated by beta-catenin in WT, in addition to upstream Wnt signaling inhibitors such as *WIF1* and *PRDC*. Not surprisingly, muscle-related genes were highly upregulated in *beta-catenin* mutated tumors, consistent with the frequent myogenic changes found histologically in such tumors (Zirn et al. 2006). While such differential gene expressions were attributed to *beta-catenin* mutation status, additional genome wide expression profiling of WT have demonstrated Wnt activation in both *WT1/beta-catenin* mutated as well as non-mutated tumors, with additional Wnt pathway genes (*BCL9*, *CTNNBIP1*, and *CBY1*) participating in Wnt activation (Corbin et al. 2009).

The development of robust Wnt-beta-catenin pathway inhibitors continues (Barker and Clevers 2006; Takahashi-Yanaga and Sasaguri 2007; Herbst and Koligs 2007; Shan et al. 2005; Emami et al. 2004; Eguchi et al. 2005; Ma et al. 2005), with more recent focus attempting to target distal effects at the level of beta-catenin-Tcf (Lepourcelet et al. 2004; Dehnhardt et al. 2010). Other recognizable compounds proposed to be beta-catenin pathway inhibitors include lithium, flavonoids, quercetin, ethacrynic acid, omega-3 polyunsaturated fatty acids, and curcumin (Takahashi-Yanaga and Sasaguri 2007; Ohori et al. 2006; Suh et al. 2009; Shan et al. 2009; Lu et al. 2009; Lim et al. 2009). Interestingly, curcumin has been shown to downregulate WT1 expression in various cancer models including solid tumors (Glienke et al. 2009).

Wnt-beta-catenin signaling also networks with many other pathways, including the EGF and PDGF pathways (Takahashi-Yanaga and Sasaguri 2007), as well as those pathways important for stem cell and progenitor cell homeostasis such as the Hedgehog, Notch, BMP, and FGF pathways (Katoh 2007). Additionally, beta-catenin downstream effectors include VEGF, COX-2, survivin, and cyclin D1, all current potential targets for molecular inhibition. To that end, recent reports demonstrate ubiquitous expression of COX-2 in all cases of WT and in WT neovasculature, independent of histology or compartment (Giordano et al. 2008). Similarly, sonic hedgehog (Shh) and its receptor patched (Ptch) are expressed in 71 and 100 % of WT, respectively (Giordano et al. 2008; Oue et al. 2010). Targeting the Wnt-beta-catenin pathway thus awaits the development of a testable agent, with potential therapeutic combinations easily imagined. Specific targeting of EGFR, VEGF, and cell cycle machinery is discussed elsewhere in this chapter.

10.3.3 VEGF and Angiogenesis

Vascular endothelial growth factor (VEGF) inhibitors are now available for clinical use. FDA-approved agents for the treatment of adult kidney cancer (renal cell carcinoma) include the monoclonal anti-VEGF antibody bevacizumab (Avastin) and the VEGF receptor tyrosine kinase inhibitors sorafenib (Nexavar), sunitinib (Sutent), and pazopanib (Votrient). VEGF, induced by HIF-1α among other stimuli, functions as an endothelial mitogen, and inhibition of which imparts an anti-angiogenic effect. VEGF signaling has additional biological consequences directly within cancer cells as well. All WT express both VEGF and HIF-1α, with at least one study demonstrating equivalent distribution of VEGF expression between epithelial and blastemal components (Karth et al. 2000) and other studies showing differential preference of various VEGF isoforms in the various WT compartments (Ghanem et al. 2003; Nowicki et al. 2007). Of potential clinical importance is that blastema may lack VEGFR-2 [111], as some of the anti-VEGF-targeted agents are VEGF receptor specific. Additional preclinical WT investigation has demonstrated elevated levels of bFGF in the urine and VEGF in the sera of WT patients, each correlating with tumor stage, decreasing following surgery, and increasing postoperatively in the setting of relapse or persistent disease (Lin et al. 1995; Blann et al. 2001; Skoldenberg et al. 2001). A worse prognosis has also been linked to increasing WT microvessel density, a marker of tumor vascularity (Ozluk et al. 2006). Preclinical data interrogating anti-VEGF therapies in WT are now available, as are anecdotal reports of WT patient response (Fig. 10.1). Importantly, some VEGF receptor tyrosine kinase inhibitors also target c-RET, important in early kidney embryogenesis and possibly WT tumori-

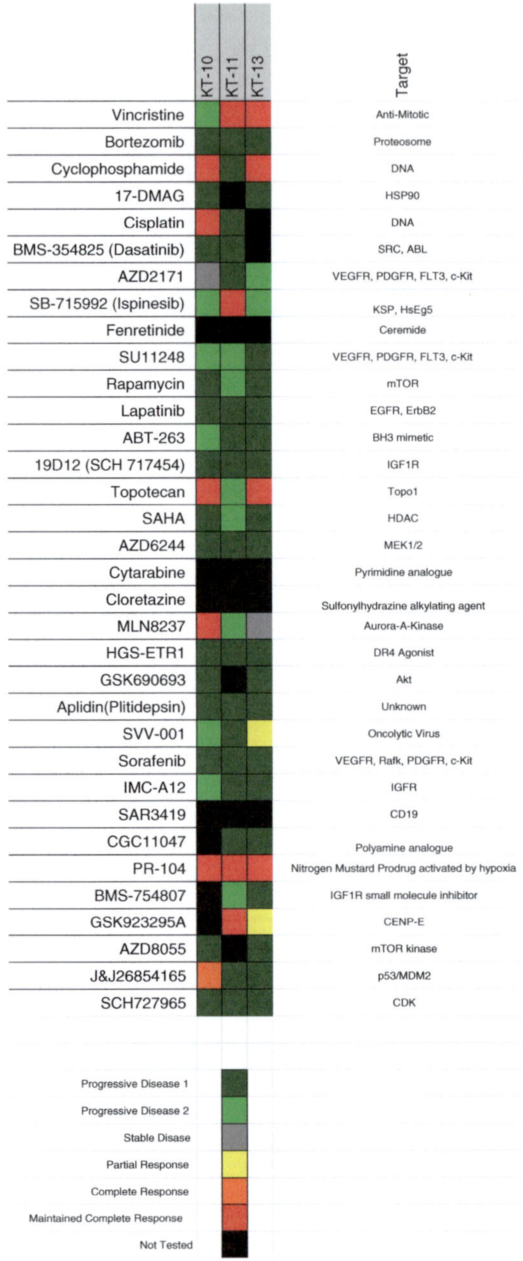

Fig. 10.1 In vivo activity data of agents tested through the PPTP (Heat Map courtesy of Drs. Peter Houghton and Malcolm Smith)

genesis. Safety data using such agents in pediatric patients is also now available. Therefore, the clinical development of anti-VEGF strategies for the treatment of pediatric high-risk renal tumors is of intense current interest.

10.3.4 EGFR Pathway

Similar to VEGF, EGFR inhibitors are currently available, FDA approved, with safety data available in pediatric solid tumor patients (gefitinib (Tarceva), erlotinib (Iressa)), and early anecdotal reports of activity in the form of disease stabilization reported in several WT patients (Daw et al. 2005). There exist limited ex vivo data available, however. EGFR is a transcriptional target of WT1, though patients with germline *WT1* mutations and Denys-Drash syndrome do not demonstrate perturbed EGFR signaling (Liu et al. 2000; Englert et al. 1995; Vicanek et al. 1997). EGFR expression is present in the various WT histological compartments, most consistently in the epithelial compartment >blastemal compartment >stromal compartment (Ghanem et al. 2001; Salem et al. 2006). EGFR expression in WT is not associated with ERBB2 gene overexpression or amplification (Vasei et al. 2009). Preclinically, anti-EGFR monoclonal antibodies demonstrate in vivo activity against WT xenografts (Pinthus et al. 2004; Yokoi et al. 2003).

10.3.5 c-Met/HGF Pathway

The HGF/c-Met pathway is involved with cell migration, differentiation, and growth, as well as with apoptosis inhibition, angiogenesis, and increased metastases (Christensen et al. 2005; Sattler and Salgia 2007). HGF/c-Met activation also leads to c-Met/beta-catenin disassociation, effectively increasing free intracellular beta-catenin (Rasola et al. 2007). Analogous to IGF and Wnt/beta-catenin signaling, HGF/cMet signaling interfaces with roles in both kidney organogenesis and oncogenesis (Vuononvirta et al. 2009). While one group of investigators have found that hepatocyte growth factor and c-Met co-localize in WT, associated with increased proliferation (Alami et al. 2002), this was not confirmed by Vuononvirta et al. who found that HGF/c-Met expression was largely linked to kidney embryogenesis and nephrogenic rests, as well as with differentiation as noted by epithelial and stromal preferential expression with only rare expression in transformed WT blastema. Using different HGF and c-Met antibodies for their studies, they could also not confirm any association between HGF/c-Met expression and increased proliferation [128]. Such findings are somewhat counterintuitive, however, as c-Met/HGF expression has been linked to more aggressive phenotypes in many other cancers. In addition, neither investigation interrogated phospho-c-Met status or downstream c-Met effectors, critically important in assessing cancer c-Met activation status. Currently, c-MET inhibitors are available for pediatric cancer patients in early phase clinical trials. Crizotinib (PF02341066) is completing initial Phase I testing in children, and tivantinib (ARQ197) Phase I testing is to begin shortly.

10.3.6 The Apoptotic Pathway and Sphingosine Metabolism

Reports assessing the prognostic impact of various apoptosis activators (Fas, caspase 8, Bid, Bak) and inhibitors (Bcl-2, survivin, Bcl-X(L/S)) in WT have had conflicting results (Alami et al. 2002; Miller et al. 2005; Fukuzawa et al. 2004; Morrison et al. 2005; Re et al. 1999; Tanaka et al. 1999). Bcl-2, the current target of several pharmaceutical agents aiming to reduce chemotherapy resistance, interestingly is under WT1-mediated transcriptional control and thus possibly involved in WT tumorigenesis (Wunsch et al. 2001). It is therefore not surprising to find notable Bcl-2 expression in nephrogenic rests. Survivin mRNA, a second IAP member subject to pharmaceutical inhibition, has been shown to be increased in WT compared with adjacent normal kidney, with one report suggesting that survivin Fas ratios demonstrate a positive and negative predictive value for WT recurrence of 85.7 and 71.4 %, respectively (Takamizawa et al. 2001). In addition to Bcl-2 and survivin, well-described WT-associated pathway perturbations such as IGF signaling (antiapoptotic) (Werner et al. 1993; Reidemann and Macaulay 2006), p53 mutation (typical of anaplastic histology WT) (Bardeesy et al. 1995), and MYCN oncogene overexpression (with resultant caspase-8 silencing via promoter methylation) have established interplay with the apoptotic program (Shaw et al. 1988; Morris et al. 2003). In addition, WT commonly express DR5, a receptor for both TNF-related apoptosis-inducing ligand (TRAIL) and pharmaceutical TRAIL agonist therapies (Alami et al. 2002).

A related and evolving field of anticancer therapeutics pertains to sphingosine metabolism. In addition to cross talk with the apoptotic program, sphingosine-1-phosphate may regulate steps critical to tumor cell proliferation, migration, and invasion. SIP1 was expressed in all 10 WT tested, particularly in the tumor associated vascular endothelial cells, and in the blastemal and epithelial tumor components. Further, SIP1 induces WiT49 cellular migration and invasion at low nanomolar concentrations, in a Gi protein, PI3kinase, and Rac1 dependent manner (Li et al. 2008, 2009).

10.3.7 Telomerase Function, Cell Cycle Machinery, and Epigenetic Mechanisms

Human telomerase is a riboprotein reverse transcriptase, present in tumor cells but largely absent in normal somatic cells, that functions to maintain telomere integrity and permit cellular immortalization (Diniz et al. 2011; Dome et al. 1999, 2005; Oh et al. 1999; Yashima et al. 1998). Early studies demonstrated that the RNA component of telomerase (hTR) is maximally expressed in immature epithelial components of WT, followed by poorly differentiated blastema. Expression of hTR in immature stroma is weak or absent and completely absent in mature kidney tubules, glomeruli, stroma, and heterologous elements present in treated WTs (Yashima et al. 1998). In 293 kidney cells and in clear cell renal cell carcinomas, WT1 can repress *hTERT* promoter and telomerase enzyme activities (the gene that encodes the catalytic component of human telomerase reverse transcriptase) (Oh et al. 1999; Sitaram et al. 2010). In addition, several case-cohort studies have now demonstrated high hTERT mRNA and protein correlating with either relapse or a worse overall prognosis in WT (Diniz et al. 2011; Dome et al. 1999). The largest case-cohort study of 291 NWTS-5 patients confirmed increased risk of relapse for WT patients maintaining tumor-specific high expression of either hTERT or hTR, but such expression was not predictive of overall survival (Dome et al. 2005). The Children's Oncology Group has just begun a pediatric Phase I study of imetelstat, a telomerase inhibitor supplied by Geron Corporation.

As telomerase permits cellular immortalization, cellular division is inescapably linked with cell cycle progression. Overexpression of cyclin/cdk complexes can abrograte WT1-mediated, possibly p21-dependent induction of G1 arrest (Kudoh et al. 1995; Englert et al. 1997). P16 expression itself is suppressed either via promoter methylation or alternative genetic or epigenetic events in WT (Arcellana-Panlilio et al. 2000; Natrajan et al. 2007b). Beta-catenin activation also readily induces increased cyclin D1 expression. In sum, *WT1* mutation, p16 silencing, and activated beta-catenin signaling all can lead to uninhibited cyclin/cdk activity, permitting rapid cell cycle transition and cellular proliferation. Importantly, CDK4, a pharmaceutically targetable CDK, has been preliminarily linked with relapse in WT (Faussillon et al. 2005). These data support the study of cell cycle inhibitors in WT.

In addition to p16, epigenetic methylation of genetic loci amenable to demethylation via clinically available demethylating agents includes caspase-8 (methylated in 43 % of WT) and O-6 methylguanine DNA methyl transferase (MGMT, methylated in 30 % of WT) (Morris et al. 2003). MGMT-mediated alkylator resistance can be targeted with currently available molecular therapy such as O-6 benzylguanine. Despite such examples of hypermethylation, 60 % of WT actually demonstrate global hypomethylation (Ehrlich et al. 2002, 2003), and thus, the net effect of demethylating agents on WT is challenging to predict.

10.4 Wilms' Tumor Xenograft Testing

In vivo agent testing in WT xenografts were somewhat limited prior to the development of the Pediatric Preclinical Testing Program (PPTP, Houghton et al. 2007). In 1989, Gansler et al.

demonstrated statistically significant response in two favorable histology WTs and one anaplastic WT when treated with a human anti-IGFR1 antibody (αIR-3) (Gansler et al. 1989). Similarly, Pinthus et al. and Yokoi et al. demonstrated in vivo WT growth suppression with N29 anti-erb2 monoclonal antibody and anti-her2/neu monoclonal antibody, respectively (Pinthus et al. 2004; Yokoi et al. 2003). Halofuginone, a collagen type I synthesis inhibitor, decreased angiogenesis in WT xenograft models, accompanied by a reduction of collagen synthesis, reduced hepatocyte growth factor, and increased WT1 levels (Pinthus et al. 2005).

The overwhelming majority of preclinical in vivo new agent testing in WT xenograft models has come out of the laboratory of Dr. Peter Houghton, either via individual laboratory testing or though the PPTP. Outside the auspices of the PPTP, depsipeptide, ABT-751, and ixabepilone demonstrated response in WT models (Peterson et al. 2005; Graham et al. 2006; Morton et al. 2007). The histone deacetylase inhibitor depsipeptide induced tumor regression and tumor stabilization in 1 WT model each, accounting for 2 of the 7 sensitive models out of a total 39 pediatric solid tumor cancer models tested (Graham et al. 2006). The novel antimitotic ABT-751 (binds tubulin at the colchicine binding site) demonstrated tumor regression in 1/6 WT models (Morton et al. 2007). Ixabepilone induced WT regressions in 5/6 WT models at 10 mg/kg (mouse MTD) and 1/5 models at 4.4 mg/kg given every fourth day, revealing a steep dose response curve. Pharmacokinetic correlative studies showed that a dose of 10 mg/kg provided an AUC/dose of 5.8 μmol/l-h, approximating that achieved in adult patients receiving 40 mg/m^2/dose (Peterson et al. 2005).

The PPTP is an initiative supported by the National Cancer Institute to help identify novel therapeutic agents that may have activity against childhood cancers. The PPTP panel includes two favorable histology WT (KT-10 and KT-11) and one anaplastic WT (KT-13). Such models have undergone microarray characterization to supplement in vivo activity with scientific insight, and all experiments are designed in as controlled a fashion as possible (Houghton et al. 2007). At the time of drafting this chapter, data is available for 34 tested compounds. The agents, target, and activities are summarized in Fig. 10.1. Robust responses have been seen with conventional cytotoxic agents as well as with camptothecin exposure. Importantly, the anaplastic WT model demonstrated partial responses to CENP-E (a centromere-targeting agent) as well as SVV-001 (an oncolytic therapy that typically is tropic for neuroendocrine tumors). The favorable histology WTs experienced some growth delay from anti-VEGF treatment and more notable responses with many antimitotic agents. Several caveats worth mentioning are 1. the PPTP and xenograft testing at large is research; 2. subcutaneous models, as utilized by the PPTP for WT testing, may not be ideal for antiangiogenic testing where tumor microenvironment may be a key factor in modulating response; and 3. all three WT models tested for anti-IGFR1 sensitivity lack IGFR1 expression, revealing limitations of such models, and the power of model characterization.

10.5 Early Phase Wilms' Tumor Clinical Trials

Several agents that inhibit targets discussed thus far have either accrued pediatric WT patients to early phase clinical trials, have clinical trials currently open, or are the subject of future planned early phase clinical study. For example, two WT patients were treated on the Phase I study of depsipeptide, and like all other patients on study, neither responded (Fouladi et al. 2006). Phase I study of gefitinib, a small molecule EGFR inhibitor, included 2 WT patients and each achieved disease stabilization for 8 to >60 weeks (Daw et al. 2005). At least one WT patient treated on the Phase I study of sorafenib demonstrated short-term imaging response (James Geller, 2014). An ixabepilone Phase II study (drug administered at 8 mg/m^2/day for 5 days) accrued 10 WT patient, with one achieving stable disease lasting 38 cycles (114 weeks) (Jacobs et al. 2010). Importantly, as mentioned previously, in vivo modeling suggested a steep dose response curve with improved response demonstrated when exposures correlate to that expected from 40 mg/m^2/dose (the alternative ixabepilone regimen in clinical use). Thus, it is possible that the COG Phase II study underestimates the possible efficacy of ixabepilone in WT patients if given on a different schedule. More recently, Phase II study of the IGFR monoclonal antibody inhibitor, IMCA12, completed a ten-patient WT strata. Data have not yet been released. Currently, a Phase I study of SVV-001 is open to accrual and includes WT as an eligible diagnosis, and an open accruing Phase II study of the aurora-A-kinase inhibitor, MLN8237, includes a WT strata, open at participating COG centers. Planned Phase II studies of WT patients to be conducted through the COG includes the combination of IMCA12 and temsirolimus (IGFR plus mTOR inhibition), as well as sorafenib.

10.6 Other Pediatric Renal Tumors

Recent investigations have provided new molecular insights into the pathogenesis of both rhabdoid tumors and pediatric renal cell carcinomas, unveiling sorely needed rationale therapeutic targets. In the case of rhabdoid tumor, the biology of *SMARCB1/INI1/Baf47*, mutated in all rhabdoid tumors and part of the SWISNF complex incorporating histone deacetylase function, has pointed to epigenetic phenomena as critical for rhabdoid tumor behavior (Gadd et al. 2010; Roberts and Bigel 2009; McKenna et al. 2008). Additional preclinical investigation of histone deacetylase inhibitors and methylation inhibitors (including new specific histone methylation inhibitors) is currently underway in several laboratories. Data also support the role of cyclin D as well as aurora-A-kinase in rhabdoid tumor pathogenesis (Smith et al. 2011; Lee et al. 2011). Importantly, the PPTP includes rhabdoid tumor models, with evidence of in vivo activity against rhabdoid tumors demonstrated for VEGF RTKs and aurora-A-kinase inhibition (Keir et al. 2010; Maris et al. 2008a, b, 2010). In turn, the COG Phase II study of MLN8237 is being amended to include a "rhabdoid" strata, inclusive of rhabdoid tumor of the kidney, non-CNS nonrenal malignant rhabdoid tumors, and CNS atypical teratoid rhabdoid tumors, representing the first salvage Phase II study for rhabdoid tumors available through a cooperative group mechanism.

Unlike rhabdoid tumors which are all hypothesized to be driven by a common mutation and common biology, pediatric renal cell carcinoma is a heterogenous group of cancers. Recent study has demonstrated that approximately 50 % of such cancers harbor enhanced TFE function, however, typically through translocations involving TFE3 with various fusion partners (Geller et al. 2008). TFE3 demonstrates functional overlap with MITF, and thus translocation renal cell carcinomas share biology with other microphthalmia-associated transcription factor (MITF)-associated cancers such as alveolar soft part sarcoma and clear cell sarcoma of soft parts (Rehli et al. 1999). Binding of TFE3 and MITF to the c-MET promoter, with increased c-MET signaling attenuated by c-MET inhibition, has prompted the recent Phase II study of the c-MET inhibitor ARQ197 (tivantinib) in this group of cancers (Tsuda et al. 2007). The limited number of TFE RCCs enrolled on study did not produce objective responses, however (Goldberg et al. 2009). Anecdotal evidence of response of TFE RCCs to VEGF RTKIs is growing (Malouf et al. 2010; Choueiri et al. 2010), and additional preclinical investigation of the defined TFE-associated translocations holds promise to reveal additional targets for clinical study.

10.7 Future Challenges

New agent development for WT and other pediatric renal cancers faces challenges beyond the typical "correct target, functional drug, and appropriate patient." Firstly, target identification has been hampered by an historic lack of validated WT cell culture systems available to investigators. Once targets are identified, solicitation of pharmaceutical industry support, acquisition of necessary preclinical data, engagement of appropriate clinical pathways for trial implementation, and patient enrollment each present obstacles. To overcome some of these barriers, the COG Renal Tumor Committee has developed collaborations with the PPTP and COG Developmental Therapeutics Committee (DVL) in order to facilitate preclinical testing of targets of interest and early clinical development of appropriate agents in WT models and patients, respectively. For Phase III study of new agents in WT, cooperative international trials including both COG and SIOP will likely be necessary to secure appropriate patient numbers.

Limitations notwithstanding, improved WT models, and the mysteries of WT biology continue to be explored. Hopefully, in addition to ongoing research in laboratories worldwide, with the advancement of the NIH sponsored TARGET initiative (Therapeutically Applicable Research to Generate Effective Treatments) for high-risk WT, applying array-based methods and next generation sequencing, recurrent targetable WT mutations, translocations, and/or high frequency copy number gains and losses will become more readily apparent in relapsed and anaplastic WT (protocol AREN03B2). WT profiling holds additional promise to improve prognostication and stratification as well as contribute to expanding our understanding of relevant signaling pathways in various WT subtypes. Trials are now being designed to include appropriate pharmacodynamics and correlative studies, and access for WT patients is available in some countries. As a final step, through international collaboration incorporating the study of molecularly targeted agents, children with WT may soon realize maximized cure with minimal short- and long-term toxicity.

10.8 Latest Updates

Since initial draft of this chapter, several notable reports have become available. With respect to the developmental aspects of WT, a large expression analysis study of 224 tumors identified 5 subgroups of tumors with apparent different developmental stages of origin (Gadd et al. 2012). The *WT1/CTNNB1* mutant subgroup was still the best recognizable group and is believed to have the earliest stage of origin. WT1 itself was shown to be directly involved in the mesenchymal to epithelial transition by directly activating the expression of *WNT4* (Essafi et al. 2011). A marker signature for WT cancer stem cells was identified as NCAM^{+}/ALDH1^{+}, and targeting of these cells in nude mice was found to be efficient (Pode-Shakked et al. 2013). Much progress was made on the generation of WT mouse models, with the publication of the first WT model through a combination of *Wt1* loss and *Igf2* activation (Hu et al. 2011) and, more serendipitous, in an overexpression model of Lin28, subsequently also found overexpressed in a significant number of human tumors (Urbach et al. 2014). Finally, a *Wtx* knockout model was described (Moisan et al. 2011), but its phenotype in the developing kidney was not conclusive nor informative for its role in WT.

The phase 2 trial of IMCA12 (IGFR inhibitor) in 10 WT patients unfortunately did not generate objective clinical responses, and allotment of a WT stratum to the IMCA12+temsirolimus trial was not advanced (Weigel et al. 2014). Further investigation into various mechanisms of IGF-pathway perturbation in WT as well as various mechanisms to modify IGF-pathway signaling still seems warranted given the preponderance of pre-clinical data and inherent limitations of this small 10-patient specific inhibitor study. The phase 2 trial of MLN8237 (aurora-A-kinase inhibitor) enrolled 10 WT patients with one complete response noted. The MLN8237 study was also amended to include rhabdoid tumor patients, though only 4 enrolled (0 responses) (MLN8237: ADVL0921 Spring 2014 study progress report). The sorafenib phase 2 trial enrolled 10 WT patients and while 2 patients maintained stable disease for 6 and 8 cycles, respectively, no RECIST-based imaging responses were noted (Sorafenib: ADVL1121 Spring 2014 study progress report). The CDK4/6 inhibitor, LEE011, is in phase I investigation in pediatric patients with perturbed RB/CyclinD1/CDK4/6 pathway signaling, with specific focus on rhabdoid tumor (NCT01747876). Lastly, the COG Renal Tumor Committee has recently endorsed formal study of the dual c-Met/VEGF multityrosine kinase inhibitor, cabozantinib, for formal Phase 2 study in WT patients.

Additional ongoing Phase I trials of interest to pediatric renal tumors conducted through the COG, with pre-clinical rationale as demonstrated through the PPTP or alternative *in vivo* WT and/or rhabdoid tumor xenograft studies, include studies ADVL1211 (cabozantinib – RP2D defined at 40 mg/m^2), (Cabozantinib: ADVL1211 Spring 2014 study progress report; Smith et al. 2013a) ADVL1011 (ruxolitinib (inhibitor of Jak) – RP2D defined at 50 mg/m^2 BID), (Ruxolitinib: ADVL1011 Spring 2014 study progress report; Houghton et al. 2014) ADVL1312 (MK1775 (wee1 inhibitor) in combination with irinotecan), and ADVL1411 (BMN673 (poly-(ADP-ribose) polymerase (PARP)) inhibitor in combination with temozolomide) (Smith et al. 2014). Upcoming Phase I trials of interest to pediatric renal tumors include ADVL1314 (eribulin – antimitotic) (Kolb et al. 2013), ADVL1315 (axitinib – second generation VEGF multi-tyrosine kinase inhibitor, with a planned Phase 2 trial in translocation renal cell carcinoma via a collaboration between COG and ECOG in development), and ADVL1412 (nivolumab – anti-PD1 immune checkpoint).

Pre-clinically, in addition to robust *in vivo* activity (complete responses) now demonstrated with ruxolitinib, eribulin and the combination of BMN673 with temozolomide (Ruxolitinib: ADVL1011 Spring 2014 study progress report; Houghton et al. 2014; Smith et al. 2014), lorvotuzumab (IMGN901), an antibody-drug conjugate fusing the CD56 target with a maytansinoid antimitotic, resulted in complete responses in both WT models tested (Wood et al. 2013). Additionally, RG7112, an MDM2 inhibitor, demonstrated complete responses in both WT and rhabdoid models (Carol et al. 2013), and a novel selective inhibitor of nuclear export (XPO1/CRM1 inhibitor KPT-330) induced a maintained remission in the KT-10 WT model (Houghton et al. 2013a). A novel histone deacetylase inhibitor, quisinostat (JNJ-26481585), resulted in growth delay of the anaplastic WT PPTP model and no effect in the single rhabdoid model tested *in vivo* (Carol et al. 2014). Agents considered to have a more conventional mechanism of action demonstrating interesting results include the topoisomerase II inhibitor, pixantrone, with potential less risk of inducing cardiomyopathy and demonstrating a complete response in one of two WT xenografts tested, and temozolomide, demonstrating a complete response in a WT model (Kurmasheva et al. 2014; Keir et al. 2013). More recently, a novel purine analog, NSC750854, demonstrated robust activity against both WT and rhabdoid tumor xenografts (Smith et al. 2013b). Finally, the antimicrotubule agent cabazitaxel seemed to demonstrate superior *in vivo* response compared with docetaxel in the KT-10 WT model, suggesting that not all taxanes may demonstrate equal clinical effect (Houghton et al. 2013b).

References

Alami J, Williams BR, Yeger H (2002) Expression and localization of HGF and met in Wilms' tumours. J Pathol 196:76–84

Alami J, Williams BR, Yeger H (2003a) Derivation and characterization of a Wilms tumor cell line, WiT 49. Int J Cancer 107:365–374

Alami J, Williams BR, Yeger H (2003b) Differential expression of E-cadherin and beta catenin in primary and metastatic Wilms tumours. Mol Pathol 56:218–225

Arcellana-Panlilio MY, Egeler RM, Ujack E, Pinto A, Demetrick DJ, Robbins SM et al (2000) Decreased expression of the INK4 family of cyclin-dependent kinase inhibitor in Wilms tumor. Genes Chromosomes Cancer 29:63–69

Bardeesy N, Beckwith B, Pelletier J (1995) Clonal expansion and attenuated apoptosis in Wilms tumors are associated with p53 gene mutations. Cancer Res 55:215–219

Barker N, Clevers H (2006) Mining the Wnt pathway for cancer therapeutics. Nat Rev Drug Discov 5:997–1014

Basson MA (2005) Sprouty1 is a critical regulator of GDNF/RET-mediated kidney induction. Dev Cell 8:229–239

Beckwith JB (1998) Nephrogenic rests and the pathogenesis of Wilms tumor: developmental and clinical considerations. Am J Med Genet 79:268–273

Birney E (2007) Identification and analysis of functional elements in 1% of the human genome by the ENCODE pilot project. Nature 447:799–816

Blann AD, Li JL, Li C, Kumar S (2001) Increased serum VEGF in 13 children with Wilms' tumour falls after surgery but rising levels predict poor prognosis. Cancer Lett 28:183–186

Brown KW, Shaw AP, Poirier V, Tyler SJ, Berry PJ, Mott MG et al (1989) Loss of chromosome 11p alleles I cultured cell derived from Wilms tumors. Br J Cancer 60:25–29

Burn SF, Webb A, Berry RL, Davies JA, Ferrer-Vaquer A, Hadjantonakis AK, Hastie ND, Hohenstein P (2011) Calcium/NFAT signalling promotes early nephrogenesis. Dev Biol 352(2):288–298. Epub 2011 Feb 3

Cabozantinib: ADVL1211 Spring 2014 Study Progress report, Children's Oncology Group

Carol H, Reynolds CP, Kang MH, Keir ST, Maris JM, Gorlick R, Kolb EA, Billups CA, Geier B, Kurmasheva RT, Houghton PJ, Smith MA, Lock RB (2013) Initial testing of the MDM2 inhibitor RG7112 by the pediatric preclinical testing program. Pediatr Blood Cancer 60(4):633–41

Carol H, Gorlick R, Kolb EA, Morton CL, Manesh DM, Keir ST, Reynolds CP, Kang MH, Maris JM, Wozniak A, Hickson I, Lyalin D, Kurmasheva RT, Houghton PJ, Smith MA, Lock R (2014) Initial testing (stage 1) of the histone deacetylase inhibitor, quisinostat (JNJ-26481585), by the pediatric preclinical testing program. Pediatr Blood Cancer 61(2):245–52

Carroll TJ, Park JS, Hayashi S, Majumdar A, McMahon AP (2005) Wnt9b plays a central role in the regulation of mesenchymal to epithelial transitions underlying organogenesis of the mammalian urogenital system. Dev Cell 9:283–292

Caspary T (1999) Oppositely imprinted genes p57(Kip2) and igf2 interact in a mouse model for Beckwith-Wiedemann syndrome. Genes Dev 13:3115–3124

Chang H (2008) Wt1 negatively regulates beta-catenin signaling during testis development. Development 135:1875–1885

Choueiri TK, Lim ZD, Hirsch MS, Tamboli P, Jonasch E, McDermott DF et al (2010) Vascular endothelial growth factor-targeted therapy for the treatment of adult metastatic Xp11.2 translocation renal cell carcinoma. Cancer 116:5219–5225

Christensen JG, Burrows J, Salgia R (2005) c-Met as a target for human cancer and characterization of inhibitors for therapeutic intervention. Cancer Lett 8:1–26

Corbin M, de Reynies A, Rickman DS, Berrebi D, Boccon-Gibod L, Cohen-Gogo S et al (2009) WNT/beta-catenin pathway activation in Wilms tumors: a unifying mechanism with multiple entries? Genes Chromosomes Cancer 48(9):816–827

Davies JA (2004) Development of an siRNA-based method for repressing specific genes in renal organ culture and its use to show that the Wt1 tumour suppressor is required for nephron differentiation. Hum Mol Genet 13:235–246

Daw NC, Furman WL, Stewart CF, Iacono LC, Krailo M, Bernstein ML et al (2005) Phase I and pharmacokinetic study of gefitinib in children with refractory solid tumors: a Children's Oncology Group Study. J Clin Oncol 23:6172–6180

Daw NC, Gregornik D, Rodman J, Marina N, Wu J, Kun LE et al (2009) Renal function after ifosfamide, carboplatin and etoposide (ICE) chemotherapy, nephrectomy and radiotherapy in children with Wilms tumour. Eur J Cancer 45:99–106

DeChiara TM, Efstratiadis A, Robertson EJ (1990) A growth-deficiency phenotype in heterozygous mice carrying an insulin-like growth factor II gene disrupted by targeting. Nature 345:78–80

DeChiara TM, Robertson EJ, Efstratiadis A (1991) Parental imprinting of the mouse insulin-like growth factor II gene. Cell 64:849–859

Dehnhardt CM, Venkatesan AM, Chen Z, Ayral-Kaloustian S, Dos Santos O, Santos ED et al (2010) Design and synthesis of novel diaminoquinazolines with vivo efficacy for B-Catenin/T-Cell transcriptional factor 4 pathway inhibition. J Med Chem 53:897–910

Desbois-Mouthon C, Cadoret A, Vlivet-Van Eggelpoel M-J, Bertrand F, Cherqui G, Perret C et al (2001) Insulin and IGF-1 stimulate the b-catenin pathway through two signalling cascades involving GSK-3b inhibition and Ras activation. Oncogene 20: 252–259

Diniz G, Aktas S, Turedi A, Temir G, Ortac R, Vergin C (2011) Telomerase reverse transcriptase catalytic subunit expression and proliferation index in Wilms tumor. Tumour Biol 32(4):761–767

Dome JS, Chung S, Bergemann T, Umbricht CB, Saji M, Carey LA et al (1999) High telomerase reverse transcriptase (hTERT) messenger RNA level correlates with tumor recurrence in patients with favorable histology Wilms' tumor. Cancer Res 59:4301–4307

Dome JS, Blockhold CA, Li SM, Baker SD, Green DM, Perlman EJ et al (2005) High telomerase RNA expression level is an adverse prognostic factor for favorable-histology Wilms' tumor. J Clin Oncol 23:9138–9145

Dome J, Cotton C, Perlman E, Breslow N, Kalapurakal J, Ritchey M et al (2006) Treatment of anaplastic histology Wilms' tumor: results from the Fifth National Wilms' Tumor Study. J Clin Oncol 24:2352–2358

Dressler GR (2006) The cellular basis of kidney development. Annu Rev Cell Dev Biol 22:509–529

Drummond IA, Madden SL, Rohwer-Nutter P, Bell GI, Sukhatme VP, Rauscher FJ 3rd (1992) Repression of the insulin-like growth factor II gene by the Wilms tumor suppressor WT1. Science 31:674–678

Eggenschwiler J (1997) Mouse mutant embryos overexpressing IGF-II exhibit phenotypic features of the Beckwith-Wiedemann and Simpson-Golabi-Behmel syndromes. Genes Dev 11:3128–3142

Eguchi M, Nguyen C, Lee SC, Kahn M (2005) ICG-001, a novel small molecule regulator of TCF/beta-catenin transcription. Med Chem 1:467–472

Ehrlich PF (2009) Bilateral Wilms' tumor: the need to improve outcomes. Expert Rev Anticancer Ther 9:963–973

Ehrlich D (2010) Nuclear accumulation of beta-catenin protein indicates activation of wnt signaling in chemically induced rat nephroblastomas. Pediatr Dev Pathol 13:1–8

Ehrlich M, Jiang G, Fiala E, Dome JS, Yu MC, Long TI et al (2002) Hypomethylation and hypermethylation of DNA in Wilms tumors. Oncogene 26:6694–6702

Ehrlich M, Hopkins NE, Jiang G, Dome JS, Yu MC, Woods CB et al (2003) Satellite DNA hypomethylation in karyotyped Wilms tumors. Cancer Genet Cytogenet 141:97–105

Emami KH, Nguyen C, Ma H, Kim DH, Jeong KW, Eguchi M et al (2004) A small molecule inhibitor of beta-catenin/CREB-binding protein transcription [corrected]. Proc Natl Acad Sci U S A 101:12682–12687

Englert C, Hou X, Maheswaran S, Bennett P, Ngwu C, Re GG et al (1995) WT1 suppresses synthesis of the epidermal growth factor receptor and induces apoptosis. EMBO J 14:4662–4675

Englert C, Maheswaran S, Garvin AJ, Kreidberg J, Haber DA (1997) Induction of p21 by the Wilms' tumor suppressor gene WT1. Cancer Res 15:1429–1434

Essafi A, Webb A, Berry RL, Slight J, Burn SF et al (2011) A Wt1-controlled chromatin switching mechanism underpins tissue-specific Wnt4 activation and repression. Dev Cell 21:559–574

Faussillon M, Moonier L, Junien C, Jeanpierre C (2005) Frequent overexpression of cyclin D2/cyclin-dependent kinase 4 in Wilms tumor. Cancer Lett 18:67–75

Fouladi M, Furman WL, Chin T, Freeman BB 3rd, Dudkin L et al (2006) Phase I study of depsipeptide in pediatric patients with refractory solid tumors: a Children's Oncology Group report. J Clin Oncol 1:3678–3685

Fukuzawa R, Heathcott RW, Sano M, Morison IM, Yun K, Reeve AE (2004) Myogenesis in Wilms tumors is associated with mutations of the WT1 gene and activation of Bel-2 and the Wnt signaling pathway. Pediatr Dev Pathol 7:668–669

Gadd S, Sredni ST, Huang CC, Perlman EJ (2010) Rhabdoid tumor: gene expression clues to pathogenesis and potential therapeutic targets. Lab Invest 90:724–738

Gadd S, Huff V, Huang CC, Ruteshouser EC, Dome JS et al (2012) Clinically relevant subsets identified by gene expression patterns support a revised ontogenic model of Wilms tumor: a Children's Oncology Group Study. Neoplasia 14:742–756

Gansler T, Allen KD, Burant CF, Inabnett T, Scott A, Buse MG et al (1988) Detection of type 1 insulin-like growth factor (IGF) receptors in Wilms tumors. Am J Pathol 130:431–435

Gansler T, Furlanetto R, Gramling TS, Robinson KA, Blocker N, Buse MG et al (1989) Antibody to type I insulinlike growth factor receptor inhibits growth of Wilms' tumor in culture and athymic mice. Am J Pathol 135:961–966

Garvin AJ, Re GG, Tarnowski BI, Hazen-Martin DJ, Sens DA (1993) The G401 cell line utilized for studies of chromosomal changes in Wilms tumor, is derived from a rhabdiod tumor of the kidney. Am J Pathol 142:375–380

Geller JI, Argani P, Adeniran A, Hampton E, De Marzo A, Hicks J et al (2008) Translocation renal cell carcinoma: lack of negative impact due to lymph node spread. Cancer 112:1607–1616

Ghanem MA, Van Der Kwast TH, Den Hollander JC, Sudaryo MK, Mathoera RB, Van den Heuvel MM et al (2001) Expression and prognostic value of epidermal growth factor receptor, transforming growth factor-alpha, and c-erb B-2 in nephroblastoma. Cancer 92(12):3120–3129

Ghanem MA, van Steenbrugge GJ, Sudary MK, Mathoera RB, Nijman JM, van der Kwast TH (2003) Expression and prognostic relevance of vascular endothelial growth factor (VEGF) and its receptor (FLT-1) in nephroblastoma. J Clin Pathol 56:107–113

Giordano G, Campanini N, Donofrio V, Bertolini P, Falleti J, Grassani C et al (2008) Analysis of Cox-2 expression in Wilms' tumor. Pathol Res Pract 204: 875–882

Glienke W, Maute L, Wicht J, Bergmann L (2009) Wilms' tumour gene 1 (WT1) as a target in curcumin treatment of pancreatic cancer cells. Eur J Cancer 45:874–880

Goldberg J, Demetri GD, Choy E, Rosen L, Pappo A, Dubois S et al (2009) Preliminary results from a phase II study of ARQ 197 in patients with microphthalmia transcription factor family (MiT)-associated tumors. J Clin Oncol 27:10502

Graham C, Tucker C, Creech J, Favours E, Billups CA, Liu T et al (2006) Evaluation of the antitumor efficacy, pharmacokinetics, and pharmacodynamics of the histone deacetylase inhibitor depsipeptide in childhood cancer models in vivo. Clin Cancer Res 1:223–234

Grundy P, Telzerow P, Breslow N, Moksness J, Huff V, Paterson M et al (1994) Loss of heterozygosity for chromosomes 16q and 1 p in Wilms tumors predicts an adverse outcome. Cancer Res 54:2331–2333

Hammes A (2001) Two splice variants of the Wilms' tumor 1 gene have distinct functions during sex determination and nephron formation. Cell 106:319–329

Harada N (1999) Intestinal polyposis in mice with a dominant stable mutation of the beta-catenin gene. EMBO J 18:5931–5942

Herbst A, Koligs FT (2007) Wnt signaling as a therapeutic target for cancer. Methods Mol Biol 361:63–91

Hohenstein P, Hastie ND (2006) The many facets of the Wilms' tumour gene, WT1. Hum Mol Genet 15:R196–R201

Houghton PJ, Morton CL, Tucker C, Payne D, Favours E, Cole C et al (2007) The pediatric preclinical testing program: description of models and early testing results. Pediatr Blood Cancer 49:928–940

Houghton PJ, Kang M, Reynolds CP, Gorlick R, Kolb EA, Maris JM, Keir ST, Carol H, Lock RB, Billups CA, Kurmasheva RT, Landesman Y, Shacham S, Kauffman M, Smith MA (2013a) Pediatric Preclinical Testing Program (PPTP) stage 1 evaluation of the XPO1/CRM1 inhibitor KPT-330. AACR (abstract LB-354)

Houghton PJ, Kang M, Reynolds CP, Lock RB, Carol H, Gorlick R, Kolb EA, Maris JM, Keir ST, Billups CA, Kurmasheva RT, Smith MA (2013b) Pediatric Preclinical Testing Program (PPTP) stage 1 evaluation of the antimicrotubule agents cabazitaxel and docetaxel. AACR (abstract 2767)

Houghton PJ, Kurmasheva RT, Lyalin D, Maris JM, Kolb EA, Gorlick R, Reynolds CP, Kang MH, Keir ST, Wu J, Smith MA (2014) Initial solid tumor testing (stage 1) of AZD1480, an inhibitor of Janus kinases 1 and 2 by the pediatric preclinical testing program. Pediatr Blood Cancer. 2014 Nov;61(11):1972–1979. doi:10.1002/pbc.25175. Epub 2014 Aug 17.

Hu Q, Gao F, Tian W, Ruteshouser EC, Wang Y, Lazar A, Stewart J, Strong LC, Behringer RR, Huff V (2011) Wt1 ablation and Igf2 upregulation in mice result in Wilms tumors with elevated ERK1/2 phosphorylation. J Clin Invest 121(1):174–183

Hueber PA, Fukuzawa R, Elkares R, Chu L, Blumentkrantz M, He SJ et al (2009) PAX3 is expressed in the stromal compartment of the developing kidney and in Wilms tumors with myogenic phenotype. Pediatr Dev Pathol 12:347–354

Ishiwata I, Ono I, Ishiwata C, Soma M, Nakaguchi T, Ohara K et al (1991) Carcinoembryonic proteins produced by Wilms' tumor cells in vitro and in vivo. Exp Pathol 41:1–9

Jacobs S, Fox E, Krailo M, Hartley G, Navid F, Wexler L et al (2010) Phase II trial of ixabepilone administered daily for five days in children and young adults with refractory solid tumors: a report from the children's oncology group. Clin Cancer Res 16:750–754

Jagt CT, Zuckermann M, Ten Kate F, Taminiau JA, Dijkgraaf MG, Heij H et al (2009) Veno-occlusive disease as a complication of preoperative chemotherapy for Wilms tumor: a clinic-pathological analysis. Pediatr Blood Cancer 53:1211–1215

Jenkins ZA (2009) Germline mutations in WTX cause a sclerosing skeletal dysplasia but do not predispose to tumorigenesis. Nat Genet 41:95–100

Karth J, Ferrer FA, Perlman E, Hanrahan C, Simons JW, Gearhart JP et al (2000) Coexpression of hypoxia-inducible factor 1-alpha and vascular endothelial growth factor in Wilms' tumor. J Pediatr Surg 35:1749–1753

Katoh M (2007) Networking of WNT, FGF, Notch, BMP, and Hedgehog signaling pathways during carcinogenesis. Stem Cell Rev 3:30–38

Keir ST, Maris JM, Lock R, Kolb EA, Gorlick R, Carol H et al (2010) Initial testing (stage 1) of the multi-targeted kinase inhibitor sorafenib by the pediatric preclinical testing program. Pediatr Blood Cancer 55:1126–1133

Keir ST, Maris JM, Reynolds CP, Kang MH, Kolb EA, Gorlick R, Lock R, Carol H, Morton CL, Wu J, Kurmasheva RT, Houghton PJ, Smith MA (2013) Initial testing (stage 1) of temozolomide by the pediatric preclinical testing program. Pediatr Blood Cancer 60(5):783–90

Kobayashi A (2008) Six2 defines and regulates a multipotent self-renewing nephron progenitor population throughout mammalian kidney development. Cell Stem Cell 3:169–181

Koesters R (1999) Mutational activation of the beta-catenin proto-oncogene is a common event in the development of Wilms' tumors. Cancer Res 59:3880–3882

Koesters R, Niggli F, von Knebel Doeberitz M, Stallmach T (2003) Nuclear accumulation of beta-catenin protein in Wilms' tumours. J Pathol 1:68–76

Kolb EA, Gorlick R, Reynolds CP, Kang MH, Carol H, Lock R, Keir ST, Maris JM, Billups CA, Desjardins C, Kurmasheva RT, Houghton PJ, Smith MA (2013) Initial testing (stage 1) of eribulin, a novel tubulin binding agent, by the pediatric preclinical testing program. Pediatr Blood Cancer 60(8):1325–32

Kreidberg JA (1993) WT-1 is required for early kidney development. Cell 74:679–691

Kudoh T, Ishidate T, Moriyama M, Toyoshima K, Akiyama T (1995) G1 phase arrest induced by Wilms tumor protein WT1 is abrogated by cyclin/CDK complexes. Proc Natl Acad Sci USA 92:4517–4521

Kumar S, Harrison CJ, Heighway J, Marsden HB, West DC, Jones PM (1987) A cell line from Wilms tumor with deletion in short arm of chromosome II. Int J Cancer 15:499–504

Kurmasheva RT, Houghton PJ (2006) IGF-I mediated survival pathways in normal and malignant cells. Biochim Biophys Acta 1766:1–22

Kurmasheva RT, Reynolds CP, Kang MH, Allievi C, Houghton PJ, Smith MA (2014) Initial testing (stage 1) of the topoisomerase II inhibitor pixantrone, by the pediatric preclinical testing program. Pediatr Blood Cancer 61(5):922–4

Lee SB (1999) The Wilms tumor suppressor WT1 encodes a transcriptional activator of amphiregulin. Cell 98:663–673

Lee S, Cimica V, Ramachandra N, Zagzag D, Kalpana GV (2011) Aurora A is a repressed effector target of the chromatin remodeling protein INI1/hSNF5 required for rhabdoid tumor cell survival. Cancer Res 71:3225–3235

Leighton PA, Ingram RS, Eggenschwiler J, Efstratiadis A, Tilghman SM (1995) Disruption of imprinting caused by deletion of the H19 gene region in mice. Nature 375:34–39

Lepourcelet M, Chen YN, France DS, Wang H, Crews P, Peterson F (2004) Small-molecule antagonists of the oncogenic Tcf/beta-catenin protein complex. Cancer Cell 5:91–102

Li CM (2002) Gene expression in Wilms' tumor mimics the earliest committed stage in the metanephric mesenchymal-epithelial transition. Am J Pathol 160:2181–2190

Li CM (2004) CTNNB1 mutations and overexpression of Wnt/beta-catenin target genes in WT1-mutant Wilms' tumors. Am J Pathol 165:1943–1953

Li W, Kessler P, Yeger H, Alami J, Reeve AE, Heathcott R et al (2005) A gene expression signature for relapse of primary wilms tumors. Cancer Res 65:2592–2601

Li MH, Sanchez T, Pappalardo A, Lynch KR, Hla T, Ferrer F (2008) Induction of anti-proliferative connective tissue growth factor expression in Wilms tumor cells by sphingosine 1-phosphate receptor 2. Mol Cancer Res 6:1649–1656

Li MH, Sanchez T, Yamase H, Hla T, Oo ML, Pappalardo A et al (2009) S1P/S1P1 signaling stimulates cell migration and invasion in Wilms tumor. Cancer Lett 276:171–179

Li MH, Yamase H, Ferrer F (2010) Characterization of a WiT49 cell line derived orthotopic model of Wilms tumor. Pediatr Blood Cancer 54:316–318

Lim K, Han C, Dai Y, Shen M, Wu T (2009) Omega-3 polyunsaturated fatty acids inhibit hepatocellular carcinoma cell growth through blocking beta-catenin and cyclooxygenase-2. Mol Cancer Ther 8:3046–3055

Lin RY, Argenta PA, Sullivan KM, Adzick NS (1995) Diagnostic and prognostic role of basic fibroblast growth factor in Wilms' tumor patients. Clin Cancer Res 1:327–331

Liu XW, Gong LJ, Guo LY, Katagiri Y, Jiang H, Wang ZY et al (2000) The Wilms' tumor gene product WT1 mediates the down-regulation of the rat epidermal growth factor receptor by nerve growth factor in PC12 cells. J Biol Chem 16:5068–5073

Lu D, Liu JX, Endo T, Zhou H, Yao S, Willert K et al (2009) Ethacrynic acid exhibits selective toxicity to chronic lymphocytic leukemia cells by inhibition of the Wnt/beta-catenin pathway. PLoS One 4:e8294

Ma H, Nguyen C, Lee KS, Kahn M (2005) ICG-001, a novel small molecule regulator of TCF/beta-catenin transcription. Med Chem 1(5):467–472

Maiti S, Alam R, Amos CI, Huff V (2000) Frequent association of beta-catenin and WT1 mutations in Wilms tumors. Cancer Res 60:6288–6292

Major MB (2007) Wilms tumor suppressor WTX negatively regulates WNT/beta-catenin signaling. Science 316:1043–1046

Malouf GG, Camparo P, Oudard S, Schleiermacher G, Theodore C, Rustine A et al (2010) Targeted agents in metastatic Xp11 translocation/TFE3 gene fusion renal cell carcinoma (RCC): a report from the Juvenile RCC Network. Ann Oncol 21:1834–1838

Maris JM, Courtright J, Houghton PJ, Morton CL, Gorlick R, Kolb EA et al (2008a) Initial testing of the VEGFR inhibitor AZD2171 by the pediatric preclinical testing program. Pediatr Blood Cancer 50:581–587

Maris JM, Courtright J, Houghton PJ, Morton CL, Kolb EA, Lock R et al (2008b) Initial testing (stage 1) of sunitinib by the pediatric preclinical testing program. Pediatr Blood Cancer 51:42–48

Maris JM, Morton CL, Gorlick R, Kolb EA, Carol H, Keir ST et al (2010) Initial testing of the aurora kinase A inhibitor MLN8237 by the Pediatric Preclinical Testing Program (PPTP). Pediatr Blood Cancer 55:26–34

Martinez-Estrada OM (2010) Wt1 is required for cardiovascular progenitor cell formation through transcriptional control of Snail and E-cadherin. Nat Genet 42:89–93

McKenna ES, Sansam CG, Cho YJ, Greulich H, Evans JA, Thom CS et al (2008) Loss of the epigenetic tumor suppressor SNF5 leads to cancer without genomic instability. Mol Cell Biol 28:6223–6233

Menke AL (2003) The wt1-heterozygous mouse; a model to study the development of glomerular sclerosis. J Pathol 200:667–674

Miller MA, Karacay B, Breslow NE, Li S, O'Dorisio MS, Grundy PE, Sandler AD (2005) Prognostic value of quantifying apoptosis factor expression in favorable histology wilms tumors. J Pediatr Hematol Oncol 27:11–14

Miyagawa K (1998) Loss of WT1 function leads to ectopic myogenesis in Wilms' tumour. Nat Genet 18:15–17

MLN8237: ADVL0921 Spring 2014 Study Progress report, Children's Oncology Group

Moisan A, Rivera MN, Lotinun S, Akhavanfard S, Coffman EJ, Cook EB, Stoykova S, Mukherjee S, Schoonmaker JA, Burger A, Kim WJ, Kronenberg HM, Baron R, Haber DA, Bardeesy N (2011) The WTX tumor suppressor regulates mesenchymal progenitor cell fate specification. Dev Cell 20(5): 583–596

Morris MR, Hesson LB, Wagner KL, Morgan NV, Astuti D, Lees RD et al (2003) Multigene methylation analysis of Wilms tumour and adult renal cell carcinoma. Oncogene 22:6794–6801

Morrison DJ, English MA, Licht JD (2005) WT1 induces apoptosis through transcriptional regulation of the proapoptotic Bcl-2 family member Bak. Cancer Res 15:8174–8182

Morton CL, Favours EG, Mercer KS, Boltz CR, Crumpton JC, Tucker C et al (2007) Evaluation of ABT-751 against childhood cancer models in vivo. Invest New Drugs 25:285–295

Moulton T (1994) Epigenetic lesions at the H19 locus in Wilms' tumour patients. Nat Genet 7:440–447

Natrajan R, Reis-Filho JS, Little SE, Messahel B, Brundler MA, Dome JS et al (2006) Blastemal expression of type I insulin-like growth factor receptor in Wilms' tumors is driven by increased copy number and correlates with relapse. Cancer Res 66:11148–11155

Natrajan R, Little SE, Sodha N, Reis-Filho JS, Mackay A, Fenwick K et al (2007a) Analysis by array CGH of genomic changes associated with the progression or relapse of Wilms tumor. J Pathol 21:52–59

Natrajan R, Williams RD, Grigoriadis A, Mackay A, Fenwick K, Ashworth A et al (2007b) Delineation of a 1MB breakpoint region at 1p13 in Wilms tumor by fine –tilling oligonucleotide array CGH. Genes Chromosomes Cancer 46:607–615

Nicholson G (1950) Studies on tumour formation. Butterworth, London

Nowicki M, Ostalska-Nowicka D, Kaczmarek M, Miskowiak B, Witt M (2007) The significance of VEGF-C/VEGFR-2 interaction in the neovascularization and prognosis of nephroblastoma (Wilms' tumour). Histopathology 50:358–364

Ogawa O (1993) Relaxation of insulin-like growth factor II gene imprinting implicated in Wilms' tumour. Nature 362:749–751

Oh S, Song Y, Yim J, Kim TK (1999) The Wilms' tumor 1 tumor suppressor gene represses transcription of the human telomerase reverse transcriptase gene. J Biol Chem 274:37473–37478

Ohori H, Yamakoshi H, Tomizawa M, Shibuya M, Kakudo Y, Takahashi A et al (2006) Synthesis and biological analysis of new curcumin analogues bearing an enhanced potential for the medicinal treatment of cancer. Mol Cancer Ther 5:2563–2571

Oue T, Yoneda A, Uehara S, Yamanaka H, Fukuzawa M (2010) Increased expression of the hedgehog signaling pathway in pediatric solid malignancies. J Pediatr Surg 45:378–392

Ozluk Y, Kilicaslan I, Gulluoglu MG, Ayan I, Uysal V (2006) The prognostic significance of angiogenesis and the effect of vascular endothelial growth factor on angiogenic process in Wilms' tumour. Pathology 38:408–414

Patek CE (1999) A zinc finger truncation of murine WT1 results in the characteristic urogenital abnormalities of Denys-Drash syndrome. Proc Natl Acad Sci U S A 96:2931–2936

Perner B, Englert C, Bollig F (2007) The Wilms tumor genes wt1a and wt1b control different steps during formation of the zebrafish pronephros. Dev Biol 309:87–96

Perotti D (2008) Functional inactivation of the WTX gene is not a frequent event in Wilms' tumors. Oncogene 27:4625–4632

Peterson JK, Tucker C, Favours E, Cheshire PJ, Creech J, Billups CA et al (2005) In vivo evaluation of exabepilone (BMS247550), a novel epothilone B derivative, against pediatric cancer models. Clin Cancer Res 1:6950–6958

Pinthus JH, Fridman E, Dekel B, Goldberg I, Kaufman-Francis K, Eshhar Z et al (2004) ErbB2 is a tumor associated antigen and a suitable therapeutic target in Wilms tumor. J Urol 172:1644–1648

Pinthus JH, Sheffer Y, Nagler A, Fridman E, Mor Y, Genina O et al (2005) Inhibition of Wilms tumor xenograft progression by halofuginone is accompanied by activation of WT-1 gene expression. J Urol 174:1527–1531

Piva R, Pellergrion E, Mattioli M, Agnelli L, Lombard L, Boccalatte F et al (2006) Functional validation fo the ana plastic lymphoma kinase signature identifies CEBPB and BCL2A1 as critical target genes. J Clin Invest 6:3171–3182

Pode-Shakked N, Shukrun R, Mark-Danieli M, Tsvetkov P, Bahar S et al (2013) The isolation and characterization of renal cancer initiating cells from human Wilms' tumour xenografts unveils new therapeutic targets. EMBO Mol Med 5:18–37

Pritchard-Jones K, Vujanic G (2006) Multiple pathways to Wilms tumor: how much is genetic? Pediatr Blood Cancer 47:232–234

Qing RQ, Schmitt S, Ruelicke T, Stallmach T, Schooenle EJ (1996) Autocrine regulation of growth by insulin-like growth factor (IFG)-II mediated by type I IGF-receptor in Wilms tumor cells. Pediatr Res 39(1):160–165

Ramburan A, Oladiran F, Smith C, Hadley GP, Goverder D (2005) Microsatellite analysis of the adenomatous polyposis coli (APC) gene and immunoexpression of beta catenin in nephroblastoma: a study including 83 cases treated with preoperative chemotherapy. J Clin Pathol 58:44–50

Rasola A, Fassetta M, De Bacco F, D'Alessandro L, Gramaglia D, Di Renzo MF et al (2007) A positive feedback loop between hepatocyte growth factor receptor and beta-catenin sustains colorectal cancer cell invasive growth. Oncogene 15:1078–1087

Ravenel J, Broman K, Perlman E, Niemitz E, Jayawardena T, Bell D et al (2001) Loss of imprinting of insulin-like growth factor-II (IGF2) gene in distinguishing specific biologic subtypes of Wilms tumor. J Natl Cancer Inst 93:1698–1703

Re GG, Hazen-Martin DJ, El Bahtimi R, Brownlee NA, Willingham MC, Garvin AJ (1999) Prognostic significance of Bcl-X(L) in rare tumor cases. Int J Cancer 20:192–200

Rehli M, Den Elzen N, Cassady A, Ostrowski MC, Hume DA (1999) Cloning and characterization of the murine genes for bHLH-ZIP transcription factors TFEC and TFEB reveal a common gene organization for all MiT subfamily members. Genomics 56:111–120

Reidemann J, Macaulay VM (2006) IGF1R signaling and its inhibition. Endocr Relat Cancer 13:33–43

Rivera MN (2007) An X chromosome gene, WTX, is commonly inactivated in Wilms tumor. Science 315:642–645

Rivera MN, Haber DA (2005) Wilms' tumour: connecting tumorigenesis and organ development in the kidney. Nat Rev Cancer 5:699–712

Roberts CW, Bigel JA (2009) The role of SMARCB1/INI1 in development of rhabdoid tumor. Cancer Biol Ther 8:412–416

Royer-Pokora B, Busch M, Beier M, Duhme C, de Torres C, Mora J et al (2010) Wilms tumor cells with WT1 mutations have characteristic features of mesenchymal stem cells and express molecular markers of paraxial mesoderm. Hum Mol Genet 19:1651–1668

Ruteshouser EC, Robinson SM, Huff V (2008) Wilms tumor genetics: mutations in WT1, WTX, and CTNNB1 account for only about one-third of tumors. Genes Chromosomes Cancer 47:461–470

Ruxolitinib: ADVL1011 Spring 2014 Study Progress report, Children's Oncology Group

Salem M, Kinoshita Y, Tajiri T, Souzaki R, Tatsuta K, Higashi M et al (2006) Association between the HER2 expression and histological differentiation in Wilms tumor. Pediatr Surg Int 11:891–896

Sattler M, Salgia R (2007) c-Met and hepatocyte growth factor: potential as novel targets in cancer therapy. Curr Oncol Rep 9:102–108

Schmitt S, Ren-Qiu Q, Torresani T, Doebeli M, Zapf J, Schoenle J (1997) High molecular weight forms of IGF-II (big-IGF-II) released by Wilms tumor cells. Eur J Endocrinol 137:396–401

Shan J, Shi DL, Wang J, Zheng J (2005) Identification of a specific inhibitor of the dishevelled PDZ domain. Biochemistry 29:15495–15503

Shan BE, Wang MX, Li RQ (2009) Quercetin inhibit human SW480 colon cancer growth in association with inhibition of cyclin D1 and surviving expression through Wnt/beta-catenin signaling pathway. Cancer Invest 27:604–612

Sharma PM, Bowman M, Yu BF, Sukumar S (1994) A rodent model for Wilms tumors: embryonal kidney neoplasms induced by N-nitroso-N′-methylurea. Proc Natl Acad Sci U S A 91:9931–9935

Shaw AP, Poirier V, Tyler S, Mott M, Berry Y, Maitland NJ (1988) Expression of the N-myc oncogene in Wilms' tumour and related tissues. Oncogene 3(2):143–149

Sitaram RT, Degerman S, Liungberg B, Andersson E, Oji Y, Sugiyama H et al (2010) Wilms' tumor 1 can suppress hTERT gene expression and telomerase activity in clear cell renal cell carcinoma via multiple pathways. Br J Cancer 103(8):1255–1262

Skoldenberg EG, Christiansson J, Sandstedt B, Larsson A, Lackgren G, Christofferson R (2001) Angiogenesis and angiogenic growth factors in Wilms tumor. J Urol 165:2274–2279

Smith MA, Morton CL, Phelps D, Girtman K, Neale G, Houghton PJ (2008) SK-NEP-1 and Rh1 are Ewing family tumor lines. Pediatr Blood Cancer 50:703–706

Smith ME, Cimica V, Chinni S, Jana S, Koba W, Yang Z et al (2011) Therapeutically targeting cyclin D1 in primary tumors arising from loss of Ini1. Proc Natl Acad Sci U S A 108:319–324

Smith MA, Kang M, Reynolds CP, Gorlick G, Kolb EA, Maris JM, Keir ST, Billups CA, Kurmasheva RT, Houghton PJ (2013a) Pediatric Preclinical Testing Program (PPTP) stage 1 evaluation of cabozantinib. AACR (abstract LB-353)

Smith MA, Kang M, Reynolds CP, Gorlick R, Kolb EA, Maris JUM, Keir ST, Billups CA, Kurmasheva RT, Houghton PJ, Collins J (2013b) Pediatric Preclinical Testing Program (PPTP) stage 1 evaluation of NSC750854, a sulfated purine analog with a distinctive anticancer activity profile. AACR (abstract 2752)

Smith MA, Kang M, Reynolds CP, Gorlick R, Kolb EA, Maris JM, Lock RB, Carol H, Keir ST, Billups CA, Kurmasheva RT, Houghton PJ (2014) Pediatric Preclinical Testing Program (PPTP) Evaluation of BMN 673, an Inhibitor of Poly-ADP Ribose Polymerase (PARP), with Temozolomide (TMZ). AACR (abstract)

Sorafenib: ADVL1121 Spring 2014 Study Progress report, Children's Oncology Group

Stanhope-Baker P, Kessler PM, Li W, Agarwal ML, Williams BR (2004) The Wilms tumor suppressor-1 target gene podacalyxin is transcriptionally repressed by p53. J Biol Chem 6:33357–33385

Stark K, Vainio S, Vassileva G, McMahon AP (1994) Epithelial transformation of metanephric mesenchyme in the developing kidney regulated by Wnt-4. Nature 372:679–683

Steenman MJ (1994) Loss of imprinting of IGF2 is linked to reduced expression and abnormal methylation of H19 in Wilms' tumour. Nat Genet 7:433–439

Stefanowicz J, Kosiak M, Kosiak W, Korbus-Kosiak A, Sierota D, Owczuk R (2010) Cystatin C and parenchymal thickness/kidney length ratio in Wilms tumor survivors. Pediatr Blood Cancer 54:41–46

Suh Y, Afaq F, Johnson JJ, Mukhtar H (2009) A plant flavonoid fisetin induces apoptosis in colon cancer cells by inhibition of COX2 and Wnt/EGFR/NF-kappaB-signaling pathways. Carcinogenesis 30:300–307

Sun FL, Dean WL, Kelsey G, Allen ND, Reik W (1997) Transactivation of Igf2 in a mouse model of Beckwith-Wiedemann syndrome. Nature 389:809–815

Takahashi-Yanaga F, Sasaguri T (2007) The Wnt/B-catein signaling pathway as a target in drug discovery. J Pharmacol 104:293–302

Takamizawa S, Scott D, Wen J, Grundy P, Bishop W, Kimura K et al (2001) The survivin: fas ratio in pediatric renal tumors. J Pediatr Surg 36:37–42

Talts JF, Aufderheide E, Sorokin L, Ocklind G, Mattson R, Ekblom P (1993) Induction of mouse tenascin expression by a human sarcomatiod Wilms tumor cell line growing in nude mice. Int J Cancer 54:868–874

Tanaka K, Granata C, Wang Y, O'Briain DS, Puri P (1999) Apoptosis and bcl-2 oncogene expression in Wilms' tumor. Pediatr Surg Int 15:243–247

Tanigawa S, Wang H, Yang Y, Sharma N, Tarasova N, Ajima R, Yamaguchi TP, Rodriguez LG, Perantoni AO (2011) Wnt4 induces nephronic tubules in metanephric mesenchyme by a non-canonical mechanism. Dev Biol 352(1):58–69. Epub 2011 Jan 21

Timofeeva QA, Plisov S, Evseev AA, Peng S, Jose-Kampfner M, Lovvorn HN et al (2006) Serine-phosphorylated STAT1 is a prosurvival factor in Wilms tumor pathogenesis. Oncogene 25:7555–7564

Tsuda M, Davis IJ, Argani P, Shukla N, McGill GG, Nagai M et al (2007) TFE3 fusions activate MET signaling by transcriptional up-regulation, defining another class of tumors as candidates for therapeutic MET inhibition. Cancer Res 67:919–929

Urbach A, Yermalovich A, Zhang J, Spina CS, Zhu H et al (2014) Lin28 sustains early renal progenitors and induces Wilms tumor. Genes Dev 28:971–982

Vasei M, Modjtahedi H, Ale-Booyeh O, Mosallaei A, Kajbafzadeh AM, Shahriari M et al (2009) Amplification and expression of EGFR and ERBB2 in Wilms tumor. Cancer Genet Cytogenet 194:88–95

Vicanek C, Ferretti E, Goodyer C, Torban E, Moffett P, Pelletier J et al (1997) Regulation of renal EGF receptor expression is normal in Denys-Drash syndrome. Kidney Int 52(3):614–619

Vize PD, Woolf AS, Bard JB (2003) The kidney. From normal development to congenital disease. Academic, London

Vuononvirta R, Sebire NJ, Messahel B, Perusinghe N, Reis-Filho JS, Pitchard-Jones K et al (2009) Expression of hepatocyte growth factor and its receptor met in Wilms' tumors and nephrogenic rests reflects their roles in kidney development. Clin Cancer Res 15:2723–2730

Weigel B, Malempati S, Reid JM, Voss SD, Cho SY, Chen HX, Krailo M, Villaluna D, Adamson PC, Blaney SM (2014) Phase 2 trial of cixutumumab in children, adolescents, and young adults with refractory solid tumors: a report from the Children's Oncology Group. Pediatr Blood Cancer 61(3):452–6

Weksberg R, Shen DR, Fei YL, Song Q, Squire J (1993) Disruption of insulin-like growth factor 2 imprinting in Beckwith-Wiedemann syndrome. Nat Genet 5:143–150

Werner H, Re GG, Drummond IA, Sukhatme VP, Frank J et al (1993) Increase expression of the insulin-like growth factor I receptor gene, IGF1R, in Wilms tumor is correlated with modulation of IGF1R promoter activity by the WT1 Wilms tumor gene product. Proc Natl Acad Sci U S A 90:5828–5832

White YA, Kyle JT, Wood AW (2009) Targeted gene knockdown in zebrafish reveals distinct intraembryonic functions for insulin-like growth factor II signaling. Endocrinology 150:4366–4375

Wood AC, Maris JM, Gorlick R, Kolb EA, Keir ST, Reynolds CP, Kang MH, Wu J, Kurmasheva RT, Whiteman K, Houghton PJ, Smith MA (2013) Initial testing (Stage 1) of the antibody-maytansinoid conjugate, IMGN901 (Lorvotuzumab mertansine), by the pediatric preclinical testing program. Pediatr Blood Cancer 60(11):1860–7

Wright KD, Green DM, Daw NC (2009) Late effects of treatment for wilms tumor. Pediatr Hematol Oncol 26:407–413

Wunsch L, Flemming P, Gluer S (2001) Expression of MIB and BCL-2 in patients with nephrogenic rest with and without associated Wilms tumors. Eur J Pediatr Surg 11:105–109

Xu YQ, Grundy P, Polychronakos C (1997) Aberrant imprinting of the insulin-like growth factor II receptor gene in Wilms' tumor. Oncogene 14(9): 1041–1046

Yashima K, Maitra A, Timmons CF, Rogers BB, Pinar H, Shay JW et al (1998) Expression of the RNA component of telomerase in Wilms tumor and nephrogenic rest recapitulates renal embryogenesis. Hum Pathol 29:536–542

Yokoi A, McCrudden KW, Huang J, Kim ES, Soffer SZ, Frischer JS et al (2003) Human epidermal growth factor receptor signaling contributes to tumor growth via angiogenesis in her2/neu-expressing experimental Wilms' tumor. J Pediatr Surg 38:1569–1573

Zirn B, Samans B, Wittmann S, Pietsch T, Leuschner I, Graf N et al (2006) Target genes of the WNT/beta-catenin pathway in Wilms tumors. Genes Chromosomes Cancer 45:565–574

Zumkeller W, Schwander J, Mitchell CD, Morrell DJ, Scholfield PN, Preece MA (1993) Insulin-like growth factor (IGF)-I,_II and IGF binding protein-2 (IGFBP-2) in the plasma of children with Wilms tumor. Eur J Cancer 14:1973–1977

11 Surgical Consideration for Wilms' Tumors and Other Neoplastic Renal Lesions

Peter F. Ehrlich and Jan Godzinski

Contents

P.F. Ehrlich, MD, MSc (✉)
Department of Pediatric Surgery, C.S. Mott Children's Hospital 4-945, 1540 East Hospital Drive SPC 4211, Ann Arbor, MI 48109-4211, USA
e-mail: pehrlich@med.umich.edu

J. Godzinski, MD, PhD
Department of Paediatric Surgery, Marciniak Hospital and Chair of Emergency Medicine, Medical University, Wroclaw, Poland
e-mail: jgodzin@wp.pl

Abstract

Wilms' tumor (WT) of the kidney, or nephroblastoma, represents one of the great success stories in pediatric cancer therapy. Outcomes for children with Wilms' tumor have improved dramatically over the last 50 years with long-term survival in both North America and European trials approaching 85 %. Furthermore, many of the low-stage tumors have survival rates between 95 and 99 %. WT is named after Carl Max Wilhelm Wilms (November 5, 1867–May 14, 1918), a German pathologist and surgeon. He published his findings in 1897 in an influential 1899 monograph titled Die Mischgeschwülste der Niere.

K. Pritchard-Jones, J.S. Dome (eds.), *Renal Tumors of Childhood: Biology and Therapy*, Pediatric Oncology, DOI 10.1007/978-3-662-44003-2_11, © Springer-Verlag Berlin Heidelberg 2014

11.1 History of Surgery for Wilms' Tumor

Wilms' tumor (WT) of the kidney, or nephroblastoma, represents one of the great success stories in pediatric cancer therapy. Outcomes for children with Wilms' tumor have improved dramatically over the last 50 years with long-term survival in both North America and European trials approaching 85 %. Furthermore, many of the low-stage tumors have survival rates between 95 and 99 % (Grundy et al. 2005; Kalapurakal et al. 2004). WT is named after Carl Max Wilhelm Wilms (November 5, 1867–May 14, 1918), a German pathologist and surgeon. He published his findings in 1897 in an influential 1899 monograph titled Die Mischgeschwülste der Niere (Wilms 1897, 1899).

Surgery was the first effective treatment for nephroblastoma and continues to be the backbone of successful multimodality therapy. Although Wilms is credited with describing the tumor, anecdotal reports on successful excision of renal tumors in children and their possible cure appeared in the end of the nineteenth century. Dr. Thomas Jessop (1837–1903), on June 7, 1877, probably performed the first successful nephrectomy on a 2-year-old child with hematuria and a tumor of the kidney (Willets 2003; Gross 1953). At the beginning of the 1900s, survival for a child with WT was 5 %. Surgery carried with it a high operative mortality. In the late 1930s, Ladd and Gross described removing renal tumors in selected children and increase in survival. This technique included large transverse transabdominal approach and early ligation of the renal vessels. This modification improved the outcome in children with nonmetastatic nephroblastoma up to 32.2 % at 3 years. In addition, operative mortality was reduced from 23 to 7 %. Today the current oncological nephrectomy currently used for Wilms' tumor is still very similar to that postulated by Ladd and Gross (Gross 1953; Kung and Nyhan 1982; Othersen et al. 1999).

Over the last 50 years, large clinical trials using surgery in combination with chemotherapy and radiotherapy have improved survival and reduced morbidity from WT. The majority of the randomized clinical studies for the treatment of children with WT have been conducted by two large clinical cooperative groups. These are the Children Oncology Group (COG – formerly the National Wilms' Tumor Study Group [NWTS]) and the Société Internationale d'oncologie Pédiatrique (SIOP). The COG/NWTS is primarily based in North America whereas SIOP is a European consortium. Since 1969 the COG/NWTS in North America and since 1971 the SIOP in Europe tested several aspects of the multimodal risk-adapted therapy. One of the primary philosophical differences is that COG/NWTS recommends primary nephrectomy in nearly all unilateral patients. The SIOP advocates preoperative chemotherapy following imaging-based diagnosis which could be supplemented with fine or core needle biopsy in case of doubts, then nephrectomy. Interestingly, nearly the same results were achieved using different policy of the initial approach (Ehrlich 2001, 2007a; de Kraker et al. 2001; D'Angio et al. 1976; Lemerle et al. 1983; Tournade et al. 2001).

11.2 Surgical Implications of Primary Nephrectomy and Primary Chemotherapy

Although similar cure rates are achieved by both SIOP and COG/NWTS studies, there are differences between these two groups that affect staging and classification that is critical to understand when interpreting outcome studies for children with Wilms' tumor. The approach used by each group affects the staging and the subsequent risk-based therapy. For example, stage III patients on COG protocols are different than those on SIOP protocols.

11.2.1 The Philosophical Arguments for Primary Nephrectomy

Primary nephrectomy (when possible) has the following potential advantages. First, the primary tumor burden is removed. The morbidity and mortality in the modern age associated with renal surgery is low. Second, the pathology of the tumor will be determined before initiating adjuvant therapy. When treatment is started without tumor pathology, benign tumors or nonneoplastic lesions will be encountered. Misdiagnosis rates as high as 8 % and using the wrong chemotherapy in 5.2 % have been reported although this has dropped to below 1 % recently (de Kraker et al. 1999; Schenk et al. 2006; Vujanic et al. 2009). It is also important to consider that not all tumors respond to chemotherapy. Although removing big tumors is challenging, the size of the tumor does not always mean the risk of metastatic disease. In COG/NWTS protocols, if the tumor is not removed primarily, the patient will be stage III and receive three drug chemotherapy and radiation. A primary nephrectomy with a stage I or II tumor would avoid this increased therapy. Another consideration is that in a child less than two with a tumor less than 550 g who is stage I may not require any adjuvant therapy for a cure. Chemotherapy also changes tumor pathology, and the COG/NWTS staging system does not at present take this into account. Primary nephrectomy allows for initial assessment of lymph node status. This is very important in the COG/NWTS protocols. The treatment regimens for the COG protocols is risk based using age, stage, and LOH as key determinants. Preoperative chemotherapy results in a loss of important staging data, particularly lymph node status. For example, patients with favorable histology WT treated on SIOP 9301 and 2001 who were stage III and LN positive after preoperative chemo have a 5-year EFS of 82 %. Those that were stage III LN negative after preoperative chemotherapy, 5-year EFS is 82 %. Alternatively, the COG/NWTS data shows that stage III patients who are LN positive also have a 5-year survival of 81 %. In contrast, the COG/NWTS patients who are stage III but LN negative have a 5-year EFS of 91 % (Grundy 2009).

11.2.2 The Philosophical Arguments for Preoperative Chemotherapy

Preoperative chemotherapy, historically, proved its importance in decreasing the tumor rupture rate and inducing very favorable stage distribution at secondary surgery (Fig. 11.1). Also, the rate of surgery-related complications is low. The problem appears in very extensive or very fragile tumors. Heroic resections are followed more frequently by surgery-related complications. Incomplete resection implies more aggressive and also more toxic postoperative chemotherapy and radiotherapy. Surgical complications appear to be lower in pretreated patient. SIOP-9 reported an 8 % surgical complication rate as compared to NWTS-3 which had a 19.8 % complication rate. However, for NWTS-4 the complication

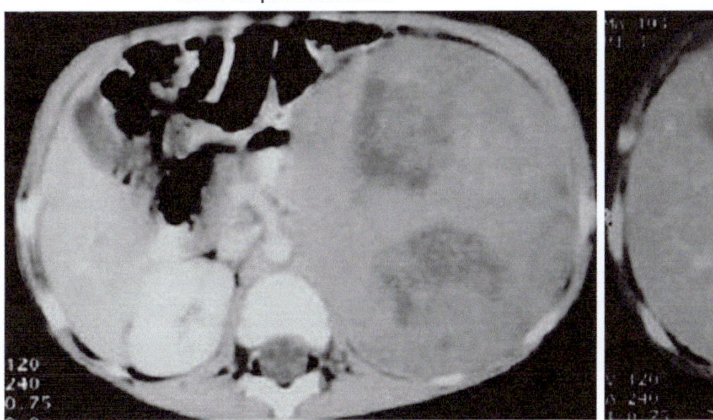

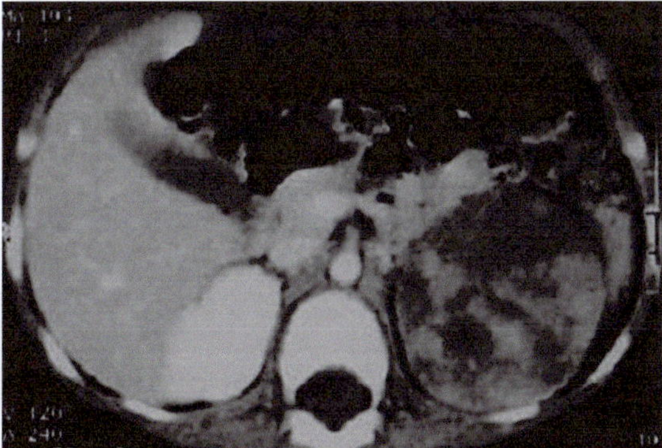

Fig. 11.1 Computed tomography scans demonstrating a picture of a Wilms' tumor at presentation and following 4 weeks of chemotherapy

rate was 12.7 %. It is also important to consider that what is considered as rupture or spill under SIOP is different in the COG/NWTS protocols. For example, in SIOP protocols, preoperative or intraoperative tru-cut or fine-needle punctures are not considered as spill, whereas in the COG/NWTS, they are considered spill. One relevant point is to look at whether a surgical spill resulted in patient being upstaged due to that spill. For NWTS-5 that was 1.4 % and for SIOP-9 that was 2.8 %, statistically there is no difference (Ehrlich et al. 2005; Godzinski et al. 1998). Tumor rupture and spillage during surgery is undoubtedly a bad event and needs to be avoided supporting an argument for pretreatment (Shamberger et al. 1999).On the other hand, those who have initially low staged tumor can benefit from lesser therapy if operated on primarily (D'Angio et al. 1976; Godzinski et al. 1998; Shamberger et al. 1999; Ritchey et al. 1992a, 2001; Kaste et al. 2008). Another argument for preoperative chemotherapy is that tumor staging does not occur until after initial chemotherapy and this results in lower rate of flank radiation in SIOP studies as compared to the COG/NWTS studies. This is an important consideration due to the late effects of radiotherapy.

Preoperative chemotherapy also preselects patients responding well to chemotherapy. That influences the histological classification which includes favorable 100 % necrotic subtype of nephroblastoma and unfavorable patients with blastema persisting the pretreatment. Also, initial extension of the disease has probably limited impact on final outcome if it regresses under the pretreatment, and, according to the SIOP experience, postoperative part of the therapy may be based upon the situation found at secondary surgery. That implies less aggressive postoperative therapy and avoidance of radiotherapy in a number of patients. On the other hand, primary chemotherapy for renal tumor diagnosed by imaging only implies certain number of treatments given to nonmalignant conditions or tumors other than nephroblastoma. Initial surgical biopsy is not recommended; however, fine-needle aspiration and tru-cut are the methods which decrease the risk of misdiagnosis (Godzinski et al. 1998, 1999; Shamberger et al. 1999; Ritchey et al. 1992a, 2001; Ritchey 1999).

11.3 Staging Aspects and the Problem of Comparing Outcomes

It is important when thinking about the potential advantages and disadvantages of each strategy to remember that outcomes are similar, but comparing patients is difficult due to the staging of patients prior to and after chemotherapy. Rather than thinking about which is better, it is more important to look at how each therapy addresses and answers some of the problems faced by any multidisciplinary groups that treat children with WT. The SIOP stages are induced by chemotherapy and separate good responders from poor responders, whereas the COG/NWTS staging systems are based on disease state prior to therapy using molecular markers such as LOH. These differences complicate markedly any direct comparisons of results, which in general should only be done very carefully and thoughtfully (Kaste et al. 2008; Godzinski et al. 1999, 2005; Brisse et al. 2006)

11.4 Nephrectomy

Surgery plays an important part of the multidisciplinary therapy for children with Wilms' tumor (WT). Regardless of timing of the renal surgery, there are several key issues that all surgeons must remember when performing operations on children with WT. These are: (a) perform safe operation, (b) understand what constitutes a complete procedure, and (c) recognize that the surgeon plays an important role in accurately staging the disease which is essential in directing future therapy. Under-staging can increase a child's risk of relapse, and over-staging could result in unnecessary chemotherapy or radiation. Intraoperative events that negatively affect patient survival include tumor spill, deficient operations, incomplete tumor removal, not assessing for extrarenal tumor extension, and surgical complications (Ehrlich et al. 2005; Shamberger et al. 1999; Ritchey et al. 2001).

The surgeon must document everything she/he does or finds in the operative note. This includes any tumor spill or rupture. Studies have shown a higher risk of recurrence in patients who had tumor spills or ruptures irrespective of the cause or extent of the soiling (Ehrlich et al. 2005; Shamberger et al. 1999; Ritchey et al. 2001). "Spill" refers to a break in the tumor capsule during operative removal whether accidental, unavoidable, or by design. Spill is also considered to have occurred if the renal vein or ureter was transected when they contain tumor. *(In the Children Oncology Group [COG] protocols, spill is also considered to have occurred if a preoperative or intraoperative needle/open biopsy was performed. This is not the case for those patients treated following Société Internationale d'Oncologie Pédiatrique protocols.)* "Rupture" refers to either the spontaneous or posttraumatic rupture of the tumor preoperatively with the result that tumor cells are disseminated throughout the peritoneal or retroperitoneal space (Grundy et al. 2007). Bloody peritoneal fluid is considered a sign of rupture, whether or not gross or microscopic tumor is identified in the fluid. Rupture is also considered to have occurred if the tumor penetrates the kidney capsule, with open raw neoplastic tissue surface being in free communication with the peritoneal cavity. All of these situations must be carefully documented in the operative note.

11.5 Technical Considerations

For a child with two normal kidneys and a unilateral renal tumor, the recommended surgical procedure is a unilateral radical ureteronephrectomy with lymph node sampling (Grundy et al. 2006; Ladd 1938). The incisions associated with the best exposure and lower complication rates are transverse transabdominal, transperitoneal, or thoracoabdominal (Ritchey et al. 1992a, b, 2001; Fuchs et al. 2009a). Large tumors or for those that come off the superior pole and extend up to the diaphragm, a thoracic extension of the incision through the eighth or ninth rib helps with exposure, although this is rarely required (Fig. 11.2). After entering the peritoneal cavity, evaluation of the peritoneal surfaces, liver, renal vein, and IVC for tumor extension is needed. Routine exploration of the contralateral kidney was originally mandated. Due to improvement in imaging, especially spiral CT scans, this is not necessary if imaging is satisfactory and does not suggest a bilateral process (Ritchey et al. 1995, 2005). If the initial imaging studies were suggestive of a possible lesion on the contralateral kidney, the contralateral kidney should be formally explored to rule out bilateral involvement. This should be done prior to nephrectomy. In addition, any evidence of a preoperative or intraoperative tumor rupture should be clearly documented in the operative report. *(In the past, the COG/NWTSG made a distinction a local and a diffuse spill. For COG protocols, this distinction is no longer made* (Shamberger et al. 1999; Kalapurakal et al. 2010). *For COG protocols, in any preoperative or intraoperative tumor biopsy, preoperative*

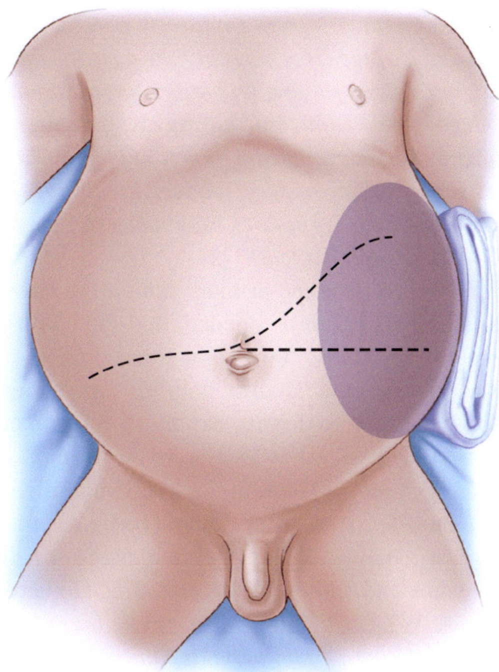

Fig. 11.2 A sketch showing patient positioning and typical abdominal incisions used for Wilms' tumor surgery

or intraoperative tumor rupture is considered a spill and is stage III. This is not the case for those patients treated following Société Internationale d'Oncologie Pédiatrique protocols: fine-needle punction or tru-cut needle punction is allowed in this study; however, surgical incisional biopsies are considered as ruptures, automatically staged III and contraindicated.)

To help expose the primary tumor, the lateral peritoneal reflection is opened, and the colon is reflected medially. For right-sided tumors, a Kocher procedure is also helpful. An attempt should be made to dissect, expose, and ligate the renal vessels in order to lessen the chance of hematogenous spread of tumor before mobilizing the tumor. The renal artery should be ligated first, then the renal vein. That prevents increasing the intrarenal and tumor blood pressure. However, because WT can be quite large, *preliminary ligation should not be pursued if technically difficult or dangerous*. For tumors that are pretreated with chemotherapy and respond, ligation of the renal vessels is often easy (Fig. 11.1). WT, as opposed to neuroblastomas, tends to displace vessels and organs. When dividing the vessels it is important for the surgeon to make sure the contralateral renal vessels, aorta, vena cava, iliac, and superior mesenteric arteries have not been ligated (Ritchey et al. 1992b). The adrenal gland may be left in place if it is not abutting the tumor, but if the mass arises in the upper pole of the kidney, the adrenal gland should be removed with the neoplasm. The ureter is ligated and divided as low as conveniently possible (Ritchey et al. 2008). The tumor and the uninvolved portion of the kidney are mobilized and removed intact. The tumor and kidney should be handled gently to avoid tumor spill as this results in a increase in local abdominal relapse (Shamberger et al. 1999, 2001; D'Angio et al. 1989).The renal vein and IVC should be palpated to look for tumor. Any suspicious areas that could represent metastases should be biopsied and marked with titanium clips. Although it is recognized that with improved CT and MRI imaging, the use of marking titanium clips may not be necessary. In addition, there is concern that clips may lead to artifacts on imaging.

WT can be large; however, in most cases there is no invasion by the tumor into contiguous organs, but typically the tumor displaces or is adherent to adjacent organs. This allows the tumor to be separated from the organs in most cases. When the surgeon does encounter a clinical situation with invasion, radical en bloc resection, e.g., partial hepatectomy, or colectomy is not warranted as a primary therapy and is associated with an increased frequency of complications (Shamberger et al. 1999; Ritchey et al. 2001). A small section of diaphragm, psoas muscle, or tip of the pancreas is acceptable. WT is very chemosensitive, and in these situations prior adjuvant therapy will allow for a safer resection.

There are clinical situations where it is agreed that primary nephrectomy poses too great a risk. These are (a) when there is extension of tumor thrombus above the level of the hepatic veins, (b) the tumor involves contiguous structures whereby the only means of removing the kidney tumor requires removal of the other structures (e.g., spleen, pancreas, colon but excluding the adrenal gland), (d) bilateral tumors, (e) or if there is pulmonary compromise due to extensive pulmonary metastases, (f) and if it is the surgeons' judgment that nephrectomy would result in significant or unnecessary morbidity/mortality, diffuse tumor spill, or residual tumor. Studies conducted by the large cooperative groups have shown that pretreatment with chemotherapy almost always reduces the bulk of the tumor (Lemerle et al. 1983; Mitchell et al. 2006; Tournade et al. 1993, 2001). This makes tumor removal easier and may reduce the incidence of surgical complications (Godzinski et al. 1998). Preoperative chemotherapy does not result in improved survival rates, and it may result in the loss of staging information and changes the histology of the tumor as noted above (Green et al. 1993; Weirich et al. 2001). It is a very rare situation when a tumor cannot be removed if pretreated. Some exceptions, however, happen. Inoperability for pretreated tumor implies a very poor outcome. In the COG protocols, a biopsy is recommended first for unilateral tumors. In SIOP protocols, this is not always the case. The COG/NWTS biopsies can be performed open, tru-cut, or imaged guided. The SIOP protocols do not recommend open biopsy. Tru-cut, under "eye control" or US guided, but still rather from posterior side and passing via portion of uninvolved kidney (if exists) is SIOP options for tumors which appeared intraoperatively impossible to remove.

11.6 Lymph Node Documentation

Pathological assessment of hilar and regional lymph nodes is critical to accurately stage a child with renal tumor (Ehrlich et al. 2005; Shamberger et al. 1999). Unfortunately, failure to sample lymph nodes (*whether dealing with a unilateral or bilateral tumor*) is the major technical errors noted in Wilms' tumor surgery (Ehrlich et al. 2005). Furthermore, studies have demonstrated a higher risk of recurrence in children who did not have lymph node status documented at the time of nephrectomy (Shamberger et al. 1999). Routine lymph node sampling from the renal hilum, the pericaval, or the para-aortic areas must be performed. Simply looking at the lymph nodes to determine whether they are positive is highly inaccurate (Othersen et al. 1990).

11.7 Management of Tumor Extension in the Renal Vein, Inferior Vena Cava, and Atrium

WT patients may present with tumor extension through the renal vein to the IVC and even up to the right atrium. This is found in between 4 and 11 % of children. Surgical treatment is dependent on the extent of vascular invasion. These are usually clinically asymptomatic, and many are detected preoperatively by US, CT, and/or MRI scans. However, those that extend just into the renal vein may only be detected at operation, reinforcing the need to palpate the renal vein and IVC at the time of nephrectomy (Shamberger et al. 2001; Ritchey et al. 1993, 1994). As noted above, a primary resection when tumor thrombus extends into the inferior vena cava at the level of the liver or higher is contraindicated. We recommend that these patients be managed initially with preoperative chemotherapy. This approach will often achieve significant shrinkage of the intravascular thrombus facilitating subsequent surgical removal (Shamberger et al. 2001; Ehrlich 2007b). Although the outcomes of the patients with vascular extension is similar with a primary or delayed resection, the severity and number of operative complications are reduced with preoperative chemotherapy for those with vascular extension above the hepatic veins. Alternatively, if the tumor extends only into the renal vein or renal vein and IVC below the level of the liver, the tumor and tumor thrombus can in most cases be removed en bloc with the kidney (Fig. 11.3).

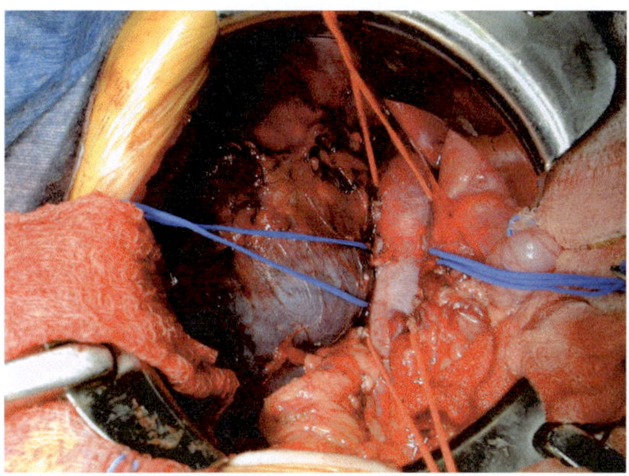

Fig. 11.3 This is an operative photo of a Wilms' tumor with vascular extension. Vessel loops are around the major vascular structures

An accurate description of the technique of removal should be given in the operative note. Control of renal veins and caval above and below the tumor with vessel loops is necessary using standard vascular surgery techniques. The tumor should not be transected, if possible, as this will result in spill and upstaging of the patient. In some cases, the tumor may be fixed to the vascular lumen. A similar technique used for removing plaque for a carotid endarterectomy is helpful to lift the tumor off the vein wall. It must be stated in the operative report if the intravascular tumor extension was removed en bloc or if tumor was transected, as well as if the tumor thrombus is removed completely and if there is evidence of either adherence or invasion of the vein wall. If after preoperative chemotherapy the tumor still extends above the hepatic veins, cardiopulmonary bypass is needed to remove the vascular extent of the tumor.

11.8 Management of Tumor Extension in the Ureter

Extension of Wilms' tumor into the ureter is a rare event (Ritchey et al. 2008). In NWTS-5, the incidence of ureteral extension was 2 %. In only 30 % of these patients did preoperative imaging detect ureteral extension; the rest were discovered at operation. Clinical presentations included gross hematuria, passage of tissue per urethra, hydronephrosis, and a urethral mass. The diagnosis should be suspected in these patients, and cystoscopy with retrograde ureterogram may aid in preoperative diagnosis in these patients. If ureteric extension is detected or suspected, the ureter should be with clear margins.

11.9 Horseshoe Kidneys, Single Kidneys, and Nonfunctioning Kidneys

Resection of a WT in a child with a horseshoe kidney presents unique challenges (Fig. 11.4). Children with horseshoe kidneys and WT must be carefully imaged prior to any surgery (Ritchey 2005). The blood supply to a horseshoe kidney can be variable and must be documented prior to any surgical procedure. At the time of operation, the blood supply to the kidney as well as the ureters must be identified and isolated. Exposure and mobilization of the kidney on the side of the tumor is carried out as if one is performing a unilateral resection. The side of the kidney containing the tumor, the isthmus, and the ipsilateral ureter are resected. As with other unilateral procedures, the lymph node groups are sampled for staging purposes. Children with a single kidney, or a situation where a tumor occurs in one kidney but the second kidney is nonfunctioning, should be managed using a renal-sparing approach with

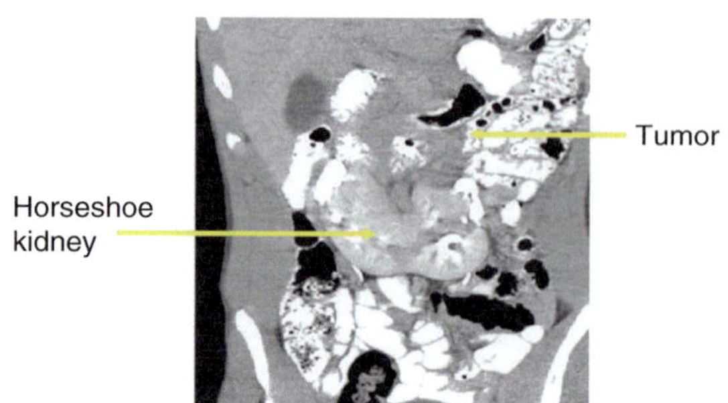

Fig. 11.4 A computed tomography scan showing a horseshoe kidney and a tumor in the upper pole of the left kidney

preoperative chemotherapy to facilitate surgery and save more renal tissue.

11.10 Surgical Management in Metastatic and Recurrent Disease

Metastatic disease (stage IV) is recognized as a poor prognostic factor for children with Wilms' tumor (Dome et al. 2006a). The primary sites of metastatic spread are to the liver and lungs. An important surgical point to remember is that the presence of lung or other site metastasis does not make the renal tumor unresectable. The abdominal tumor should be removed and staged locally as appropriate.

Lung metastases are the most common site of stage IV disease in children with Wilms' tumor. Depending on the treatment protocol, children with lung disease may be treated with just chemotherapy or both chemotherapy and radiation therapy. Historically, patients treated on COG/NWTS studies have been treated with radiotherapy in combination with either two or three drug therapy. Event-free survival for patients treated on NWTS-5 with lung metastasis was 76 % (72 %, 80 % CI 95 %). Review of the SIOP material by Jan de Kraker and co-workers evidenced overall survival and event-free survival of 83 % at 4 years for patients with pulmonary metastasis. Best outcomes were observed in those in whom metastasis disappeared after preoperative chemotherapy (23/27 alive and in CR) or were completely

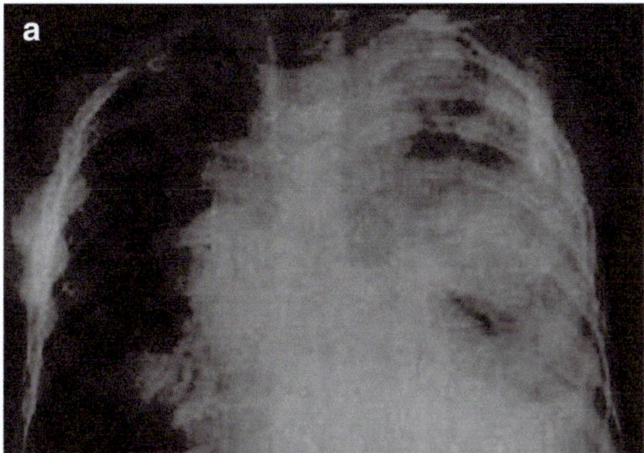

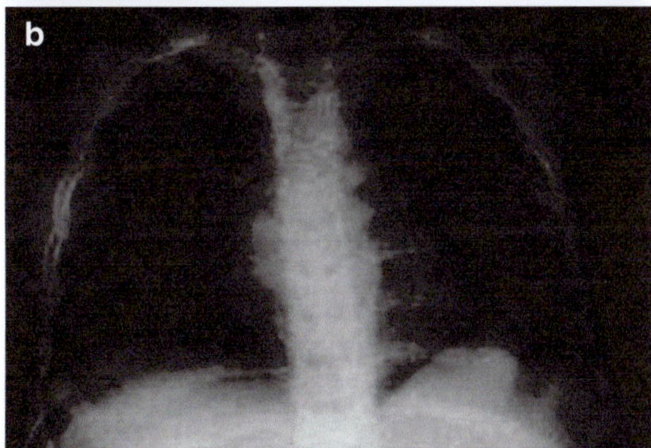

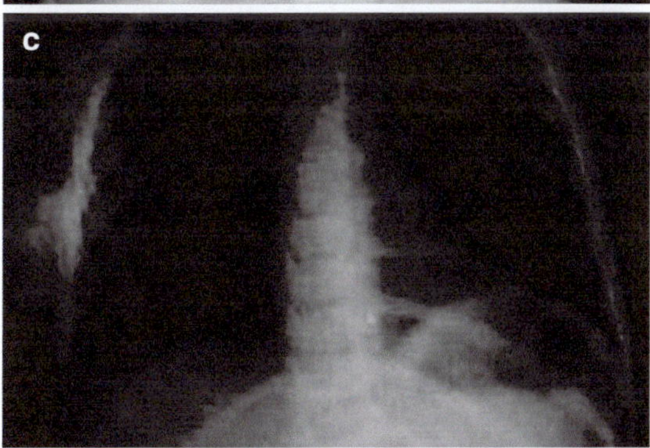

Fig. 11.5 (**a**) A chest radiograph in a patient with Wilms' tumor presenting with pulmonary disease. (**b**) The same patient's chest radiograph after 4 weeks of chemotherapy with vincristine, actinomycin D, and doxorubicin. (**c**) The same patient's chest radiograph after 4 more weeks of chemotherapy and radiotherapy

resected (5/5 CR) (de Kraker et al. 1990) (Fig. 11.5). Nearly the same results were reported by Steven Warmann and colleagues recently (Warmann et al. 2009).

Early treatment protocols assessed lung disease through a chest radiograph. However, current studies use CT and lesions are found on CT scan that are not found on CXR (Mankowski et al. 2004; Green 2002). These lesions have been managed in a variety of ways. The COG/NWTS analyzed these patients, and an inferior relapse-free survival was seen when children were treated with vincristine and actinomycin D only, whether or not they received pulmonary irradiation, compared to those who received doxorubicin. Thus, there appears to be no additional beneficial effect of lung irradiation on the outcome of some of these children when chemotherapy was taken into consideration. A second study examined the pathology of lung lesions seen only on CT scan in children from the NWTS-4/5 study (Owens et al. 2002). The results demonstrated that small lesions are usually but not invariably tumor. Based on these and other results, a current COG trial (ARENO533) for children with pulmonary lesions gives upfront chemotherapy followed by imaging at 6 weeks. If the lesions are still present, more intensive therapy including radiotherapy will be given.

There may be several times a surgeon may be asked to intervene in a child with a pulmonary lesion. The first is at diagnosis if there is uncertainty about pulmonary lesions. The second may occur after the first round of chemotherapy if lesions shrink but do not go away completely. If there is a concern about a lesion, it would be valuable to assess the histology of the lesion prior to giving radiotherapy. The third situation is if tumor remains after both chemotherapy and radiotherapy requiring surgical resection for cure. In the current SIOP 2001 protocol, if lesions remained after pretreatment, a metastasectomy is recommended. The suggested technical modalities include wedge resections or, rarely, lobectomies. Most WT metastases are peripheral and superficial, and many of these lesions can now be fully excised by video-assisted thoracic surgery (Fig. 11.6). Neither heroic, very extensive resections as bilobectomy or pneumonectomy nor surgery on progressing patients is recommended (de Kraker et al. 2001; Kaste et al. 2008; Ehrlich et al. 2006).

The approach to liver disease is less straightforward. Recent reports suggested that liver involvement at diagnosis in infants and children with Wilms' tumor indicated a worse prognosis than lung or other sites of stage IV disease (Varan

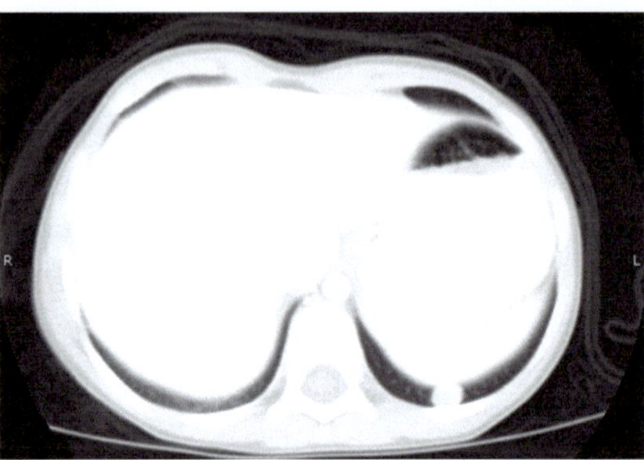

Fig. 11.6 Computed tomography scan showing peripheral lung lesions

et al. 2005; Szavay et al. 2006; Fuchs et al. 2008). The International Society of Pediatric Oncology (SIOP) and the German Pediatric Oncology Group (GPOH) studied 29 patients with liver metastasis at diagnosis (Szavay et al. 2006). The overall survival was less than 60 %, but all patients who had complete resection of the hepatic lesions survived. Another report from Varan et al. of 18 patients with liver metastases also noted a poorer outcome than for patients with pulmonary disease (50.2 % vs. 16.6 %) (Varan et al. 2005). These authors suggested, based on the poor outcomes of patients with liver metastases, that more intensive chemotherapy and more aggressive surgical treatment were warranted.

The COG also recently published their results of patients presenting with liver disease at diagnosis (Ehrlich et al. 2009). The estimated 5-year EFS (95 % confidence interval [CI]) for 634 patients with metastatic FH Wilms' tumor was 75 % (71, 78 %). The 5-year EFS (95 % CI) by stage IV category was: lung only 76 % (72, 80 %) (513 patients); liver, not lung, 76 % (58, 87 %) (34 patients); liver and lung 70 % (57, 80 %) (62 patients); and other sites 64 % (42, 79 %) (25 patients). There were no significant differences among stage IV categories ($p=0.60$). Event-free survival was not different for the patients with liver metastases and a primary resection of the liver metastases compared to those who did not undergo primary resection of the liver metastases. The COG conclusion was that an initial aggressive approach to liver disease was not warranted. All agree that those patients whose disease does not completely go away or does not respond to therapy should undergo a liver resection (Ehrlich et al. 2009).

Metastases locate mainly in lungs and in liver. Other locations are rare (Kaste et al. 2008; Godzinski et al. 1991, 2001). Patients on SIOP-9 with extrapulmonary and hepatic metastasis have been reviewed. For SIOP-9 patients, the key variable appears to be the pathology variant, with very poor outcome for anaplastic nephroblastoma (Godzinski et al. 2001). More data and study is needed to help determine the role and timing of surgery in the management of extrapulmonary and extrahepatic metastasis.

11.11 Relapse

One of the major challenges in the treatment of children with WT is the management of a child who relapses. Although the overall relapse rate for children with WT has decreased to less than 15 %, the long-term survival for patients with recurrent disease remains between 30 and 45 %. The role of surgery in the treatment of relapsed disease has not been elucidated. For NWTS-5 a specific treatment protocol for relapsed patients was available. The study design was to determine if alternating cycles of cyclophosphamide/etoposide and carboplatin/etoposide improved the event-free survival (EFS) of children with WT who relapsed after chemotherapy with VAD and radiation therapy (DD-4A). All patients received induction therapy. Those who showed at least minimal response to therapy went on to have surgical resection of the tumor followed by radiation therapy of all sites of disease. Four-year event-free survival (EFS) and overall survival (OS) were 42.3 and 48.0 %, respectively, for all patients and were 48.9 and 52.8 % for those who relapsed in the lungs only. Sixty were analyzed. Unfortunately, details of the surgical procedure and extent of resection as well as complications have not been published. In 2008 the SIOP published their outcome of relapses of nephroblastoma patients registered in the SIOP/GPOH trials. One hundred and seventy relapses were evaluated, 28 % were local, metastatic in 57 %, and combined in 15 %. No specific treatment protocol was used, but patients with isolated distant metastasis had a significantly better outcome than those with local and combined relapses ($p = 0.001$). Similar to the COG/NWTS study, the details of the surgical treatment for these patients have not been analyzed. Taken together, it makes it too difficult to determine what role and how aggressive surgeons should be in the treatment of relapsed disease.

11.12 Nephron-Sparing Surgery (NSS) and Minimal Invasive Nephrectomy (MIN) for Unilateral Nephroblastoma

Partial nephrectomy for unilateral tumors is an area of controversy. The goal of preserving renal tissue is laudable, but it is balanced against reducing survival and coupled with the knowledge that the long-term renal failure in patients after nephrectomy is exceedingly low. Nevertheless, experience gained in the treatment of bilateral tumors indicates that partial nephrectomy may be sufficient local therapy (Fuchs et al. 2009b; Herrera et al. 1996; Gentil Martins and Espana 1989; Moorman-Voestermans et al. 1994, 1998; Cozzi and Zani 2006).

Better pediatric care with wide access to imaging sometimes allows for very early discovery of low staged renal tumors. Some of those, if submitted to the preoperative chemotherapy, appear limited to polar or peripheral parts of the kidney. Currently, available CT or MRI makes possible precise imaging of the involved kidney and planning or excluding the patient as a candidate for NSS. On the other hand, status of the regional lymph nodes and pathology variant of tumor, incorrect interpretation, or technical problems at NSS which is more complicated than classical nephrectomy, all elevate the risk of relapse in this otherwise favorable group of patients. In what subset of patients the benefits of conservative surgery leaving more functional renal tissue outweighs the risk of the oncological failure is still an unanswered question. The SIOP started to register unilateral patients submitted to NSS in 2001. The safety measures included the list of contraindications which had to be respected to include the case in the study. Protocol clearly suggested to consider this technique in patients suffering from contralateral nephrological or urological disorders and syndromes of an increased risk of Wilms' tumor rather than in classical unilateral nephroblastoma (de Kraker et al. 2001; Kaste et al. 2008; Cozzi and Zani 2006).

11.13 Contraindications for NSS in Unilateral Nephroblastoma (de Kraker et al. 2001)

- Preoperative tumor rupture or biopsy
- Tumor infiltrating extrarenal structures
- Intra-abdominal metastases or lymph nodes seen on preoperative imaging
- Thrombus in the renal vein or vena cava
- Tumor involving more than 1/3 of the kidney (at least 50 % of renal tissue should be spared after the tumor resection with a margin of healthy tissue, to give any worthwhile protection against hyper perfusion)
- Multifocal tumor
- Central location
- Involvement of calyces
- Hematuria
- Little experience in partial nephrectomy.

The interim analysis made on cases registered thus far seems to emphasize the role of tumor stage. Preliminarily, of 41 analyzed patients submitted to NSS, 5 relapsed at 24-month follow-up but none of the 18 who were staged 1. Regarding pathology variants, of 6 patients with anaplastic nephroblastoma, 3 relapsed, but again not the case staged 1. Those results and review of literature look encouraging but only if the adequate safety rules are applied. The central review of the preoperative imaging and qualification of the candidates for NSS by the panel of dedicated and experienced surgeons are probably the correct way to find the adequate balance between risk and benefit of conservative surgery. The oncological experience of the treating center and the experience and skills of the operating surgeon are of great value. Technique of NSS does not differ from that modalities used for bilateral tumors. The balance of risk and benefit suggests using very simple techniques of partial nephrectomy assuring adequate margin of healthy tissue. Sophisticated resections justified in bilateral tumors, if there is no other possibility to save at least a portion of the functional kidney, are not recommended for unilateral patients.

At this point the COG strongly recommends against partial nephrectomy. The outcomes are excellent with unilateral tumors. The tumors tend to be larger prior to chemotherapy and many will not fit criteria for NSS. In addition, as mention above the importance of lymph nodes sampling and the risk of relapse are too high to justify. Whether the preoperative chemotherapy may sufficiently decrease this risk in responding patients needs further studies.

11.14 Minimal Invasive Nephrectomy (MIN)

Another option currently discussed is minimally invasive nephrectomy (MIN) for renal tumors. It is not easy to see any crucial benefit of this technique over the open access surgery. The procedure is far more difficult than the classical one. It is especially important in the regional lymph nodes sampling and manipulating the larger tumors covering aorta and/or vena cava. Abdominal incision, wherever located, must be large enough to gently sort out the tumor. The potential group of candidates resemble that for NSS, but NSS offers more benefit to the child than the minimally invasive surgery. According to our experience, a limited group of relatively small, not covering central vessels and centrally located tumors, which excludes NSS, are candidates for MIN.

The place of minimal invasive surgery in metastatic patients appears a little different. Thoracoscopy or VATS may be a good and safe methods of exploring and resecting the subpleural metastatic nodules. Those, however, must be well imaged on high-quality CT to avoid missing the parenchymal metastasis. One shall remember that the metastases progressing under the treatment nearly always are not a surgical target regardless of technique used (de Kraker et al. 1990, 1997, 2001; Ehrlich et al. 2006).

11.15 Bilateral Wilms' Tumor and Surgery

Bilateral Wilms' tumors (BWT) can be synchronous or metachronous. Children with synchronous BWT account for 5–7 % of all patients with Wilms' tumor (Breslow et al. 1993; Coppes et al. 1989; Petruzzi and Green 1997; Ritchey 2008). (Fig. 11.7) They occur more frequently in girls (sex ratio 0.6:1) and at a younger age (mean age 2.5 years). There is a higher incidence of nephrogenic rests, genetic malformations, and predisposing syndromes in children with BWT (Dome et al. 2006a) Patients with metachronous bilateral WT present with unilateral WT and subsequently develop contralateral disease. The incidence of metachronous bilateral Wilms' tumor ranges from 1.0 to 1.9 % (Coppes et al. 1989; Blute et al. 1987; Shearer et al. 1993). As in synchronous

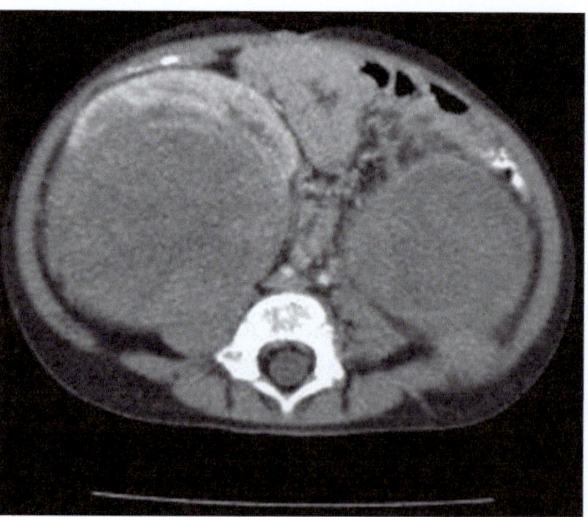

Fig. 11.7 A computed tomography scan demonstrating the typical appear of a bilateral Wilms' tumor

disease, the incidence is higher in girls and in young children (less than 12 months) with nephrogenic rests. Beckwith-Wiedemann syndrome, hemihypertrophy, or congenital aniridia seems to have a higher risk of developing a metachronous tumor than children with other syndromes or congenital anomalies known to predispose to the development of WT. (Coppes et al. 1999)

Imaging of BWT is best performed by CT or MRI. Computed tomography (CT) scan of the abdomen will confirm the renal origin of the mass and determine whether there are bilateral tumors. Early generations of CT scans missed 7–10 % of bilateral lesions, and it was always mandated to explore the contralateral side prior to doing a nephrectomy (Ritchey et al. 1995). A recent review of WT cases with modern helical CT scans demonstrated that only 0.25 % of bilateral tumors were missed, all of which were less than 1 cm (Ritchey et al. 2005). The SIOP currently recommends using MRI for all bilateral lesions, but there is no data comparing the two modalities in this situation.

The outcomes for most children with WT are outstanding. This is not the case, however, for children with bilateral Wilms' tumor (BWT) where survival is poor and the potential for late effects such as renal failure is great (Coppes et al. 1989; Shearer et al. 1993; Malogolowkin et al. 2008; Paulino et al. 1996; Weirich et al. 2004). In 1998, United Kingdom Children's Cancer Study Group (UKCCSG) published their experience with 70 BWT patients (Kumar et al. 1998). Conservative surgical treatment with initial biopsy followed by chemotherapy and delayed tumor resection was done in 57 children. Thirteen underwent primary surgical resection followed by chemotherapy. Overall survival was 69 % with similar survival in the conservatively treated and initial surgical resection groups. BWT with an unfavorable histology was associated with poorest prognosis. In 2004, Weirich reported BWT outcomes on 28 BWT patients from SIOP-9. Although therapy was individualized, all 28 patients with BWT were treated with preoperative therapy. Only three were anaplastic histology. Survival was 85.1 % for those with low-risk histology (95 % CI 71.6–98.6 %; four deaths, 2/3 anaplastics) and relapse-free survival 80.5 % (95 % CI 65.2–95.8 %; five relapses) (Weirich et al. 2004). The most recent survival for the 158 patients treated on NWTS-5 with BWT was 61 %, 80.8 % with favorable histology, and 43.8 % for a child with anaplastic histology. Data from SIOP 9301 compared bilateral partial nephrectomy with other resections used (mainly unilateral partial + total) and showed no decrease in survival in patients submitted to partial nephrectomy on both sides, although these comparisons are difficult due to possibly different extents of tumors in each group. Thus, the suggestion – do bilateral partial nephrectomy whenever "oncologically" possible – seems justified. It also reinforces the need for formal studies of BWT patients (Godzinski J, 2010, Results of surgery for bilateral Wilms tumors from SIOP 9301. Ehrlich PF, personal communication).

In addition to survival, renal failure is a major concern for patients with BWT. Factors that contribute to renal failure include progressive renal disease related to a genetic predisposition, inadequate renal parenchyma after one or more tumor resections, the nephrotoxic effects of chemotherapy and radiation, and the potential for hyperfiltration injury to the remaining renal parenchyma (Breslow et al. 2005; Feusner et al. 2008; Ritchey et al. 1996). In UKCCSG study BWT patients treated between 1980 and 1995, renal function (at follow-up) was normal in 80 % of the patients. Renal mass was 45 and 35 % in the conservatively treated and initial resection groups, respectively, with a trend toward better preservation in those treated conservatively (Kumar et al. 1998). The SIOP studies have reported renal failure in 3.8 % of all patients. A specific evaluation of stage V patients is currently being prepared. On NWTS-1–4 BWT was the greatest risk factor for renal failure (16.4 % for NWTS-1 and -2, 9.9 % for NWTS-3, and 3.8 % for NWTS-4). Other risk factors identified were: Denys-Drash syndrome, progressive tumor in the remaining kidney, and radiation nephritis (Ritchey et al. 1996). Breslow reported 20-year end-stage renal disease (ESRD) outcomes in children treated for WT (Breslow et al. 2005). Fifty-five of 379 (14.5 %) of patients with BWT developed ESRD at 20 years. The incidence of ESRD after diagnosis of bilateral Wilms' tumor was 50 % for the Denys-Drash syndrome (6 patients), 90 % for WAGR (10), 25 % for genito-urinary anomalies (25), and 11.5 % for BWT alone. Thus, preservation of renal tissue without sacrificing long-term survival is of particular importance for those with BWT.

A major factor contributing to the suboptimal outcomes for children with BWT has been lack of a formal clinical trial. This has produced a variability of treatment schemes, many with prolonged and intensified therapy. In July 2009, the COG opened the first BWT study ARENO534 – Treatment for Patients with Bilateral, Multicentric, or Bilaterally-Predisposed Unilateral Wilms' Tumor. However, results from this study will not be known for some time.

Prolongation and intensification of therapy may increase the risks of treatment-related complications and may provide the opportunity for metastasis. Shamberger et al. reviewed and highlighted the pitfalls of continued therapy in a study of progressive or nonresponsive disease (PNRD) in 38 children with BWT. (Shamberger et al. 2006) Of the 38, chemotherapy was given for a median of 7 months (range: 2–29 months) before definitive resection. Thirty-six children went on to a second regimen, and of these, 21 children received a third regimen before resection. Eleven patients received radiation to one or both kidneys. Pathology at resection revealed previously undiagnosed anaplasia in 3 patients (2 diffuse and 1 focal) treated for 14, 15, and 15 months before resection. A fourth patient developed a diffusely anaplastic tumor 13 months after therapy.

Tumor volume may not change after chemotherapy due to tumor differentiation or anaplastic tumor histology (Weirich et al. 2001; Boccon-Gibod et al. 2000; Zuppan et al. 1988). Chemotherapy can result in tumor necrosis, rhabdomyomatous differentiation, or mature stromal differentiation without significant changes in tumor size. Despite not responding to chemotherapy, children with these differentiated tumors with limited mitotic activity have good outcomes (Anderson et al. 2002). Therefore, tumors with limited mitotic activity may have minimal shrinkage with continued therapy and are best served with resection. Anaplastic tumors also respond poorly to chemotherapy. Furthermore, discordant pathology can be seen in children with BWT, and this may result in one kidney responding to chemotherapy and the other does not (Kumar et al. 1998; Dome et al. 2006b; Green et al. 1994a; Hamilton et al. 2006) Therefore, continuing therapy without reevaluating tumor pathology in both kidneys in a patient with BWT seems counterproductive. Figure 11.8 shows a case of progressive disease in a child with BWT despite prolonged chemotherapy. The pathology in this case was stromal predominant.

In both the current COG ARENO534 study and the SIOP guidelines, surgery occurs after a maximum of 12 weeks of chemotherapy. These observations highlight the issue of drawn-out therapy without response but also raise the question about how long therapy should be considered prior to biopsy or a definitive resection. Results from SIOP-9 help answer this question: patients with unilateral tumors were randomized to receive either 4 or 8 weeks of actinomycin and vincristine preoperatively. There was a 48 % reduction in tumor volume after 4 weeks that increased to 62 % after 8 weeks of chemotherapy (Tournade et al. 2001; Graf et al. 2000).

11.16 Surgical Considerations for Patients with Bilateral Wilms' Tumor

11.16.1 Renal Biopsies

Upfront biopsy of children with BWT may not be necessary before starting chemotherapy but renal biopsies play an important role in direct therapy, especially in those tumors which are nonresponsive. When considering tissue samples in children with bilateral tumors, the biopsies should be done from each kidney due to the high rate of discordant pathology (Hamilton et al. 2006). One of the reasons to perform a biopsy is to detect anaplastic tumors. This can be difficult and is often missed on percutaneous or core biopsies;

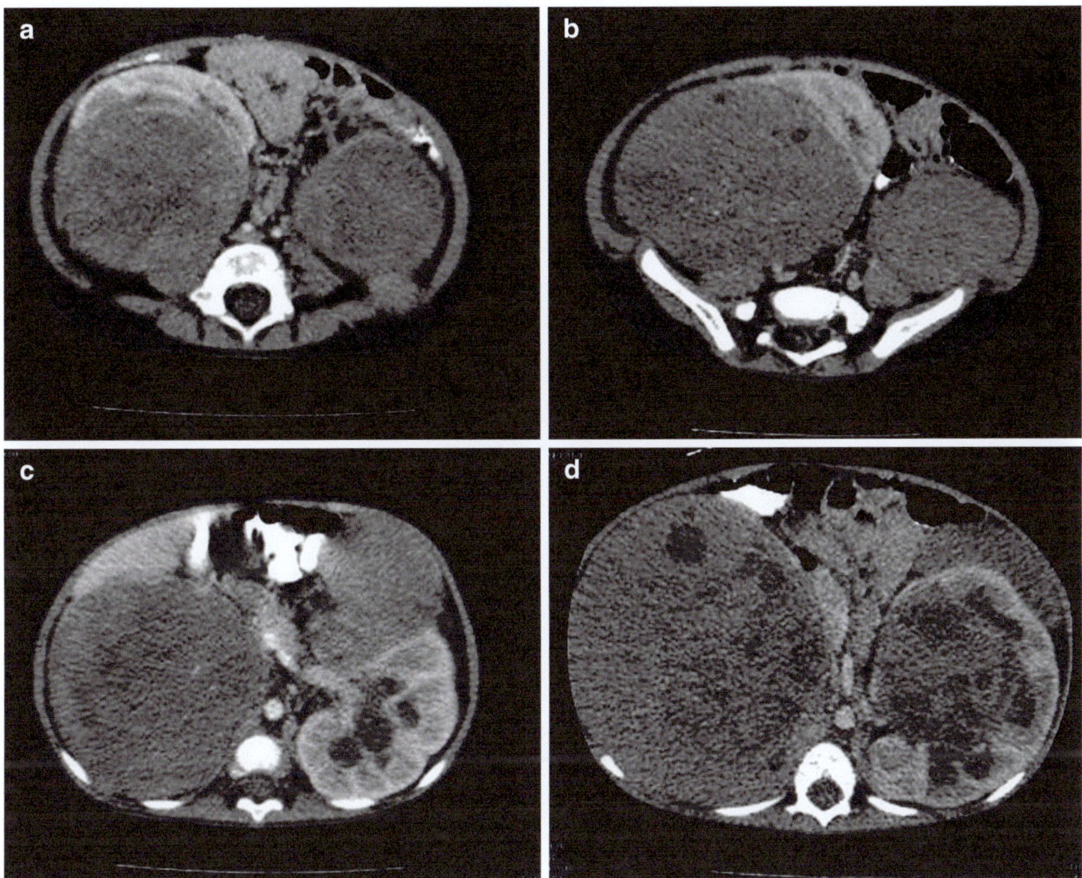

Fig. 11.8 (**a**, **b**) Computed tomography scans at presentation of a 1.5-year-old girl with aniridia and bilateral Wilms' tumor. (**c**, **d**) Comparison computed tomography scans after 8 weeks of chemotherapy demonstrating no response to therapy but pathology showed a stromal variant

thus a formal open biopsy is preferred in the COG protocol. (Hamilton et al. 2006) After 12 weeks of therapy both COG and SIOP option is to force resection rather than perform open biopsy in stage V nonresponsive cases.

11.16.2 Renal-Sparing Surgery

Despite the variability of treatment approaches, nephron-sparing surgery is an important consideration for all children with BWT. Both SIOP and COG agree that preoperative chemotherapy is the best first line of treatment for BWT followed by renal-sparing surgery. The two exceptions are those with extensive tumor thrombus that does not respond to therapy and patients with anaplastic histology where clear margins cannot be obtained. In patients with anaplastic histology where clear margins cannot be obtained with a partial nephrectomy, a complete nephrectomy is required. Anaplastic histology in BWT is difficult to diagnosis, and with preoperative chemotherapy, the pathology variant is usually unknown at surgery (Hamilton et al. 2006). This illustrates how crucial is correct planning of every nephron-sparing resection.

Preoperative imaging is valuable to help plan the operation. Three-dimensional computed tomography or MRI reconstructions are extremely useful in planning the operation. In addition, intraoperative ultrasound can be very helpful. Although by imaging large lesions may appear unresectable, they may just be

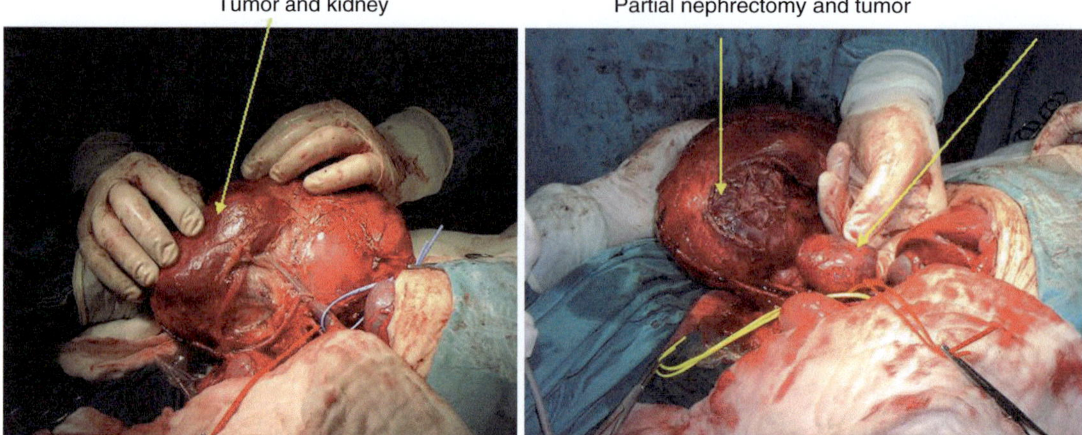

Fig. 11.9 Operative photographs of a patient with bilateral Wilms' tumor undergoing a partial nephrectomy. Spared part of the kidney (*Yellow arrow*)

compressing adjacent normal kidney where substantially more viable renal parenchyma exists than may have been anticipated by the preoperative imaging studies. This situation argues for attempting nephron-sparing surgery for all lesions (Ritchey 2008; Cozzi and Zani 2006; Davidoff et al. 2008). Figure 11.9 shows an example of partial nonanatomic renal resection.

Once the tumor is removed, the kidney volume can appear remarkably normal as these patients are followed over time. Atypical resections and unconventional tumor resections of localized lesions have also salvaged several kidneys that would have been sacrificed by traditional criteria. An interesting and promising technique of nephron-sparing resection for tumors extending to the renal hilum was proposed by Joerg Fuchs (Fuchs et al. 2009b). The technique included transection of the kidney and tumor resection performed longitudinally followed by extensive reconstruction of pyelon. Surgery was performed in vascular exclusion of the kidney and extrarenal cooling. All 5 reported cases were in CR for mean follow-up of 26.6 months (3.5–66) (Fuchs et al. 2009b).

Several different renal preservation strategies have been described and can be considered depending on the extent of resection and the location of the tumor. Clamping of the renal artery is safe with warm ischemia for approximately a half hour. Surface cooling with ice slush allows an hour of safe occlusion of renal artery. However, the layer of ice that must be packed around the kidney can interfere with the technical aspects of the surgery. Continuous in situ cold perfusion with solutions, which are in common use during organ transplantation, has also been reported in a patient with multifocal BWT. (Cozzi and Zani 2006; De Backer et al. 1995) However, the arteriotomy and the venotomy that are needed for in situ perfusion increase the risk of renal artery thrombosis and/or tumor spillage from the renal vein. Cases using ex vivo tumor dissection followed by autotransplantation in an attempt to preserve functioning renal tissue have also been described (Desai et al. 1999). In many instances, temporary vascular occlusion is not required.

The peritoneal cavity is entered through a standard transverse upper abdominal incision. Any suspicious lesion should be biopsied and frozen section obtained prior to starting the kidney resection. The kidney should be mobilized completely and elevated on its vascular pedicle without traction as it can result in vascular thrombosis, especially in very young patients. In most cases, identification of the lesions is relatively easy. If there is some concern, intraoperative ultrasound is useful. After lesions to be excised are identified, the capsule of the kidney is scored with electrocautery to outline the planned extent of resection. The most difficult lesions are those located near the hilum. A rim of normal kidney (~1 cm) should be taken around the lesion when possible.

Hemostasis in most cases can be achieved with electrocautery and digital compression but can be assisted by a ligature, harmonic scalpel, or argon-beam coagulation. Surgicel™ or another procoagulant is also helpful in maintaining hemostasis (Johnson and Johnson 2009). It is very important to remember to remove regional lymph nodes from each kidney to obtain accurate staging data, as each kidney is staged independently.

Injecting a dilute solution of methylene blue into the renal pelvis after temporarily occluding the ureter will help visualize defects in the collecting system after resection. Some leaks may benefit from placement of a double J stent. The decision to place a ureteral stent is based on the degree of disruption of the collecting system and the complexity of its closure. An open, rather than a closed, suction drain is commonly placed in surgical resection site, but this is primarily a surgeon preference issue. Closing the renal defect can often be difficult in a kidney that has been pretreated with chemotherapy as they are much less pliable than normal kidney. Perirenal fat, omentum, or oxidized cellulose can help close the renal defect.

In rare circumstances, enucleation of the tumor is possible to preserve renal function. This is only for patients with favorable histology Wilms' tumor. A problem with tumor enucleation is an unrecognized pseudocapsule penetration and spill (Green et al. 1994b; Green 1997). Furthermore, enucleation increases the risk of local tumor spillage.

Early complications from partial nephrectomy include urine leaks, pyelonephritis, renal failure, and positive surgical margins. Delayed complications have included bowel obstructions, hydronephrosis, and scar tissue causing an ureteropelvic junction obstruction and end-stage renal disease (Davidoff et al. 2008).

References

Anderson J, Slater O, McHugh K et al (2002) Response without shrinkage in bilateral Wilms tumor: significance of rhabdomyomatous histiology. J Pediatr Hematol Oncol 24:31–34

Blute ML, Kelais PP, Offord KP et al (1987) Bilateral Wilms tumor. J Urol 138:968–973

Boccon-Gibod L, Rey A, Sandstedt B et al (2000) Complete necrosis induced by preoperative chemotherapy in Wilms tumor as an indicator of low risk: report from the International Society of Pediatric Oncology(SIOP) Nephroblastoma Trial and Study 9. Med Pediatr Oncol 34:190

Breslow N, Olshan A, Beckwith JB, Green DM (1993) Epidemiology of Wilms tumor. Med Pediatr Oncol 21:172–181

Breslow N, Collins AJ, Ritchey ML et al (2005) End stage renal failure in patients with Wilms tumor: results from the national wilms tumor study group and the United States renal data system. J Urol 174:1972–1975

Brisse H, Schleiermacher G, Helfe S (2006) Evaluation of 61 nephroblastoma patients with clinical and/or radiological sign of tumor rupture- a single institution study. Pediatr Blood Cancer 47:364

Coppes MJ, de Kraker J, van Dijken PJ (1989) Bilateral Wilms' tumor: long-term survival and some epidemiological features. J Clin Oncol 7:310–315

Coppes MJ, Beckwith JB, Ritchey ML, D'Angio GJ, Green DM, Breslow N (1999) Factors affecting the risk of contralateral wilms tumor development (A report from the national Wilms tumor study group). Cancer 85:1616–1625

Cozzi DA, Zani A (2006) Nephron-sparing surgery in children with primary renal tumor: indications and results. Semin Pediatr Surg 15:3–9

D'Angio GJ, Evans AE, Breslow N, Beckwith JB et al (1976) The treatment of Wilms' tumor. Cancer 38:633–646

D'Angio GJ, Breslow N, Beckwith JB et al (1989) Treatment of Wilms' tumor. Results of the Third National Wilms' Tumor Study. Cancer 64:360

Davidoff AM, Giel GW, Jones DP et al (2008) The feasibility and outcome of nephron-sparing surgery for children with bilateral Wilms tumor. The St Jude Children's Research Hospital experience: 1999–2006. Cancer 112:2060

De Backer A, Lamote J, Keuppens F et al (1995) Bilateral Wilms' tumor: in situ cooling of the kidney facilitates curative excision of tumors, with preservation of renal function. J Pediatr Surg 30:1338–1340

de Kraker J, Lemerle J, Voute PA et al (1990) Wilms tumor with pulmonary metastases at diagnosis: the significance of primary chemotherapy. J Clin Oncol 8:1187–1190

de Kraker J, Tournade MF, Weirich A et al (1997) Wilms tumour stage IV. A report from the SIOP-9 study. Med Pediatr Oncol 29:370

de Kraker J, Delemarre JF, Lilien MR, Tournade MF (1999) Misstaging in nephroblastoma. causes and consequences. A report of the sixth nephroblastoma trial and study of the International Society of Paediatric Oncology. Eur J Pediatr Surg 9(3):153–157

de Kraker J, Graf N, Pein F et al (2001) Society of international paediatric oncology (SIOP) Wilms tumor protocol http://web.visu.uni-saarland.de/rtsg/

Desai D, Nicholls G, Duffy PG (1999) Bench surgery with autotransplantation for bilateral synchronous

Wilms tumor: a report of three cases. J Pediatr Surg 34(4):632–634

Dome JS, Perlman EJ, Ritchey ML, Coppes MJ, Kalapurakal J, Grundy PE (2006a) Renal tumors. In: Pizzo PA, Poplack DG (eds) Principles and practice of pediatric oncology. Lippincott Williams and Wilkins, Philadelphia, pp 905–932

Dome JS, Cotton CA, Perlman EJ (2006b) Treatment of anaplastic histology Wilms' tumor: results from the fifth National Wilms' Tumor Study. J Clin Oncol 24:2352–2358

Ehrlich PF (2001) Wilms tumor: progress to date and future considerations. Expert Rev Anticancer Ther 1(4):555–564

Ehrlich PF (2007a) Wilms tumor: progress and considerations for the surgeon. Surg Oncol 16:157–171

Ehrlich PF (2007b) Re: Intracaval and intracardiac extension of Wilms' tumor. The influence of preoperative chemotherapy on surgical morbidity. Int Braz J Urol 33:847–848

Ehrlich PF, Ritchey ML, Hamilton TE et al (2005) Quality assessment for Wilms' tumor: a report from the National Wilms' Tumor Study-5. J Pediatr Surg 40:208–212

Ehrlich PF, Hamilton TE, Grundy PE et al (2006) The value of surgery in directing therapy of Wilms tumor patients with pulmonary disease. A Report From The National Wilms Tumor Study Group (NWTS –5). J Pediatr Surg 41:162–167

Ehrlich PF, Ferrer F, Ritchey ML et al (2009) Hepatic metastasis at diagnosis in patients with Wilms tumor is not an independent adverse prognostic factor for stage iv Wilms tumor. A report from the children's oncology group/national wilms. Ann Surg 250:642–648

Ehrlich PF, Anderson JR, Ritchey ML et al (2013) Clinicopathologic findings predictive of relapse in children with stage III favorable-histology Wilms tumor. J Clin Oncol 20;31(9):1196–1201

Feusner JH, Ritchey ML, Norkool PA (2008) Renal failure does not preclude cure in children receiving chemotherapy for Wilms tumor: a report from the National Wilms Tumor Study Group. Pediatr Blood Cancer 50:242–245

Fuchs J, Szavay P, Luithle T et al (2008) Surgical implications for liver metastasis in nephroblastoma- data from the SIOP/GPOH study. Surg Oncol 17:33–40

Fuchs J, Kienecker K, Furtwängler R (2009a) Surgical aspects in the treatment of patients with unilateral wilms tumor: a report from the SIOP 93-01/German Society of Pediatric Oncology and Hematology. Ann Surg 249:666–671

Fuchs J, Szavay P, Scheel-Walter H et al (2009b) Longitudinal partial nephrectomy for stage V nephroblastoma with extension into the renal hilus. Pediatr Blood Cancer 53:715–716

Gentil Martins A, Espana M (1989) Partial nephrectomy for nephroblastoma – a plea for less radical surgery. Med Pediatr Oncol 17:320

Godzinski J, Tournade MF, de Kraker J et al (1991) Stage IV nephroblastoma with extra pulmonary metastatic involvement in the SIOP 6 and 9 Study. Med Pediatr Oncol 19:371

Godzinski J, Tournade MF, de Kraker J, Lemerle J, Voute PA (1998) Rarity of surgical complications after postchemotherapy nephrectomy for nephroblastoma. Experience of the International Society of Paediatric Oncology-Trial and study "SIOP-9". International Society of Paediatric Oncology Nephroblastoma Trial and Study Committee. Eur J Pediatr Surg 8(2): 83–86

Godzinski J, Tournade MF, de Kraker J et al (1999) The role of preoperative chemotherapy in the treatment of nephroblastoma -the SIOP experience. Semin Urol Oncol 17:28–32

Godzinski J, de Kraker J, Weirich A et al (2001) Local treatment for extrapulmonary metastases in the SIOP-9 initial stage IV Wilms' tumour patients. Med Pediatr Oncol 37:338

Godzinski J, Heij H, Cecchetto G et al (2005) Does pretreatment tumor rupture influence the outcome in patients with nephroblastoma submitted to preoperative chemotherapy. Pediatr Blood Cancer 45:387

Graf N, Tournade MF, de Kraker J (2000) The role of preoperative chemotherapy in the management of Wilms tumor. The SIOP studies. Urol Clin North Am 443–454

Green DM (1997) Enucleative surgery for stage I nephroblastoma with a normal contralateral kidney. J Urol 185:548–549

Green DM (2002) Use of chest computed tomography for staging and treatment of Wilms' tumor in children. J Clin Oncol 20:2763–2764

Green DM, Breslow N, D'Angio GJ et al (1993) The treatment of children with unilateral Wilms' tumor. J Clin Oncol 11:1009–1010

Green DM, Beckwith JB, Breslow N et al (1994a) Treatment of children with stages II to IV anaplastic Wilms Tumor : a report from the National Wilms' Tumor Study Group. J Clin Oncol 12:2126–2131

Green DM, Beckwith JB, Weeks D et al (1994b) The relationship between microsubstaging variables, age at diagnosis, and tumor weight of children with stage I/ favorable histology Wilms' tumor. A report from the National Wilms' Tumor study. Cancer 74:1820

Gross R (1953) Embryoma of the kidney (Wilms tumor). In: Gross R (ed) The surgery of infancy and childhood. WB Saunders, Philadelphia, pp 588–605

Grundy PE, Perlman EJ, Ehrlich PF et al (2005) Current issues in Wilms tumor management. Curr Probl Cancer 29:221–260

Grundy PE, Dome JD, Perlman EJ et al (2006) Renal tumors classification, biology, and banking study. https://members.childrensoncologygroup.org/Prot/AREN03B2/AREN03B2DOC.pdf

Grundy PE, Dome JS, Ehrlich PF (2007) Renal tumors classification, biology and banking studies. https://members.childrensoncologygroup.org/Prot/AREN03B2/AREN03B2DOC.pdf, pp 18–33

Hamilton TE, Green DM, Perlman EJ et al (2006) Bilateral Wilms' tumor with anaplasia: lessons from the National Wilms' Tumor Study. J Pediatr Surg 41:1641–1644

Herrera JM, Gauthier F, Tournade MF et al (1996) Bilateral synchronous Wilms' tumour (WT): is it a good model of conservative surgery for unilateral WT? Med Pediatr Oncol 27:219

Johnson and Johnson. Surgicel (2009) http://www.jnj.com/connect/

Kalapurakal JA, Dome JS, Perlman EJ, Malogolowkin M, Haase GM, Grundy PE, Coppes MJ (2004) Management of Wilms' tumour: current practice and future goals. Lancet Oncol 5:37–46

Kalapurakal JA, Li SM, Breslow N et al (2010) Intraoperative spillage of favorable histology Wilms tumor cells: influence of irradiation and chemotherapy regimens on abdominal recurrence. A report from the National Wilms Tumor Study Group. Int J Radiat Oncol Biol Phys 76:201–206

Kaste S, Dome JS, Babyn PS et al (2008) Wilms Tumor :prognostic factors, staging, therapy and late effects. Pediatr Radiol 38:2–17

Kumar R, Fitzgerald R, Breatnach F (1998) Conservative surgical management of bilateral wilms tumor: results of the United Kingdom children's cancer study group. J Urol 160:1450–1453

Kung FH, Nyhan WL (1982) Wilms tumor. In: Holland JF, Frei E (eds) Cancer medicine. Lea and Feiger, Philadelphia, pp 2181–2192

Ladd WE (1938) Embryoma of the kidney (Wilms' tumor). Ann Surg 108:885–902

Lemerle J, Voute PA, Tournade MF (1983) Effectiveness of preoperative chemotherapy in Wilms' tumor: results of an international society of pediatric oncology (SIOP) clinical trial. J Clin Oncol 1:604–609

Malogolowkin M, Cotton CA, Green DM et al (2008) Treatment of Wilms tumor relapsing after initial treatment with vincristine, actinomycin D, and doxorubicin. A report from the National Wilms Tumor Study Group. Pediatr Blood Cancer 50:236–241

Mankowski P, Godzinski J, Jankowski A et al (2004) Minimal invasive pulmonary metastasectomy in stage IV malignancies in children. Pediatr Blood Cancer 43:334–335

Mitchell C, Pritchard-Jones K, Shannon R (2006) Immediate nephrectomy versus preoperative chemotherapy in the management of non-metastatic Wilms' tumour: results of a randomised trial (UKW3) by the UK Children's Cancer Study Group. Eur J Cancer 42:2554–2562

Moorman-Voestermans CGM, Staalman CR, Delamarre JFM (1994) Partial nephrectomy in unilateral Wilms' tumour is feasible without local recurrence. Med Pediatr Oncol 23:218

Moorman-Voestermans CGM, Aronson DE, Staalman CR et al (1998) Is partial nephrectomy appropriate treatment for unilateral Wilms' tumour? J Pediatr Surg 33:165–170

Othersen HB, Delorimier A, Hrabovsky E, Kelalis P, Breslow N, D'Angio GJ (1990) Surgical evaluation of lymph node metastases in Wilms tumor. J Pediatr Surg 25:330–331

Othersen HB, Hebra A, Tagge E (1999) Nephroblastoma and other renal tumors. In: Grosfeld JL (ed) The surgery of childhood tumors. Arnold, Philadelphia, pp 107–139

Owens CM, Veys PA, Pritchard J et al (2002) Role of chest computed tomography at diagnosis in the management of Wilms' tumor: a study by the United Kingdom Children's Cancer Study Group. J Clin Oncol 20:2768–2773

Paulino AC, Wilimas J, Marina N et al (1996) Local Control in synchronous bilateral wilms tumor. Int J Radiat Oncol Biol Phys 36:541–548

Petruzzi MJ, Green DM (1997) Wilms tumor. Pediatr Clin North Am 44:939–952

Ritchey ML (1999) The role of preoperative chemotherapy for Wilms tumor; the NWTSG perspective. Semin Urol Oncol 17(1):21–27

Ritchey ML (2005) Renal sparing surgery for Wilms tumor. J Urol 174:1172–1173

Ritchey ML (2008) Renal sparing surgery for children with bilateral Wilms tumor. Cancer 112:1877–1878

Ritchey ML, Kelalis P, Breslow N et al (1992a) Surgical complications after nephrectomy for Wilms tumor. Surg Gynecol Obstet 175:514

Ritchey ML, Lally KP, Haase GM et al (1992b) Superior mesenteric artery injury during nephrectomy for Wilms' tumor. J Pediatr Surg 27:612–615

Ritchey ML, Kelalis P, Haase G (1993) Preoperative therapy for intracaval and atrial extension of Wilms tumor. Cancer 71:4104–4110

Ritchey ML, Pringle K, Breslow N (1994) Management and outcome of inoperable Wilms tumor: a report of the national Wilms tumor study group. Ann Surg 220:683–690

Ritchey ML, Green DM, Breslow N (1995) Accuracy of current imaging modalities in the diagnosis of synchronous bilateral Wilms tumor. A report from the National Wilms' Tumor Study Group. Cancer 75:600–604

Ritchey ML, Green DM, Thomas PRM (1996) Renal failure in Wilms tumor patients: a report from the National Wilms Tumor Study Group. Med Pediatr Oncol 26:75

Ritchey ML, Shamberger RC, Haase G, Horwitz J, Bergemann TL (2001) Surgical complications after primary nephrectomy for Wilms' tumor: report from the National Wilms' Tumor Study Group. J Am Coll Surg 192:63–68

Ritchey ML, Shamberger RC, Hamilton TE, Haase G (2005) Fate of bilateral renal lesions missed on preoperative imaging: a report from the National Wilms Tumor Study Group. J Urol 174:1519–1521

Ritchey ML, Daley S, Shamberger RC et al (2008) Ureteral extension in Wilms' tumor: a report from the National Wilms' Tumor Study Group (NWTSG). J Pediatr Surg 43:1625–1629

Schenk JP, Schrader C, Zieger B et al (2006) Reference radiology in nephroblastoma: accuracy and relevance for preoperative chemotherapy. Rofo 178:38–45

Shamberger RC, Guthrie KA, Ritchey ML, Haase G, Taskashima BA, Beckwith JB, D'Angio GJ, Green

DM, Breslow N (1999) Surgery related factors and local recurrence of Wilms tumor in the national Wilms tumor study 4. Ann Surg 229:292–297

Shamberger RC, Ritchey ML, Haase G, Bergemann TL, Loechelt-Yoshioka T, Breslow N, Green DM (2001) Intravascular extension of Wilms tumor. Ann Surg 234(1):116–121

Shamberger RC, Haase GM, Argani P (2006) Bilateral Wilms' tumors with progressive or nonresponsive disease. J Pediatr Surg 41:642–657

Shearer P, Parham DM, Fontanesi J et al (1993) Bilateral Wilms tumor. Review of Outcome, associated anomalies and late effects in 36 patients treated at a single institution. Cancer 72:1422–1426

Szavay P, Luithle T, Graf N (2006) Primary hepatic metastases in nephroblastoma–a report of the SIOP/GPOH Study. J Pediatr Surg 41:168–172

Tournade MF, Com-Nougue C, Voute PA, Lemerle J, de Kraker J (1993) Results of the sixth International Society of Pediatric Oncology Wilms' tumor trial and study: a risk-adapted therapeutic approach in Wilms' tumor. J Clin Oncol 11(6):1014–1023

Tournade MF, Com-Nougue C, de Kraker J et al (2001) Optimal duration of preoperative chemotherapy in unilateral non metastatic Wilms tumor in children older than six months. Results of the ninth International Society of Pediatric Oncology tumor trial. J Clin Oncol 19:488–500

Varan A, Büyükpamukçu N, Caglar M (2005) Prognostic significance of metastatic site at diagnosis in Wilms' tumor: results from a single center. J Pediatr Hematol Oncol 27:188–191

Vujanic G, Sandstedt B, Kelsey A, Sebire NJ (2009) Central pathology review in multicenter trials and studies: lessons from the nephroblastoma trials. Cancer 115:1977–1983

Warmann S, Nourkami N, Seitz G et al (2009) Lung metastases in children with Wilms' tumor: data from SIOP9, SIOP 93–01, and SIOP 2001/GPOH. Pediatr Blood Cancer 53(5):753

Weirich A, Leuschner I, Harms D et al (2001) Clinical impact of histologic subtypes in localized non-anaplastic nephroblastoma treated according to the trial and study SIOP-9/GPOH. Ann Oncol 12:311–319

Weirich A, Ludwig R, Graf N (2004) Survival in nephroblastoma treated according to the trial and study SIOP-9/GPOH with respect to relapse and morbidity. Ann Oncol 15(5):808–820:5–808

Willets IE (2003) Jessop and the Wilms tumor. J Pediatr Surg 38:1496–1498

Wilms M (1897) Diagnostischer und therapeutischer Werth der Lumbalpunction. Druckbestimmung mit Quicksilvermanometer. Munch Med Wochenschr 3:53–57

Wilms M (1899) Die Mischgeschwülste der Niere. Verlag von Arthur Georgi, Leipzig

Zuppan CW, Beckwith JB, Luckey DW (1988) Anaplasia in unilateral Wilms tumor. A report from the National Wilms Tumor Study Pathology Center. Hum Pathol 19:1199–1209

12 Radiotherapy for Wilms' Tumor and Other Childhood Renal Cancers

Mark N. Gaze and John A. Kalapurakal

Contents

M.N. Gaze, MD, FRCP, FRCR (✉)
University College London Hospitals
and Great Ormond Street Hospital for Children
NHS Foundation Trusts, London, UK
e-mail: mark.gaze@uclh.nhs.uk

J.A. Kalapurakal, MD
Radiation Oncology, Northwestern University
Feinberg School of Medicine Chicago,
Illinois 60611, USA
e-mail: j-kalapurakal@northwestern.edu

K. Pritchard-Jones, J.S. Dome (eds.), *Renal Tumors of Childhood: Biology and Therapy*, Pediatric Oncology,
DOI 10.1007/978-3-662-44003-2_12, © Springer-Verlag Berlin Heidelberg 2014

Abstract

Radiation therapy continues to play an important role in the multi-modality management of Wilms' tumor, the commonest renal cancer of childhood. Following clinical trials conducted in both Europe, by the International Society of Paediatric Oncology (SIOP) Renal Tumors Group and other organisations, and North America, by the National Wilms' Tumor Study (NWTS), the approach taken to radiotherapy for Wilms' tumor has been modified over time. Successive trials have refined the indications for radiation therapy, for example, in NWTS-1, the majority of children received flank irradiation with doses ranging from 18 Gy in babies to as high as 40 Gy in older patients, whereas now, only 25–30 % of children receive irradiation and to a much lower dose of 10 Gy irrespective of patient's age.

The NWTS treatment strategy for Wilms' tumor has been to perform upfront, radical nephrectomy whenever possible after initial clinical evaluation and diagnostic staging with computed tomography (CT) and ultrasound scanning. This approach without any preoperative therapy facilitates the adoption of a risk-adapted multi-modality treatment based upon a combination of factors that includes age, tumor weight, tumor staging, pathological classification and molecular prognostic factors. The radiation therapy guidelines of the Children's Oncology Group (COG) are based on the results of the NWTS protocols.

In Europe and countries taking part in SIOP protocols, preoperative chemotherapy is the norm. Radiotherapy is given: as part of initial multi-modality therapy to only a minority of patients, carefully selected on the basis of post-chemotherapy, postoperative staging and pathology; or as part of relapse treatment. Radiation doses are, as in COG protocols, lower now than were used historically. As a result of careful risk assessment, and intensification of systemic treatment for the highest risk patients, survival rates are better than before, despite the reduction in the use of radiotherapy. The incidence and severity of late effects expected in currently treated patients are less than in those treated historically, as a result of the reduction in the use of radiotherapy, the lower doses used and refinements in radiotherapy planning and delivery.

The past decade has witnessed several technological developments in radiation delivery systems and treatment planning software that has enabled the use of CT or magnetic resonance imaging (MRI)-based three-dimensional treatment planning in most modern Wilms' tumor protocols. These advances have resulted in more accurate tumor targeting and superior protection of normal tissues. Presently, research is being conducted to explore the role of newer technologies like intensity-modulated radiation therapy (IMRT) and proton therapy in primary and metastatic Wilms' tumors.

The role of radiotherapy in non-Wilms' childhood renal cancers is also briefly reviewed in this chapter.

12.1 Introduction

Radiotherapy has been an important component of multi-modality therapy for kidney cancers in children and young people for more than half a century. Collaborative multicentre research groups include the National Wilms' Tumor Study (NWTS), now part of the Children's Oncology Group (COG), and the International Society for Paediatric Oncology (SIOP) and have carried out sequential clinical trials over most of that period. As a consequence, outcomes for children with Wilms' tumor have improved significantly. For example, a population-based study of 2,697 children with Wilms' tumor in Europe showed that the 5-year survival rate increased from 78.9 % in 1983–1985 to 84.65 in 1992–1994 (Gatta et al. 2005). A better understanding of the biology and natural history of the diseases, coupled with advances in imaging and pathology, has allowed risk stratification. This has enabled the avoidance of radiotherapy, and importantly the associated treatment related morbidity, in those patients where radiotherapy may not contribute to an increased chance of survival. Evidence from these clinical trials has also made it possible to reduce the dose of radiation administered to those patients who still need it. Technical advances in the planning and delivery of radiation therapy have enabled more accurate and individualised treatment and helped to diminish morbidity further.

While the prospects for cure are similar across the world, treatment philosophies differ. In North America and areas influenced by the NWTS, primary nephrectomy with risk-adapted adjuvant treatment selected on the basis of pathology and surgical staging is still the management plan of choice in most cases. In Europe and countries influenced by SIOP, preoperative chemotherapy is preferred, with risk-adapted postoperative treatment based on the response to chemotherapy, pathological subtype and extent of disease at the time of operation. The current treatment recommendations in both America and Europe are not based on insular prejudice but have been formulated in the light of all available evidence, and there is a continuing dialogue between members of the different schools of thought. In this chapter, the key points from the principal North American and European trials have been reviewed, but not every trial has been mentioned. Except where otherwise stated, treatments and data relate to Wilms' tumor, and not to non-Wilms' renal tumors.

Table 12.1 Principal indications for radiotherapy in Wilms' tumor

1. Loco-regional disease	Reduction of risk of local recurrence
	Improved probability of cure
2. Metastatic disease	Control of lung metastases which have not responded well to initial chemotherapy
	Control of metastases at other sites, most commonly liver
3. Relapsed disease	Part of multi-modality salvage strategy

There are three main indications for radiotherapy in Wilms' tumor (Table 12.1). Firstly, to reduced the likelihood of local or loco-regional recurrence and improve the prospects for survival in patients with locally advanced disease. This includes both those with disease limited to the renal area, including adjacent involved lymph nodes, who receive flank irradiation, and also those with disease which has spread through the peritoneal cavity who require whole abdominal and pelvic radiotherapy. Both these groups would be regarded as stage III disease, which is quite a heterogeneous category. Secondly, radiotherapy is indicated in some patients with haematogenous spread at the time of diagnosis. These most commonly have pulmonary metastases, for which whole-lung irradiation is required if there is not a rapid complete response to chemotherapy. Finally, with radiotherapy forming part of the initial management protocol in only a minority of patients, irradiation may be required as part of the salvage strategy for relapsed patients.

12.2 Evidence from Studies on Radiotherapy in Wilms' Tumor

12.2.1 Radiotherapy for Local Control: The North American Experience

12.2.1.1 National Wilms' Tumor Study, Trial 1

In NWTS-1 (1969–1974), flank irradiation doses were age adjusted (birth to 18 months of age, 18–24 Gy; 18–30 months, 24–30 Gy; 31–40 months, 30–35 Gy; 41 months or older, 35–40 Gy). This study showed that flank irradiation was not necessary in group I patients younger than 2 years. However, based on the good survival outcomes in group II tumors receiving dactinomycin with vincristine without irradiation, it was postulated that postoperative vincristine with dactinomycin could substitute for postoperative irradiation with dactinomycin alone. No radiation dose–response relationship was observed for the doses ranging between 18 and 40 Gy. Delays of up to 10 days in initiating postoperative irradiation appeared acceptable. Whole-abdomen irradiation was not found to be necessary for localised tumor spills or for prior tumor biopsy. In these patients, flank radiotherapy fields were adequate (D'Angio et al. 1976, 1978; Tefft et al. 1976).

12.2.1.2 National Wilms' Tumor Study, Trial 2

In NWTS-2 (1974–1979), flank irradiation was given only in group II–IV tumors according to the age-adjusted regimen used in NWTS-1. There was no reduction in survival outcomes after omitting irradiation in group I tumors. The incidence of abdominal relapse in group 2 and 3 tumors was 4 %. Again no radiation therapy dose–response was observed. As in NWTS-1, the important prognostic factors were tumor histology and radiation therapy delay beyond 10 days after nephrectomy. Adriamycin added considerable benefit in groups II–III favourable histology tumors. The 2-year relapse-free survival rates were 88 % for group I, 78 % for group II, 70 % for group III and 49 % for group IV patients (D'Angio et al. 1981; Tefft et al. 1980).

12.2.1.3 National Wilms' Tumor Study, Trial 3

NWTS-3 (1979–1985) demonstrated that radiation therapy could also be safely omitted in stage II favourable histology tumors without compromising survival. The most significant contribution of this study was the successful reduction of the radiation dose in stage III tumors from the age-adjusted radiation dosing regimen (18–40 Gy) used in NWTS-1 and -2 to 10 Gy when given concurrently with vincristine, dactinomycin and doxorubicin. In stage III FH, 10 Gy was equivalent to 20 Gy with no difference in frequency of intra-abdominal relapse between these doses, although the trend favoured the use of doxorubicin with irradiation. The 2-year relapse-free and overall survival rates for NWTS-2 (82 and 89 %) and NWTS-3 (85 and 92 %) demonstrated that the improvements in survival were sustained in NWTS-3 despite targeted reduction in the intensity of therapy (Thomas et al. 1991; D'Angio et al. 1989).

12.2.1.4 National Wilms' Tumor Study, Trial 4

NWTS-4 (1986–1994) did not have any major radiation therapy questions in the study design. The flank or abdominal radiation dose was 10 Gy for stage III favourable histology tumors. Unfavourable histology tumors were treated according to the age-adjusted radiation dose regimen used in NWTS-1. This study established the pulse-intensive drug administration of chemotherapy as the new standard (Green et al. 1998).

12.2.1.5 National Wilms' Tumor Study, Trial 5

In NWTS-5 (1995–2001), the radiotherapy guidelines were similar to those used in NWTS-4 except for patients with anaplastic tumors for whom a dose of 10 Gy was recommended as compared to an age-adjusted schedule (18–40 Gy) used in NWTS 1-4. Patients with stage I anaplastic tumors were treated with actinomycin D and vincristine without irradiation. Patients with stage II–IV diffuse anaplastic histology were treated with regimen 'I' chemotherapy that consisted of vincristine, doxorubicin, cyclophosphamide and etoposide plus flank/abdominal radiation therapy. This study showed that the omission of radiation therapy and doxorubicin in patients with stage I anaplastic tumors resulted in inferior outcomes The 4-year event-free and overall survival for stage I anaplastic histology tumors were 70 and 83 % respectively. The 4-year event-free and overall survival in stage II, III and IV diffuse anaplastic tumors after immediate nephrectomy were 83 and 82 %, 65 and 67 % and 33 and 33 %, respectively (Dome et al. 2006). These results form the basis for the augmentation of therapy for anaplastic tumors in the current COG study.

12.2.1.6 Bilateral Wilms' Tumor

The goal of therapy in bilateral Wilms' tumor patients is to cure with maximal preservation of renal function. Radical nephrectomy should not be performed as part of the initial surgical procedure. The initial surgery should define the extent of tumors in each kidney and obtain biopsies from these tumors and suspicious lymph nodes. Subsequently, the child should be treated with chemotherapy in order to reduce the size of these tumors and facilitate nephron-sparing surgery at second-look surgery. Unpublished NWTS-3 and -4 data showed a 10-year relapse-free and overall survival of only 65 and 78 %, respectively. The factors that contributed to the poor outcomes were under-staging and/or under-treatment, delay in local tumor control with definitive surgical resection and increased incidence of anaplasia (Ritchey et al. 1996). Some centres have advocated parenchymal-sparing procedures in unilateral Wilms' tumors to reduce the risk of renal insufficiency. However, the overall incidence of renal failure following treatment in unilateral tumors is only 0.25 % (Shamberger et al. 2006). There are certain groups of children at higher risk for renal failure. Breslow et al. reported a 38 % risk of renal failure at a median of 14 years after diagnosis among certain subgroups like patients with WAGR and Denys–Drash syndromes (Breslow et al. 2000). Other groups of children that could benefit from renal parenchymal-sparing surgery are those at increased risk for development of metachronous WT such as those with aniridia and a number of overgrowth syndromes, e.g. Beckwith–Wiedemann Syndrome (BWS) and idiopathic hemihypertrophy (Coppes et al. 1999).

12.2.2 Radiotherapy for Local Control: The European Experience

12.2.2.1 Evaluation of Preoperative Therapy

The majority of European clinical trials for Wilms' tumor have not asked specific randomised questions about the place of radiotherapy. More commonly, there have been radiotherapy guidelines based on the available evidence, which have been refined from trial to trial in the light of experience and new data. The earliest studies addressed the place of preoperative therapy, initially radiotherapy and then chemotherapy. Subsequently, attempts were made to limit the use of radiotherapy through risk-adapted treatment strategies.

12.2.2.2 SIOP Nephroblastoma Study 1

The first SIOP trial, which recruited patients between 1971 and 1974, evaluated the role of preoperative radiotherapy (Lemerle et al. 1976). After the diagnosis of Wilms' tumor, 136 children were randomised either to receive preoperative radiotherapy to a dose of 20 Gy or to undergo primary nephrectomy. There was no significant difference in the likelihood of recurrence or the risk of death between the randomised arms. However, there was a major difference ($p=0.001$) in the risk of tumor rupture during surgery: this was seen in only 4 % of 73 irradiated patients but in 32 % of 63 patients who underwent operation without prior radiotherapy. Does the difference in rupture rate matter? Yes it does. Of the 19 ruptures seen in the initial surgery group, the majority, 11, were classed as massive ruptures with tumor spillage throughout the abdominal cavity. To reduce the risk of tumor regrowth, whole abdominal and pelvic radiotherapy, rather than just flank irradiation, was indicated in these patients. This is associated with a greater incidence of late effects, including subsequent infertility in the seven girls. In addition, although there was no difference in overall survival, more children, 51 %, with tumor ruptures experienced recurrence, compared with only 27 % among those without rupture ($p = 0.01$). In this study, preoperative treatment was found to downstage tumors. Following surgery alone, 33 % were stage III and just 22 % stage I. In those who received radiotherapy before surgery, the postoperative staging was 12 % stage III and 43 % stage I ($p = 0.005$).

12.2.2.3 SIOP Nephroblastoma Study 2

Similar results emerged from a subsequent study, SIOP 2, which recruited patients between 1974 and 1976. Preoperative radiotherapy 20 Gy with actinomycin D was given to 86 patients, and 52 patients underwent initial operation. This study was non-randomised, and there was a selection bias, with small tumor size being the main indication for primary nephrectomy. Nonetheless in this group in whom it might have been envisaged that the risk of a surgical complication would be less, the tumor rupture rate was still 20 %, compared with only 5 % in those with larger tumors who had received chemo-radiotherapy prior to surgery.

12.2.2.4 SIOP Nephroblastoma Study 5

With SIOP 1 and SIOP 2 having indicated a benefit from preoperative radiotherapy or chemo-radiotherapy, SIOP 5 which recruited patients between 1977 and 1979 addressed the question of whether chemotherapy alone was as good as chemo-radiotherapy (Lemerle et al. 1983). The randomisation was either to preoperative chemo-radiotherapy with radiotherapy 20 Gy and actinomycin D or to chemotherapy alone using actinomycin D with vincristine. Postoperatively, radiotherapy was given to those with stage II and III disease but omitted in those with stage I disease. A greater dose, 30 Gy, was used in those with no prior radiotherapy and just 15 Gy in those who had already received preoperative radiotherapy. Both treatment arms were found to be equivalent in terms of tumor rupture rate, which was seen in 12 of 164 patients, postoperative stage, and in relapse-free and overall survival. As following preoperative chemotherapy alone, 43 % had stage I disease and did not receive any radiotherapy at all, this strategy has been followed in all subsequent SIOP studies to minimise the incidence of late radiotherapy related morbidity.

12.2.2.5 SIOP Nephroblastoma Study 6

In this trial, which ran from 1980 to 1987, there was a randomised radiotherapy question. After initial chemotherapy and surgery, 123 patients who were stage II and node negative (or what we could now describe simply as stage II, since what used to be called node-positive stage II patients are now categorised as stage III) were randomised to receive, or not to receive, radiotherapy. The small numbers reflect the fact that this randomisation was stopped early when it seemed that there was an excess of recurrences in the unirradiated group. However, when the data matured, no significant difference was apparent with a 2-year disease-free survivals of 72 % (unirradiated) and 78 % (irradiated) (Tournade et al. 1993).

12.2.2.6 UK Wilms' Tumor Study 3

The United Kingdom did not participate in the early SIOP studies, instead national studies were coordinated initially by the Medical Research Council (MRC) and later by the United Kingdom Children's Cancer Study Group (UKCCSG, now the Children's Cancer and Leukaemia Group, CCLG). The third UKCCSG Wilms' Tumor trial, UKW3, which recruited patients between 1991 and 2001, also addressed value of preoperative chemotherapy (Mitchell et al. 2006). At the outset, there was equipoise in the minds of clinicians in the British Isles about the relative merits of the SIOP preoperative chemotherapy approach and the NWTS primary surgery strategy. A total of 205 children with newly diagnosed non-metastatic renal tumors, of which 186 had Wilms' on histology, were randomised to either initial operation or 6 weeks of preoperative chemotherapy. Event free and overall survival rates were similar for Wilms' tumor, but there were many fewer stage III patients, 9.8 % versus 29.8 % ($p=0.008$), in the group receiving chemotherapy. This meant that the requirement for radiotherapy was reduced by two thirds, from about 30 % to just 10 %, an absolute reduction of 20 %.

12.2.2.7 Should All Stage III Patients Be Treated in the Same Way?

It is clear from the definition of stage III disease (see Chaps. 4–6 and 11) that it comprises a heterogeneous range of patients. At one extreme, there are patients with multiple, gross, unresectable deposits scattered throughout the peritoneal cavity. At the other extreme, there are those who have a near complete excision of a localised tumor, with just a positive margin detected pathologically, or those with clear margins postoperatively who underwent an initial open wedge biopsy for some reason. Apart from stage, there are also other independent risk factors, such as the pathological subtype or age (Pritchard-Jones et al. 2003), which make recurrence more likely.

Patients with peritoneal implants seem to have the same probability of disease control as stage II patients without peritoneal implants (Kalapurakal et al. 2010a). Patients who have stage III disease by virtue of lymph node positivity have a worse prognosis than stage III lymph node-negative patients (Spreafico et al. 2012).

While treatment protocols have mandated a uniform treatment policy including radiotherapy for stage III Wilms' tumor, individual clinicians have withheld radiotherapy in selected circumstances.

In a small, carefully selected series of young patients who were stage III only by virtue of microscopically positive margins, radiotherapy was safely omitted (Pachnis et al. 1998).

In a review of German patients treated according to the SIOP 9 protocol, 122 of 454 patients were mandated to receive radiotherapy; however, only 98 did. Radiotherapy was omitted in 24 patients because of clinician choice for reasons including operative biopsy or young age. There were six local failures in the 24 unirradiated children (25 %), compared with 13 in the 98 irradiated patients (13 %) ($p=0.15$). All six of these local failures occurred in 8 unfavourable histology unirradiated patients. The incidence of local failure among unfavourable histology irradiated unfavourable histology patients was 9 out of 26 ($p<0.05$). With standard histology, there were no local recurrences among 16 unirradiated patients and 4 local recurrences among 73 treated patients.

These data seem to indicate that a carefully selected set of low-risk histology stage III patients may be safely treated without radiotherapy. This deserves prospective evaluation.

12.2.3 Radiotherapy for Metastatic Wilms' Tumor: The North American Perspective

12.2.3.1 Pulmonary Metastases

For patients with pulmonary metastasis detected by chest radiographs at diagnosis, the addition of whole-lung irradiation (WLI) to 12 Gy in 8 fractions is standard. Stage IV FH with lung metastases had an 80 % 4-year survival rate on NWTS-3, whereas survival for those with stage IV UH was about 55 % (D'Angio et al. 1989). Omission of WLI in patients with stage IV favourable histology tumors with complete resolution of pulmonary metastases after chemotherapy, as in the UKCCSG study (See Sect 12.2.4.1), has resulted in inferior relapse-free (50 %) and overall survival (65 %) rates (Pritchard et al. 1995).

The value of WLI in CT-only but not chest X-ray lesions has not been resolved. A report from the NWTS-3 and –4 did not demonstrate a clear benefit for whole-lung irradiation. The 4-year event-free survival rate was 89 % for patients treated with chemotherapy only and 80 % for those who received irradiation (Meisel et al. 1999).

12.2.3.2 Liver Metastases

Liver metastases may be treated by hepatic irradiation in addition to chemotherapy in patients who do not undergo upfront complete tumor resection before chemotherapy. In a report from NWTS-4 and 5, the relapse-free survival rate for 96 patients with favourable histology tumors and liver metastases was 76 %. Their survival rates were similar to that of patients with lung metastases (76 %), liver and lung metastases (70 %) and metastases to other sites (64 %). Twenty-two patients had a primary liver resection and 13 underwent resection after chemotherapy/irradiation. Eighty-two patients received abdominal radiation (Ehrlich et al. 2009).

12.2.4 Radiotherapy for Metastatic Wilms' Tumor: The European Perspective

12.2.4.1 UK Wilms' Tumor Study 1

The lungs are by far the most common site for metastases at diagnosis. In the first UKCCSG Wilms' Tumor Study (1980–1986), UKW1, the lung was the sole site of metastatic disease in 30 out of 40 stage IV patients, seven had combined lung and other site and only three has extra-pulmonary metastatic disease only. In UKW1, lung radiotherapy was only given as part of first-line treatment in stage IV patients if the metastases had not disappeared on chest radiography by 12 weeks from diagnosis (Pritchard et al. 1995). Radiotherapy, with a recommended dose of 12 Gy, was used in only four of 40 patients with favourable histology stage IV disease. In this group, the event-free and overall survival rates at 6 years were 50 and 65 %, respectively, indicating that the majority of relapsed patients could not be salvaged.

12.2.4.2 UK Wilms' Tumor Study 2

As the results for stage IV patients in UKW1 were worse than those from NWTS during the same time period, lung radiotherapy was reintroduced systematically for all patients in the second UKCCSG study, UKW2 (Mitchell et al. 2000). This recruited 60 favourable histology stage IV patients between 1986 and 1991. The event-free and overall survival rates at 4 years were 70 and 75 %, respectively. Compared with UKW1, these data demonstrate an appreciable improvement in freedom from relapse and a probable improvement in overall survival (although of course one always has to be cautious about drawing inferences from historical controls) but a smaller likelihood of successful salvage when relapse does occur after radiotherapy.

In the UKW3 trial, patients with stage IV disease were not eligible for randomisation but were registered and followed up. Guidelines advised treatment in the same way as in UKW2, that is, lung radiotherapy for all patients with pulmonary metastases visible on the chest radiograph at diagnosis, regardless of response to radiotherapy.

However, not every clinician followed these guidelines. A survey of all 102 patients with pulmonary metastatic disease enrolled in UKW2 and UKW3 has shown that only 71 % received radiotherapy as part of initial treatment (Nicolin et al. 2008). There were no discernable differences in patient characteristics or prognostic factors between those who did, and did not, receive lung irradiation. The event-free survival, with a median follow-up of 9 years, was 79.2 % for irradiated patients, compared with 53.3 % for unirradiated patients ($p=0.006$). The overall survival figures for the same groups were 84.7 and 73.2 %, respectively ($p=0.157$).

12.2.4.3 Pulmonary Metastases in SIOP Protocols

In SIOP protocols, whole-lung radiotherapy has been reserved for patients who have failed to achieve complete response to induction chemotherapy and, where necessary and feasible, surgical removal of metastases. A review of 234 stage IV (out of a denominator of 1,770) patients with Wilms' tumor, treated on these protocols, has shown that only 14 % required radiotherapy as part of first-line treatment. For the whole group of 234 patients, the event-free survival was 73 % and the overall survival was 82 %, indicating that about one in three of those relapsing could be salvaged with further treatment. Even in the presence of pulmonary metastases, local tumor stage was a strong determinant of outcome, with patients with local stages I and II tumor faring appreciably better than those with local stage III disease. Patients irradiated for multiple inoperable pulmonary metastases after chemotherapy fared significantly worse (5 year OS 48 %) than those who achieved a complete response to chemotherapy (5-year OS

Table 12.2 Outline of the SIOP postoperative pathology risk classification

1. Low-risk tumors
Mesoblastic nephroma
Cystic partially differentiated nephroblastoma
Completely necrotic nephroblastoma
2. Intermediate-risk tumors
Nephroblastoma – epithelial type
Nephroblastoma – stromal type
Nephroblastoma – mixed type
Nephroblastoma – regressive type
Nephroblastoma – focal anaplasia
3. High-risk tumors
Nephroblastoma – blastemal type
Nephroblastoma – diffuse anaplasia
Clear cell sarcoma of the kidney
Rhabdoid tumor of the kidney

For full details, and for information about pathological risk classification in patients who have not undergone chemotherapy before surgery, see Chap. 4 or Vujanic et al. 2002

Italics indicate non-Wilms' histologies

88 %) or to chemotherapy and surgery (5-year OS 92 %, $p<0.001$) (Verschuur et al. 2012). Prognosis is also worse in patients with SIOP high-risk histology (Table 12.2) (Warmann et al. 2011).

12.2.4.4 Abnormalities Visible on Chest CT But Not Chest X-Ray

In the era before computed tomography (CT) stage IV disease included patients with pulmonary metastatic disease which could be identified on plain postero-anterior and lateral chest radiographs. As CT was introduced into clinical practice, it became clear that there were some patients who had no metastatic disease detectable by chest radiography, but who had small volume lung nodules visible on CT. These patients were still regarded as having localised disease and were treated according to the extent and histology of the abdominal component of their disease. A study was undertaken of 141 patients enrolled on the second UKCCSG Wilms' Tumor Study with normal chest radiographs at diagnosis who also had thoracic CT performed. In 31 patients (22 %), small pulmonary nodules were detected. Among stage I patients, the risk of pulmonary relapse was greater in the CT-positive group (3/7, 43 %) than in the CT-negative group (5/48, 10 %) ($p=0.02$). Among stages II, III and V patients, the risk of pulmonary relapse, at 5 %, was similar in both the CT-positive and CT-negative groups. This suggests that the more intensive chemotherapy given to patients with more advanced disease is adequate to treat small volume pulmonary metastases not visible on chest radiographs but that the very limited chemotherapy given to stage I patients is not adequate in this situation (Owens et al. 2002).

12.2.5 Radiotherapy for Relapsed Disease

12.2.5.1 Relapsed Disease: The North American Perspective

Patients who had relapsed or progressive disease after initial chemotherapy with vincristine and actinomycin D and no radiation therapy were treated on stratum 'B' of the NWTS-5 relapse protocol. The relapse treatment included chemotherapy with regimen 'I' with alternating courses vincristine, doxorubicin, cyclophosphamide and etoposide/cyclophosphamide, surgery and radiation therapy. The 4-year event-free and overall survival were 71 and 81 % for all patients, 68 and 81 % for those who relapsed in the lung only and 78 and 83 % for those who relapsed in the operative bed with or without lung metastasis (Green et al. 2007) Patients who had relapsed or progressive disease after initial chemotherapy including vincristine, actinomycin and doxorubicin and radiation therapy were treated on stratum 'C' of the NWTS-5 relapse protocol. The relapse treatment included alternating courses of drug pairs (cyclophosphamide/etoposide and carboplatin/etoposide), surgery and radiation therapy. The 4-year event-free and overall survival were 42 and 48 % for all patients and 49 and 53 % for those who relapsed in the lung only (Malogolowkin et al. 2008). The radiation therapy recommendations for children with relapsed tumor in NWTS-5 are identical to the COG radiation therapy guidelines (Table 12.3).

Table 12.3 Children's oncology group radiation therapy guidelines

Treatment site	Clinical presentation and indication	Dose and modifications
Flank irradiation	Stage III, FH	*10.8 Gy*
All patients with residual tumor will receive supplemental irradiation with a *10.8 Gy boost* to the area of residual disease	Stage I-III, FA	
	Stage I-II, DA	
	Stage I*-III, CCSK	*10.8 Gy*
		*Stage I CCSK will not receive RT if complete staging, lymph node sampling and central pathology review have been performed
	Stage III, DA	*19.8 Gy*
	Stage I-III, RTK	(10.8 Gy if age ≤12 months)
	Recurrent Wilms tumor	*21.6 Gy*
		(12.6–18 Gy if age ≤12 months)
Whole abdominal irradiation (WAI)	Indicated for all histologies when Stage III due to:	*10.5 Gy*
Patients with residual tumor in the flank will receive supplemental irradiation with a 10.8 Gy boost	(a) Cytology-positive ascites	Patients with stage III DA, RTK and age >12 months will receive additional flank boost of 9 Gy
	(b) Any preoperative tumor rupture	
	(c) Diffuse surgical spillage	
	(d) Peritoneal seeding	
	Patients with diffuse and unresectable peritoneal implants	*21 Gy*
		When WAI is >10.5 Gy renal shielding is required to limit the dose to the normal kidney to <14.4 Gy)
Whole lung irradiation (WLI)	Indicated for lung metastases for:	*12 Gy*
	Favorable histology tumors not in CR at week 6	10.5 Gy if < 12 months
	All patients with higher risk tumors (LOH, multiple metastatic sites and unfavorable histology)	
Whole brain irradiation	Brain metastases	*21.6* + 10.8 Gy boost; Age <16 years
		30.6 Gy, age ≥16 years
Liver irradiation	Focal metastases	*19.8 Gy*
Patients with residual tumor will receive supplemental irradiation with *5.4–10.8 Gy*	Diffuse metastases	*19.8 Gy*
Bone irradiation	Bone metastases	*25.2 Gy*; Age <16 years
		30.6 Gy; Age ≥16 years
Lymph node irradiation	Resected LN metastases	*10.8 Gy*
	Unresected LN metastases	*19.8 Gy*
Metachronous Wilms tumor	Negative surgical margins	*No RT*
	Microscopically involved margins or nodes	*10.8 Gy*
	Diffuse spillage or abdominal involvement	*Follow WAI guidelines*
	Microscopically involved margins after partial nephrectomy	*14.4 Gy*
	Gross residual disease after partial resection or biopsy	*21.6 Gy*

FH favourable histology, *FA* focal anaplasia, *DA* diffuse anaplasia, *CCSK* clear cell sarcoma of kidney, *MRTK* malignant rhabdoid tumor of kidney, *WT* Wilms' tumor, *CR* complete response

12.2.5.2 Relapsed Disease: The European Perspective

Most published studies have addressed the initial treatment of newly diagnosed patients. In poorer prognostic groups, treatments have been intensified, with the aim of maximising relapse-free and overall survival, while in better prognostic groups, there has been a careful reduction of treatment intensity in the hope that survival rates can be maintained while reducing the morbidity of treatment. There is evidence that when early-stage patients relapse without prior radiotherapy, salvage with relapse protocols, which usually involve radiotherapy, is possible. For example, in UKW1, where radiotherapy was not given to stage I patients, the 6-year event-free and overall survival rates for favourable histology stage I patients were 89 and 96 %, respectively, implying that more than half of relapsed cased can be salvaged. By contrast in stage III disease, where radiotherapy was routinely used, the 6-year event-free and overall survival rates for favourable histology patients were 82 and 83 %, implying little chance of salvage for relapse (Pritchard et al. 1995).

12.3 Current Radiotherapy Recommendations

12.3.1 Children's Oncology Group Studies: Radiation Therapy Guidelines

12.3.1.1 Current COG Protocols

The COG renal tumor committee is the successor of the NWTS. The COG Wilms' tumor Staging System is similar to that used in NWTS-5 except in patients with local tumor spillage, who were designated as stage II in NWTS-5 but will be upstaged to stage III in COG protocols (Table 12.4). This change in the staging system was necessitated by the inferior survival rates observed in stage II patients with tumor spillage. For stage II patients (NWTS-4), the 8-year event rates, with and without spillage, respectively, were 79 and 87 % for relapse-free survival ($p=0.07$) and 90 and 95 % for overall survival ($p=0.04$) (Kalapurakal et al. 2010b). The COG risk-group classification for treatment assignment will, in addition to tumor stage, also consider patient's age, tumor weight, presence or absence of LOH at 1p and 16q and response to chemotherapy in children with favourable histology tumors and lung metastases.

AREN 0321 is the protocol for the treatment of children with high-risk renal tumors (anaplastic Wilms' tumor, clear cell sarcoma and malignant rhabdoid tumor). This protocol will determine whether a regimen of cyclophosphamide/carboplatin/etoposide alternating with vincristine/doxorubicin/ cyclophosphamide will improve the event-free and overall survival of patients with diffuse anaplastic Wilms' tumor and malignant rhabdoid tumor. For patients with stage I clear cell sarcoma of the kidney with thorough clinical and pathologic staging, the outcomes with just chemotherapy alone and without abdominal irradiation will be determined. Patients with stage I diffuse anaplastic Wilms' tumor and stages I–III focal anaplastic Wilms' tumor are treated with vincristine, dactinomycin, doxorubicin and flank radiation.

AREN0533 is the protocol for the treatment of newly diagnosed higher-risk favourable histology Wilms' tumors. This protocol will not use diagnostic imaging criteria such as chest X-ray or CT scan positivity to determine the need for whole-lung irradiation. Rather, the indication for lung irradiation will be based on the response of the lung metastases to 3-drug chemotherapy. One of the main objectives of this study is to demonstrate that patients with stage IV favourable histology Wilms' tumor with pulmonary metastases only, who have complete resolution of the pulmonary lesions after 6 weeks of regimen DD-4A chemotherapy (vincristine, dactinomycin and doxorubicin) called rapid complete responders (RCR), will have at least an 85 % 4-year event-free survival after therapy with additional chemotherapy (regimen DD-4A) and without whole-lung irradiation. For those patients who do not have resolution of pulmonary metastases by week 6, called slow incomplete responders (SIR), their therapy will be augmented with the addition of cyclophosphamide and etoposide to a modified regimen DD4-A (regimen M) and whole-lung irradiation (12 Gy). All pulmonary metastases patients with LOH at 1p and 16q, multiple sites of metastases and unfavourable histology tumors will receive whole-lung irradiation (12 Gy).

AREN0534 is the protocol for bilateral Wilms' tumor. This study recommends earlier biopsies and resection of tumors that are not responding to therapy in the hope of avoiding prolonged ineffective therapies for patients with diffuse anaplasia. The study recommends more intensive

Table 12.4 Children's Oncology Group Staging of Wilms' tumor

Stage I – Tumor limited to kidney, completely resected. The renal capsule is intact. The tumor was not ruptured or biopsied prior to removal. The vessels of the renal sinus are not involved. There is no evidence of tumor at or beyond the margins of resection. NOTE: For a tumor to qualify for certain therapeutic protocols as stage I, regional lymph nodes must be examined microscopically
Stage II – The tumor is completely resected, and there is no evidence of tumor at or beyond the margins of resection. The tumor extends beyond kidney, as is evidenced by any one of the following criteria:
There is regional extension of the tumor (i.e. penetration of the renal capsule, or extensive invasion of the soft tissue of the renal sinus, as discussed below)
Blood vessels within the nephrectomy specimen outside the renal parenchyma, including those of the renal sinus, contain tumor
Note: Rupture or spillage confined to the flank, including biopsy of the tumor, is no longer included in stage II and is now included in stage III
Stage III – Residual non-haematogenous tumor present following surgery and confined to abdomen. Any one of the following may occur:
Lymph nodes within the abdomen or pelvis are involved by tumor. (Lymph node involvement in the thorax or other extra-abdominal sites is a criterion for stage IV)
The tumor has penetrated through the peritoneal surface
Tumor implants are found on the peritoneal surface
Gross or microscopic tumor remains postoperatively (e.g. tumor cells are found at the margin of surgical resection on microscopic examination)
The tumor is not completely resectable because of local infiltration into vital structures,
Tumor spillage occurring either before or during surgery
The tumor was biopsied (whether tru-cut, open or fine-needle aspiration) before removal
Tumor is removed in greater than one piece (e.g. tumor cells are found in a separately excised adrenal gland; a tumor thrombus within the renal vein is removed separately from the nephrectomy specimen)
Stage IV – Haematogenous metastases (lung, liver, bone, brain, etc.) or lymph node metastases outside the abdomino-pelvic region are present. (The presence of tumor within the adrenal gland is not interpreted as metastasis and staging depends on all other staging parameters present)
Stage V – Bilateral renal involvement by tumor is present at diagnosis. An attempt should be made to stage each side according to the above criteria on the basis of the extent of disease

chemotherapy upfront (3-drugs) and requires second-look surgery at 6 weeks and definitive surgery at 12 weeks, and this is to be followed by chemotherapy based on histologic response after definitive surgery. The other objectives of this protocol are to prevent complete removal of at least one kidney in 50 % of patients with bilateral Wilms' tumor. This study will also determine whether partial nephrectomy in lieu of radical nephrectomy could be performed in at least 25 % of children by using preoperative chemotherapy in children with syndromic unilateral tumors who are at a high risk for developing metachronous tumors such as in patients with aniridia, Beckwith–Wiedemann syndrome (BWS) and other overgrowth syndromes. Radiation therapy in stage V Wilms' tumor is indicated when definitive surgery has been accomplished and one or both of the primary tumors are found to be stage III favourable histology, stages I–III anaplastic tumors, CCSK or rhabdoid tumor or when preoperative chemotherapy and one or two surgeries have not achieved negative resection margins. The performance of a needle biopsy or delivery of preoperative chemotherapy is not considered to be a stage III criterion in bilateral Wilms' tumor.

The COG radiation therapy guidelines (indications, volumes and dose-fractionation) are outlined in Table 12.3.

12.3.1.2 Timing of Radiation Therapy

Delayed initiation of treatment beyond 10 days after surgery has been related to higher risk of abdominal recurrence in several, but not all, studies (D'Angio et al. 1976, 1981, 1989). Most relapses related to delayed start of therapy have been in patients with unfavourable histology tumors. An analysis of patients enrolled in

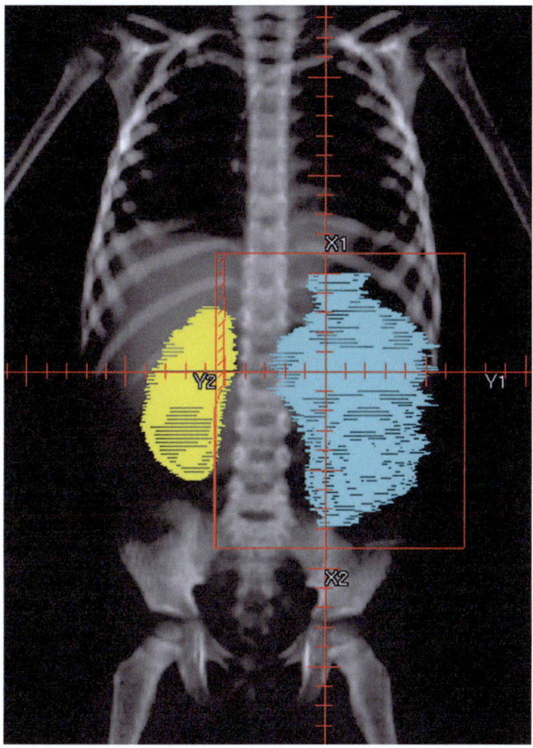

Fig. 12.1 A typical flank irradiation field in a child with left-sided Wilms' tumor. The preoperative CT scan-based tumor volume is shown in *blue* and the right kidney is shown in *yellow*

NWTS-3 and -4 looked at the influence of delay of radiation therapy on outcome in Wilms' tumor in patients with stage II–IV favourable histology tumors. The mean delay in radiotherapy was 10.9 days from surgery, and the median was 9 days; 59 % of children were treated 8–12 days postoperatively. For children who were treated 0–9 days postoperatively and those treated at least 10 days postoperatively, there was no difference in the rate of flank or abdominal recurrence. In NWTS-1 and NWTS-2, 80 % of children were treated with radiotherapy during week 1, whereas in NWTS-3 and NWTS-4, 24 % of children were treated in week 1, but 66 % were treated with radiotherapy in week 2 (Kalapurakal et al. 2003). NWTS-5 recommended that postoperative irradiation begin no later than the ninth postoperative day. In the COG protocols, it is recommended that radiation therapy be initiated by day 9 if possible, but no later than day 14 after nephrectomy.

12.3.1.3 Radiation Therapy Volumes

The classic flank irradiation treatment fields include the tumor bed that is defined as the outline of the kidney and associated tumor based on the pretreatment CT or MRI scans. The superior, inferior and lateral margins of the flank fields are placed approximately 1 cm beyond the kidney/tumor outline. The field should extend to the dome of the diaphragm only in patients in whom the tumor is known to have extended that far superiorly. Medially, the target volume should encompass the entire width of the vertebral bodies in order to avoid the development of scoliosis and to include the entire para-aortic lymph node chain but exclude the remaining kidney (Fig. 12.1).

For patients with preoperative tumor rupture and intraoperative rupture with diffuse peritoneal tumor dissemination and in patients with diffuse peritoneal implants, the irradiation fields should include the entire abdominal cavity. The target volume includes all of the peritoneal surfaces, defined superiorly by the diaphragms, laterally by the abdominal walls and inferiorly at the bottom of the obturator foramen. The acetabulum and femoral heads should be blocked (Fig. 12.2).

Whole-lung irradiation (WLI) fields must encompass the entire lungs and mediastinum including both lung apices and the costophrenic recesses. The typical WLI field extends above the clavicles and approximately down to T12–L1. The shoulders should be blocked (Fig. 12.3). When clinical situations call for WLI plus flank irradiation as in abdominal stage III patients with lung metastases, it is preferred that patients be treated with one large field rather than separate fields in order to avoid excessive irradiation of the liver in right-sided disease and heart in left-sided tumors.

12.3.2 European Recommendations

12.3.2.1 Radiotherapy Decision-Making

The most recent SIOP trial, SIOP WT 2001, has now closed. While awaiting the published results from that study, current recommendations are by

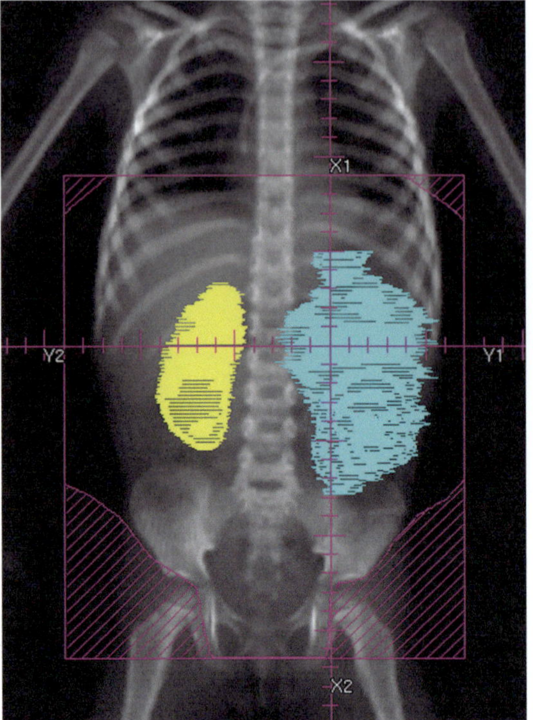

Fig. 12.2 A typical whole-abdomen irradiation field in a child with left-sided Wilms' tumor. The preoperative tumor volume is shown in *blue* and the right kidney is shown in *yellow*

Table 12.5 Outline of the SIOP postoperative staging system

Stage I
The tumor is limited to the kidney or surrounded with a fibrous pseudocapsule if outside of the normal contours of the kidney, and it has been completely resected with clear margins
Stage II
The tumor extends beyond the kidney, for example, into peri-renal fat or the vena cava, but has been completely excised with clear margins
Stage III
Incomplete excision of the tumor, which extends beyond the resection margins, i.e. microscopic or gross residual disease remains; any intra-abdominal lymph nodes are, or have been, involved; preoperative or intraoperative rupture; tumor has penetrated through the peritoneum; presence of peritoneal deposits; tumor thrombi present at resection margins in veins or ureter, transected or removed piecemeal; or the tumor has been surgically biopsied
Stage IV
Presence of haematogenous metastases in lungs, liver, or other organs, irrespective of the 'local' stage (i.e. I, II or III)
Stage V
Bilateral renal tumors, irrespective of their 'local' stage

For full details, refer to Chaps. 4, 8 and 11

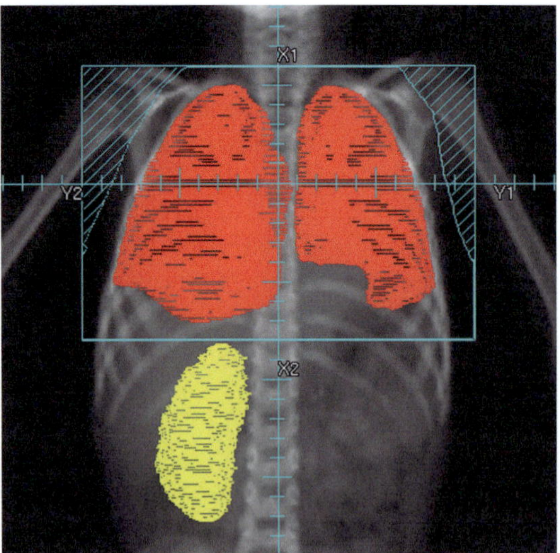

Fig. 12.3 A typical whole-lung irradiation field in a child with left-sided Wilms' tumor and lung metastases. The total lung volume is shown in *red* and the right kidney is shown in *yellow*

and large those recommended in the SIOP WT 2001 protocol, which were themselves based the evidence reviewed briefly above, and in the section on the North American approach to radiotherapy in Wilms' tumor.

The decision, on whether or not to use radiotherapy in any particular patient, should be made at a multidisciplinary team meeting involving, as a minimum, the paediatric (medical) oncologist, the paediatric clinical (radiation) oncologist, the paediatric (urological) surgeon, the paediatric radiologist and the paediatric pathologist. This team should review the imaging at diagnosis and preoperatively the operative findings and the postoperative pathology. The SIOP staging system, based on imaging and postoperative pathology, and the postoperative pathological risk classification are discussed in detail elsewhere in this book, but as a reminder, they are outlined in Tables 12.2 and 12.5.

12.3.2.2 Stage I

Radiotherapy is not indicated in stage I disease of any histological subtype.

12.3.2.3 Stage II

Radiotherapy is not indicated for low-risk or intermediate-risk histology stage II disease. Patients with high-risk histology stage II (except blastemal type) should receive flank radiotherapy.

12.3.2.4 Stage III

Stage III disease with intermediate- or high-risk histology indicates the need for radiotherapy.

In stage II disease, and in disease which is stage III by virtue of localised positive margins, localised residual tumor, localised tumor rupture or lymph node positivity, radiotherapy is limited to the ipsilateral flank. This encompasses the tumor bed and immediately surrounding area and the renal hilar and adjacent para-aortic lymph node areas. If there has been gross intra-abdominal contamination by preoperative or intraoperative tumor rupture or if there is diffuse intraperitoneal spread, then whole abdominal and pelvic radiotherapy is given.

12.3.2.5 Stage IV

In stages IV and V disease, radiotherapy to the primary site is indicated by the local stage (I, II or III) of the primary tumor and its postoperative histological subtype.

In stage IV disease, whole-lung irradiation will be given if a complete remission on CT scan has not been achieved after 4 weeks of preoperative chemotherapy and complete surgical resection of residual or doubtful pulmonary lesions. Hepatic radiotherapy will be given if there are residual liver lesions after chemotherapy and surgery. Radiotherapy will be given to other involved distant sites, for example, bone or brain, regardless of the response to chemotherapy and, if feasible, surgery. In stage IV disease, local or abdominal radiotherapy is given according to the local extent of tumor (i.e. stage I, II or III). It is advisable to give radiotherapy to the flank or abdomen and metastatic sites concurrently.

12.3.2.6 Stage V

Following chemotherapy and surgery for stage V disease, radiotherapy is usually given according to the local extent of tumor on each side. If the only remaining renal tissue is part of one kidney, it is advisable to avoid irradiating this to a high dose to prevent renal failure. Two healthy kidneys can safely tolerate a dose of around 15 Gy. When one kidney is removed, the remaining one undergoes a period of compensatory hypertrophy, during which time it is more sensitive to radiation damage. The recommended maximum dose to a solitary kidney is 12 Gy. When a patient has undergone a total nephrectomy and a partial nephrectomy, the renal remnant will also undergo compensatory hypertrophy to some degree, and it will be more vulnerable to radiation damage in the period of 6–8 weeks after surgery. Even when this process is complete, the renal function as measured by glomerular filtration rate will be much less than normal, and even a mild reduction in function could have major deleterious effects. There are no very good data on the maximum 'safe' dose in this situation. While a dose in the region of 10 Gy, as used in COG protocols is possibly safe, it is probably better to avoid radiotherapy if at all possible. However, it is important to cure the cancer, so very occasionally, radiotherapy encompassing all residual renal tissue may be undertaken in the face of high-risk disease. This should be done in the knowledge that renal failure may result, and renal replacement therapy with dialysis and transplantation may become necessary. Nephrotoxicity is a late radiation effect, so renal failure may take 18 months to 2 years or longer to develop.

12.3.2.7 The Paediatric Radiotherapy Department

In the modern era, radiotherapy for Wilms' tumor will be given in a radiotherapy department recognised for paediatric radiotherapy, by appropriately trained staff experienced in the delivery of radiotherapy to children, with the support of a paediatric anaesthetic team in many cases.

Before radiotherapy planning commences, informed consent for planning and treatment should be obtained from the parents or guardians of the child. Discussions should be supplemented by written information and documented. The rationale for radiotherapy, and the risks of not giving radiotherapy, should be explained. The practicalities of treatment planning and delivery, including anaesthesia, if needed, should be outlined. The likely short-term side effects, including the risks of anaesthesia, and possible long-term complications must be explained. These include the effect on bone and soft tissue growth, the effect on reproductive capacity and the possibility of second malignant neoplasms (Taylor et al. 2008). It should be stated that nowadays, as a result of research, fewer patients with Wilms' tumor – only those with adverse prognostic factors – receive radiotherapy and a lower dose is used than was the case historically. This means that the incidence and severity of late effects related to radiotherapy will be less than was historically the case. Nonetheless, all irradiated patients will be kept under long-term surveillance in a late effects clinic.

12.3.2.8 Target Volume Definition

Target volume definition will be performed on a planning CT scan, taking into account the post-chemotherapy, presurgery magnetic resonance imaging or CT scans. The surgeon may have placed clips to mark the extent of the tumor or any areas suspicious for residual disease. The clinical target volume (CTV) is defined as the preoperative extent of disease plus the remaining ipsilateral kidney, as defined on imaging, plus a 1 cm margin. This may be modified by additional information from the operation note, position of clips and pathology report. The CTV will be extended medially to cover the full width of the vertebral bodies. Any definite residual disease should be volumed as a separate CTV. The remaining kidney and liver should be volumed as organs at risk (OAR).

The planning target volume (PTV) is defined as the CTV, plus a margin, informed by a periodic departmental audit of movement, to cover errors and uncertainties in positioning. Usually, anterior and posterior parallel opposed fields will be used to cover the PTV. The superior and inferior field margins should pass through intervertebral spaces, rather than through vertebral bodies. Fields will be shaped by multi-leaf collimators, or blocks, to exclude any nontarget tissues. Dosimetrists will then produce a plan, which may be optimised by the addition of segment fields, and dose volume histograms of the target volumes and OAR, for approval.

If the whole abdomen and pelvis requires treatment, care should be taken to ensure that the whole peritoneal cavity is included from the dome of the diaphragm in expiration to the pelvic floor. Care should be taken to shield the femoral heads and hip joints.

For whole-lung radiotherapy, the CTV should cover from the lung apices, to the base of the lungs, in the full range of respiratory motion. The shoulder joints should be shielded from the treated volume, and the heart should be volumed as an OAR.

If multiple areas are to be treated, for example, flank or whole abdomen and pelvis plus the lungs or lungs and liver, a composite volume should be treated as one. This avoids the risk of an overlap, for example, between left flank and the thoracic fields, which may result in an excessive cardiac dose.

12.3.2.9 Treatment and Verification

For treatment, megavoltage irradiation from a linear accelerator, usually 6 MV, will be used. Imaging for geometric verification, and in vivo dosimetry, should be used as per national or departmental guidelines to ensure accuracy of treatment delivery.

12.3.2.10 Time, Dose and Fractionation

The fraction size should not exceed 1.8 Gy for flank radiotherapy but should be lowered to 1.5 or 1.25 Gy if large volumes are treated, for example, whole lungs or whole abdomen and pelvis and in very young children, for example, less than 2 years old.

The total dose is determined by the stage and pathological risk group (see Table 12.2). The prescribed dose for flank radiotherapy in intermediate-risk disease should be 14.4 Gy in 8 fractions or 15 Gy in 10 fractions if it is to be treated in continuity with the lungs or in children less than 2 years old. With high-risk histology, a dose of 25.2 Gy in 14 fractions (or 25.5 Gy in 17 fractions if treated in continuity with the lungs or in a very young child) should be prescribed. If there is definite macroscopic disease, a boost of an additional 10.8 Gy 6 fractions (or 10.5 Gy in 7 fractions) may be considered. Formerly a boost to the para-aortic nodes was advised if there was evidence of lymph node involvement, but as there is no evidence to support this practice, it is not currently recommended. For whole abdominal and pelvic radiotherapy, 15 Gy in 10 fractions is recommended for intermediate-risk disease. In very young children, the dose can be limited to 10.5 Gy in 7 fractions. In high-risk histology, the dose to the whole abdomen should be limited to 21 Gy in 14 fractions, with an additional 4.5 Gy in 3 fractions to the flank. The dose received by the remaining kidney should be limited to 12 Gy.

For metastatic disease, the recommendation for whole-lung (with lung correction) or whole-liver radiotherapy is 15 Gy in 10 fractions. While a boost of, say, 10.5 Gy in 6 fractions may be considered for an area of bulk residual disease, surgical excision of any large pulmonary metastases still present after chemotherapy is preferred. The volume of lung receiving in excess of 15 Gy should be limited to less than 25 %. Radiotherapy for bone or brain metastases present at the time of initial presentation is only very rarely required and may be individualised.

The prescription point is to the 100 % isodose or to the midplane if simple parallel opposed fields are used. In accordance with ICRU recommendations, the dose variation should be between 95 and 107 %.

Radiotherapy should be commenced as soon after surgery as practicable. As it usually takes at least a week for the pathology to be reported and reviewed at a multidisciplinary team meeting, and because the process of preparation for radiotherapy including gaining informed, preparation of the child and planning is now more complex than previously, this duration usually exceeds the 10 days previously recommended by NWTS. However, in contrast to the case with primary nephrectomy, there is no evidence that after initial chemotherapy, this longer time period is harmful. There is evidence, however, that surgery to radiotherapy intervals exceeding 30 days has an adverse effect on outcome (Spreafico et al. 2012).

Once commenced, radiotherapy should be delivered in five daily fractions per week without interruption. If an interruption is inevitable, this should, if possible, be compensated for by hyperfractionation so that the overall treatment time isn't extended.

12.3.2.11 Relapse Treatment

When patients with good prognosis disease relapse after initial limited chemotherapy and surgery, without having had radiotherapy, their disease is by definition less chemo-sensitive than the cohort of patients with similar stage and pathology who do not relapse. Salvage protocols therefore almost always include radiotherapy as well as additional chemotherapy and surgery. Abdominal radiotherapy doses are likely to be higher for relapsed disease, for example, 20 to 30 Gy depending on histology, than are used for initial therapy, but the lung dose at 15 Gy is unchanged. A good proportion of patients may expect to be cured.

When worse prognosis patients relapse after more intensive chemotherapy and radiotherapy, the likelihood of cure is much smaller, especially if the recurrence is within the previously irradiated volume. It is not safe to re-irradiate the lungs following the initial 15 Gy treatment. Local recurrences in the flank may be re-irradiated with care taken to respect normal tissue tolerance, for example, liver and spinal cord. When there is an abdominal recurrence outside the irradiated flank, further radiotherapy is possible, but again care must be taken not to exceed the tolerance of critical normal structures from the combined treatments. Treatments are individualised, taking into account many factors such as site of recurrence, volume and dose of prior radiation treatment, age, elapsed time since the previous treatment, histology and co-morbidity. Doses of up to 30 Gy may be considered, depending on histology.

Table 12.6 Dose/fractionation recommendations used in SIOP trials

Site	Intermediate-risk histology	Intermediate-risk histology, younger children	High-risk histology	High-risk histology, younger children
Flank	Stage III (localised)	Stage III (localised)	Stage II or III (localised)	Stage II or III (localised)
	14.4 Gy 8 fractions	15 Gy 10 fractions	25.2 Gy 14 fractions	25.5 Gy 17 fractions
Whole abdomen and pelvis	Stage III (widespread)	Stage III (widespread)	Stage III (widespread)	Stage III (widespread)
	15 Gy in 10 fractions	10.5 Gy 7 fractions	21 Gy in 14 fractions (plus 4.5 Gy in 3 fractions to flank)	15 Gy in 10 fractions (plus 4.5 Gy in 3 fractions to flank)
Whole lungs or whole liver	15 Gy in 10 fractions	Up to 15 Gy in 10 fractions	15 Gy in 10 fractions	Up to 15 Gy in 10 fractions
Consider boost for inoperable macroscopic residual disease	10.8 Gy in 6 fractions	10.5 Gy in 7 fractions	Up to 10.8 Gy in 6 fractions	Up to 10.5 Gy in 7 fractions

See text for full details and caveats. The SIOP Renal Tumors Study Group is currently considering adopting the reduced doses used by COG

12.3.2.12 Non-Wilms' Histologies

The majority about 90 % of children with renal tumors have Wilms' tumor. A variety of histologies comprise the remainder: congenital mesoblastic nephroma (most commonly diagnosed in the first 6 months of life, although the majority of renal tumors presenting under the age of 6 months are still Wilms' tumor (van den Heuvel-Eibrink et al. 2008)), clear cell sarcoma of the kidney (sometimes called the bone metastasising renal tumor of childhood), malignant rhabdoid tumor of the kidney (which has a similar biology and natural history to malignant rhabdoid tumor arising at other sites) and renal adenocarcinoma (presenting in the adolescent years) and others types seen too infrequently to merit a mention. As all childhood renal tumors tend to present in similar ways, and as the various non-Wilms' childhood renal tumors are too rare for individual clinical trials, non-Wilms' renal tumors have historically been treated within clinical trials designed for Wilms' tumor. With the exception of mesoblastic nephroma which usually has a benign clinical course and requires surgery only, they have usually been lumped together with anaplastic Wilms' tumor as 'unfavourable' or 'high-risk' histology. Over the years, and with increasing clinical experience, the differences between the two principal malignant non-Wilms' histologies, clear cell sarcoma and malignant rhabdoid tumor and Wilms' have become apparent.

Malignant rhabdoid tumor is often very chemo-sensitive initially, but it is characterised by a tendency to CNS metastasis and early progression which is chemo-resistant. The best outcomes have been seen in patients with localised disease who have early surgery and postoperative radiotherapy. It is recommended that if a malignant rhabdoid tumor is found on biopsy of a renal tumor, screening for metastatic spread should include neuroimaging and treatment should be given according to non-rhabdomyosarcoma soft tissue sarcoma guidelines for the treatment of malignant rhabdoid tumor arising at any site. Radiotherapy forms an important component of treatment for localised disease.

Outcomes for patients with clear cell sarcoma of the kidney have improved over the years with more aggressive treatment, and in particular, the recognition that patients with stage III disease treated with radiotherapy had a lower risk of recurrence than patients with stage II disease treated without radiotherapy. Current treatment recommendations therefore include radiotherapy to the primary site in all patients except those with stage I disease, to the higher doses for high-risk histology mentioned above and in Table 12.6. All metastatic sites should be systematically irradiated, regardless of response to chemotherapy.

Patients with renal adenocarcinoma should be managed in conjunction with adult oncologists experienced in the management of this disease in adults.

12.4 Future Developments

12.4.1 Late Effects

Important lessons on radiation and chemotherapy-induced toxicities such as second malignancies, congestive heart failure and adverse pregnancy outcomes are being learned from the data being gathered by the long-term follow-up studies conducted by the NWTS and others (Breslow et al. 1988; Green et al. 2001, 2002). These reports will continue to challenge current treatment paradigms in order to maximise not only short- and intermediate-term outcomes but also long-term outcomes extending into several decades after therapy.

The incidence and severity of radiation-related late effects in survivors of Wilms' tumor have been reduced by a combination of (1) reduction of the proportion of patients irradiated through risk stratification, (2) reduction of the prescribed radiation doses and (3) replacement of older techniques such as rectangular fields based on anatomical landmarks with current ones including CT planning and accurate delineation of target volumes.

12.4.2 Radiotherapy Technology

Radiotherapy technology is continually evolving. Can newer technologies improve the outlook for future patients with Wilms' tumor further? Intensity-modulated radiotherapy (IMRT) is now widely available. This offers the possibility of greater conformality of the high-dose volume to the target volume, thereby reducing the volume of nontarget tissues receiving the full prescribed dose, usually at the expense of a greater volume of healthy normal tissue being exposed to low radiation doses (Fig. 12.4). This may reduce the risk of some late effects, and IMRT is considered

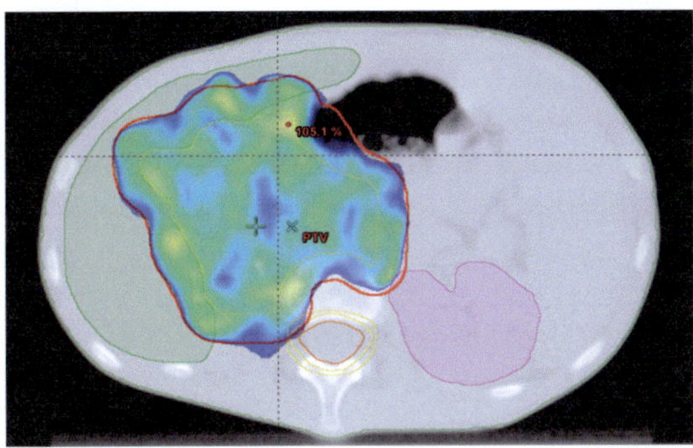

Fig. 12.4 Example of IMRT used to treat a localised abdominal recurrence in a previously irradiated area and spare adjacent normal tissue

especially valuable where high prescribed doses are required to volumes situated close to dose-limiting critical normal structures, as is often the case with brain tumors and various head and neck cancers. There is a concern that there may be an increased risk of second cancers because of the low-dose bath effect. IMRT has been demonstrated to show improved dose distributions in Wilms' tumor (Hillbrand et al. 2008; Fogliata et al. 2007), but concerns about the possible increase in second cancer risk remain. Given the low dose required for Wilms' tumor, the benefits of IMRT in routine treatment remain unclear. There may be occasions, however, such as for the re-treatment of recurrent disease in previously irradiated patients, where the advantages may outweigh any concerns.

Proton beam therapy, although not universally available, has clear advantages in terms of normal tissue sparing in a variety of circumstances, for example, brain tumors and head and neck cancers. Dosimetric studies including Wilms' tumor have demonstrated improvement over standard photon treatment, particularly with regard to the second cancer risk (Hillbrand et al. 2008; Fogliata et al. 2009). Clinical practice shouldn't be changed on this basis without meticulous prospective clinical evaluation.

Of course technology is only as good as the people using it. Significant inter-clinician variability, which may affect the possibility of late effects, has been demonstrated in radiotherapy planning for Wilms' tumor, even when the same protocol is being followed (Padovani, et al. 2009). This may be reduced through greater specialisation and better training and by national or international quality assurance programmes.

12.4.3 Biological Advances

In addition to advances in the delivery of radiotherapy to patients who may need it, there is the hope that current biological research will lead to better identification of those whose Wilms' tumor may be cured without recourse to radiation treatment and a refined risk-stratification system.

References

Breslow NE, Norkool PA, Olshan A et al (1988) Second malignant neoplasms in survivors of Wilms tumor: a report from the National Wilms' Tumor Study. J Natl Cancer Inst 80:592–595

Breslow NE, Takashima JR, Ritchey ML et al (2000) Renal failure in the Denys-Drash & Wilms tumor aniridia syndromes. Cancer Res 60:4030–4032

Coppes MJ, Arnold M, Beckwith JB et al (1999) Factors affecting the risk of contralateral Wilms tumor development. Cancer 85:1616–1625

D'Angio GJ, Evans AE, Breslow N et al (1976) The treatment of Wilms tumor: results of the National Wilms' Tumor Study. Cancer 38:633–646

D'Angio GJ, Tefft M, Breslow N et al (1978) Radiation therapy of Wilms' tumor: results according to dose, field, post-operative timing and histology. Int J Radiat Oncol Biol Phys 4:769–780

D'Angio GJ, Evans A, Breslow N et al (1981) The treatment of Wilms' tumor: results of the Second National Wilms' Tumor Study. Cancer 47:2302–2311

D'Angio GJ, Breslow N, Beckwith JB et al (1989) Treatment of Wilms' tumor: results of the Third National Wilms' Tumor Study. Cancer 64:349–360

Dome JS, Cotton CA, Perlman EJ et al (2006) Treatment of anaplastic histology Wilms tumor: results from the fifth National Wilms Tumor Study. J Clin Oncol 24:2352–2358

Ehrlich PF, Ferrerar F, Ritchey M et al (2009) Hepatic metastasis at diagnosis in favorable histology Wilms tumor is not an independent adverse prognostic factor. A report from the National Wilms Tumor Study Group. Ann Surg 250:642–648

Fogliata A, Nicolini G, Alber M et al (2007) On the performances of different IMRT treatment planning systems for selected paediatric cases. Radiat Oncol 2:7

Fogliata A, Yartsev A, Nicolini G et al (2009) On the performances of intensity modulated protons, RapidArc and helical tomotherapy for selected paediatric cases. Radiat Oncol 4:2

Gatta G, Capocaccia R, Stiller C et al (2005) Childhood Cancer Survival Trends in Europe: a EUROCARE Working Group Study. J Clin Oncol 23:3742–3751

Green DM, Breslow NE, Beckwith JB et al (1998) Comparison between single-dose and divided-dose administration of dactinomycin and doxorubicin for patients with Wilms' tumor: a report from the National Wilms' Tumor Study Group. J Clin Oncol 16: 237–245

Green DM, Grigoriev YA, Nan B et al (2001) Congestive heart failure after treatment for Wilms tumor: a report from the National Wilms Tumor Study Group. J Clin Oncol 19:1926–1934

Green DM, Peabody EM, Nan B et al (2002) Pregnancy outcome after treatment for Wilms tumor: a report from the National Wilms' Tumor Study Group. J Clin Oncol 20:2506–2513

Green DM, Cotton CA, Malogolowkin M et al (2007) Treatment of Wilms tumor relapsing after initial treatment with vincristine and Actinomycin D: a report from the National Wilms tumor Study Group. Pediatr Blood Cancer 48:493–499

Hillbrand M, Georg D, Gadner H, Pötter R, Dieckmann K (2008) Abdominal cancer during early childhood: a dosimetric comparison of proton beams to standard and advanced photon radiotherapy. Radiother Oncol 89:141–149

Kalapurakal JA, Li AM, Breslow NE et al (2003) Influence of radiation therapy delay on abdominal tumor recurrence in patients with favorable histology Wilms' tumor treated on NWTS-3 and NWTS-4: a report from the National Wilms' Tumor Study Group. Int J Radiat Oncol Biol Phys 57:495–499

Kalapurakal JA, Green DM, Haase G, Anderson JR, Dome JS, Grundy PE (2010a) Outcomes of children with favorable histology wilms tumor and peritoneal implants treated in National Wilms Tumor Studies-4 and -5. Int J Radiat Oncol Biol Phys 77:554–558

Kalapurakal JA, Li SM, Breslow NE et al (2010b) Intraoperative spillage of favorable histology Wilms tumor cells: Influence of irradiation and chemotherapy on abdominal recurrence. A report from the National Wilms Tumor Study Group. Int J Radiat Oncol Biol Phys 76:201–206

Lemerle J, Voute PA, Tournade MF et al (1976) Preoperative versus postoperative radiotherapy, single versus multiple courses of Actinomycin D in the treatment of Wilms' tumors. Preliminary results of a controlled clinical trial conducted by the International Society for Paediatric oncology (S.I.O.P.). Cancer 38:647–654

Lemerle J, Voute PA, Tournade MF et al (1983) Effectiveness of preoperative chemotherapy in Wilms' tumor: results of an International Society of Paediatric Oncology (SIOP) clinical trial. J Clin Oncol 1: 604–609

Malogolowkin M, Cotton CA, Green DM et al (2008) Treatment of Wilms tumor relapsing after initial treatment with vincristine, actinomycin D and doxorubicin. A report from the National Wilms tumor Study Group. Pediatr Blood Cancer 50:236–241

Meisel JA, Guthrie KA, Breslow NE et al (1999) Significance and management of computed tomography detected pulmonary nodules: a report from the National Wilms Tumor Study Group. Int J Radiat Oncol Biol Phys 44:579–585

Mitchell C, Morris Jones P, Kelsey A et al (2000) The treatment of Wilms' tumour: results of the United Kingdom Children's Cancer Study Group (UKCCSG) second Wilms' Tumour study. Br J Cancer 85: 602–608

Mitchell C, Pritchard-Jones K, Shannon R et al (2006) Immediate nephrectomy versus preoperative chemotherapy in the management of non-metastatic Wilms' tumour: results of a randomised trial (UKW3) by the UK Children's Cancer Study Group. Eur J Cancer 42:2554–2562

Nicolin G, Taylor R, Baughan C, Shannon R, Stevens S, Richardson D, Kelsey A, Pritchard-Jones K, Mitchell C (2008) Outcome after pulmonary radiotherapy in Wilms' tumor patients with pulmonary metastases at diagnosis: a UK Children's Cancer Study Group, Wilms' Tumour Working Group Study. Int J Radiat Oncol Biol Phys 70:175–180

Owens CM, Veys PA, Pritchard J, Levitt G, Imeson J, Dicks-Mireaux C (2002) Role of chest computed tomography at diagnosis in the management of Wilms' tumor: a study by the United Kingdom Children's Cancer Study Group. J Clin Oncol 20: 2768–2773

Pachnis A, Pritchard J, Gaze MN, Levitt G, Michalski A (1998) Radiotherapy omitted in the treatment of selected children under three years of age with Stage III favourable histology Wilms' Tumor. Med Pediatr Oncol 31:150–152

Padovani L, Huchet A, Claude L et al (2009) Inter-clinician variability in making dosimetric decisions in paediatric treatment: a balance between efficacy and late effects. Radiother Oncol 93:372–376

Pritchard J, Imeson J, Barnes J et al (1995) Results of the United Kingdom Children's Cancer Study Group First Wilms' Tumor Study. J Clin Oncol 13:124–133

Pritchard-Jones K, Kelsey A, Vujanic G et al (2003) Older age is an adverse prognostic factor in Stage I, favourable histology Wilms' tumor treated with vincristine monochemotherapy: a study by the United Kingdom Children's Cancer Study group, Wilms' Tumour Working Group. J Clin Oncol 21:3269–3273

Ritchey ML, Green DM, Thomas P et al (1996) Renal failure in Wilms tumor. Med Pediatr Oncol 26:75–80

Shamberger RC, Haase GC, Argani P et al (2006) Bilateral Wilms tumors with progressive or nonresponsive disease. J Pediatr Surg 41:652–657

Spreafico F, Gandola L, D'Angelo P, Terenziani M, Collini P, Bianchi M, Provenzi M, Indolfi P, Pession A, Nantron M, Di Cataldo A, Marchianò A, Catania S, Fossati Bellani F, Piva L (2012) AIEOP Wilms Tumor Working Group. Heterogeneity of disease classified as stage III in Wilms tumor: a report from the Associazione Italiana Ematologia Oncologia Pediatrica (AIEOP). Int J Radiat Oncol Biol Phys 82:348–354

Taylor AJ, Winter DL, Pritchard-Jones K et al (2008) Second primary neoplasms in survivors of Wilms' tumour – a population based cohort study from the British Childhood Cancer Survivor Study. Int J Cancer 122:2085–2093

Tefft M, D'Angio GJ, Grant W et al (1976) Post-operative radiation therapy for residual Wilms' tumor: review of group III patients in the National Wilms' Tumor Study. Cancer 37:2768–2772

Tefft M, D'Angio GJ, Beckwith B et al (1980) Patterns of intra-abdominal relapse in patients with Wilms' tumor who received radiation: analysis by histopathology, a report of National Wilms' Tumor Studies 1 and 2. Int J Radiat Oncol Biol Phys 6:663–667

Thomas PR, Tefft M, Compaan PJ et al (1991) Results of two radiation therapy randomizations in the third National Wilms' Tumor Study. Cancer 68:1703–1707

Tournade MF, Com-Nougué C, Voûte PA et al (1993) Results of the International Society of Paediatric Oncology 6 Wilms' tumor trial and study: a risk-adapted therapeutic approach in Wilms' tumor. J Clin Oncol 11:1014–1023

Van den Heuvel-Eibrink MM, Grundy P, Graf N et al (2008) Characteristics and survival of 750 children diagnosed with a renal tumour in the first seven months of life: a collaborative study by the SIOP/GPOH/SFOP, NWTSG, and UKCCSG Wilms Tumor Study Groups. Pediatr Blood Cancer 50:1130–1134

Verschuur A, Van Tinteren H, Graf N, Bergeron C, Sandstedt B, de Kraker J (2012) Treatment of pulmonary metastases in children with stage IV nephroblastoma with risk-based use of pulmonary radiotherapy. J Clin Oncol 30(28):3533–3539, Epub 2012 Aug 27

Vujanic GM, Sandstedt B, Harms D et al (2002) Revised International Society of Paediatric Oncology (SIOP) working classification of renal tumours of childhood. Med Pediatr Oncol 38:79–82

Warmann SW, Furtwängler R, Blumenstock G, Armeanu S, Nourkami N, Leuschner I, Schenk JP, Graf N, Fuchs J (2011) Tumor biology influences the prognosis of nephroblastoma patients with primary pulmonary metastases: results from SIOP 93-01/GPOH and SIOP 2001/GPOH. Ann Surg 254:155–162

Late Effects and QOL Chapter 13

Gill A. Levitt and Daniel M. Green

Contents

G.A. Levitt (✉)
Department of Oncology and Haematology, Great Ormond Street Hospital for Children NHS Trust, London WCIN3JH, UK
e-mail: gill.levitt@gosh.nhs.uk

D.M. Green
Department of Epidemiology and Cancer Control, St. Jude Children's Research Hospital, 262 Danny Thomas Place Mail Stop 735, Memphis, TN 38105-2794, USA
e-mail: daniel.green@stjude.org

Abstract

The use of multimodality regimes in the treatment of renal tumors has been very successful over the last two decades. The good overall survival has made available a large number of survivors who have been carefully studied leading to information on the late consequences of treatment. Late mortality due to treatment received was reported in 20 % of deaths. Morbidity studies have highlighted problems, in particular life threatening cardiac disease and the development of second malignant neoplasms. Other problems noted are pulmonary dysfunction, renal disease, reproductive issues particularly in abdominally irradiated females and reduced quality of life. This information can be used to inform future protocols to reduce late sequelae and surveillance follow-up programmes to identify and treat sequelae.

13.1 Introduction

Cancer treatment, designed to be cytotoxic, is not specific to cancer cells, and therefore, normal tissue damage may occur. The late effects of treatment are defined as clinical or subclinical consequences that persist or appear more than 5 years after diagnosis.

Late sequelae of cancer treatment have become an important issue as survival rates have improved. This is particularly pertinent for childhood renal

K. Pritchard-Jones, J.S. Dome (eds.), *Renal Tumors of Childhood: Biology and Therapy*, Pediatric Oncology, DOI 10.1007/978-3-662-44003-2_13, © Springer-Verlag Berlin Heidelberg 2014

tumors where the overall survival has been consistently high over the last two decades (Ries et al. 2008).

The extent of the damage depends on many factors including the demographics of the patient, genetic factors and the treatment modalities and doses required to cure the cancer. The majority of renal tumors occur in young children with the commonest, Wilms tumor, presenting at a mean age of 3 years. These young patients therefore are more vulnerable to tissue damage because of the effect on the potential growth and development which still needs to occur.

The main constituents of treatment for common renal tumors include nephrectomy, combination chemotherapy and, for some, radiation of the chest and/or abdomen. Studies on long-term outcome of patients treated during the 1980/1990s are relevant to survivors of present-day protocols.

The information on treatment-related late effects comes from a variety of studies including large epidemiological (population/multicentre) and single/multicentre studies from a disease perspective or a particular organ function, and the results need to be viewed with an understanding of the aims and limitations of the studies.

In this chapter, we will address the clinically significant late sequelae that occur in survivors of childhood renal tumors, including late mortality; cardiovascular, pulmonary, renal, musculoskletal and reproductive function; the development of benign and malignant second neoplasms; and quality of life.

13.2 Late Mortality

Late mortality studies ascertain the number and causes of death in survivors who enter the study cohort at 5 years from diagnosis. The most frequent cause of death is the primary tumor, but 20 % of deaths are due to the cancer treatment.

Treatment-induced mortality has been studied in a number of countries. These studies give an indication of the systems damaged by treatment and the prevalence of such damage. In America, there are two recent studies in which patient participation partially overlaps, but which give a good overview. The Childhood Cancer Survivor Study (CCSS) is a multi-institutional study of over 20,000 5-year survivors (Armstrong et al. 2009). The initial cancers were diagnosed between 1970 and 1986 and the year of ascertainment was 2002. There were 1,735 patients with renal tumors 97 of whom died resulting in a standardised mortality ratio (SMR) of 4.6 (95 % confidence interval (CI), 3.8–5.6) and a cumulative incidence at 30 years of 8.6 %, which is a nearly fivefold increase in the risk of early death compared with their age and sex-matched peers in the general population (Armstrong et al. 2009). The causes of mortality change over the follow-up interval. Initially, recurrence of disease is the primary cause but, by 30 years from diagnosis, the occurrence of second malignant tumors becomes the leading cause of death with an SMR of 16.4 (95 % CI 10.8–23.8). Other causes of late mortality highlighted were cardiac (SMR, 12.7, 95 % CI, 6.3–22.8) and pulmonary (SMR, 4.3, 95 % CI, 0.5–15.1).

Cotton et al. studied the cause of death in 6,185 patients registered on the National Wilms Tumor Study (NWTS) between 1969 and 1995, 90 % of whom had Wilms tumor, with clear cell sarcoma and rhabdoid tumors specified. They noted that over a 30-year period the SMR fell, but remained increased in patients surviving more than 20 years from diagnosis (SMR, 12.6 after 5 years to 4.3 after 20 years). Over one-third of deaths in the 5-year survivor cohort were due to late effects (cardiac, end-stage renal disease and pulmonary) including second malignant neoplasms (SMN). The risk of death from treatment-related causes was approximately 2 % (Cotton et al. 2009).

13.3 Overall Late Morbidity

Studies conducted on large cancer survivor cohorts have highlighted the increased morbidity in patients receiving anthracyclines, alkylating agents and abdominal and/or thoracic radiation. The CCSS studied adverse outcomes declared by patients or their proxies via questionnaires across different tumor types (Oeffinger et al. 2006).

The event was defined and graded by the Common Terminology Criteria for Adverse Events (version 3) produced by the National Cancer Institute (National Cancer Institute 2006). Six hundred and seventy Wilms tumor survivors diagnosed between 1970 and 1986 were compared with sibling controls. The cumulative incidence of grade 1–5 (mild to life threatening) adverse events at 20 years was 60 %, with 20 % of patients having severe or life-threatening events such as second malignant tumors or cardiotoxicity.

Geenen et al. performed a clinical assessment on 189 survivors of Wilms tumor from a single centre diagnosed between 1966 and 1996, 29 % of whom had no adverse effects. Twelve percent demonstrated a high or severe burden of adverse effects. They highlighted the increased risk of cardiovascular problems after anthracyclines and thoracic/abdominal radiation with relative risks (RR) of 3.55 (95 % CI, 1.52–8.20) and 2.36 (95 % CI, 1.69–3.29), respectively (Geenen et al. 2007).

13.4 Treatment Modalities

13.4.1 Surgery

All patients undergo abdominal surgery which can rarely cause adhesions with some children requiring operative intervention. Small bowel obstruction seems to be the commonest with rates varying between 2.9 and 14.3 % (Paulino et al. 2000; Ritchey et al. 1992; Taylor 1997; Weirich et al. 2004). In the later two series, abdominal radiotherapy appeared to be a contributory factor. Surgery for removal of the primary renal tumor and for diagnosis/resection of lung disease will be discussed under the relevant section.

13.4.2 Radiotherapy

Radiation causes injury to tissues within the radiation field. The degree of damage and the ability to recover from radiation induced injury is dependent on tissue characteristics including cell differentiation, cell turnover and renewal potential. Acute effects occur in tissues with rapid cell turnover (such as mucosal membranes and intestine) and healing occurs within a few weeks. Tissues with poor mechanisms for repair present with late toxicities and the extent of damage is related to dose per fraction and total dose. However, many radiation-associated late effects are probably mediated by damage to the vasculature causing tissue ischaemia (Hopewell 1980).

The fields generally used in the treatment of renal tumors are designed to maximise local and distant control. The abdominal field is usually a single flank or the whole abdominal. The upper and lower borders depend on the position of the tumors. Upper limits may require areas of lung and heart to be included within the field (Fig. 13.1a, b). Lower limits may necessitate radiation including ovaries and the uterus.

Metastatic spread is most frequently to the lungs but can be to the liver and, in the case of clear cell sarcoma, bony metastases may develop which may necessitate the use of local radiotherapy. Therefore, vulnerable normal tissues include soft tissues, spine, chest wall, lungs, heart, remaining kidney and ovaries/uterus. The effects of exposure to radiation will be discussed further under organ dysfunction.

The doses of radiation have been reduced over the last decades. Initially abdominal radiation doses were as high as 35 Gy but, even for unfavourable disease, the total doses given currently do not exceed 24 Gy. Lung radiation has also been reduced and in the USA doses of 12 Gy are employed.

When assessing a patient for potential late effects, there must be a clear understanding which normal tissues were in the field and the doses they received. Modern planning techniques give good dosimetry information for all exposed tissues and reduce doses to normal tissues to a minimum.

13.4.3 Chemotherapy

The late sequelae resulting from chemotherapy are varied depending on the properties of the agents used. The mainstay of Wilms tumor treatment involves three drugs: vincristine, actinomycin D and anthracyclines. Patients with

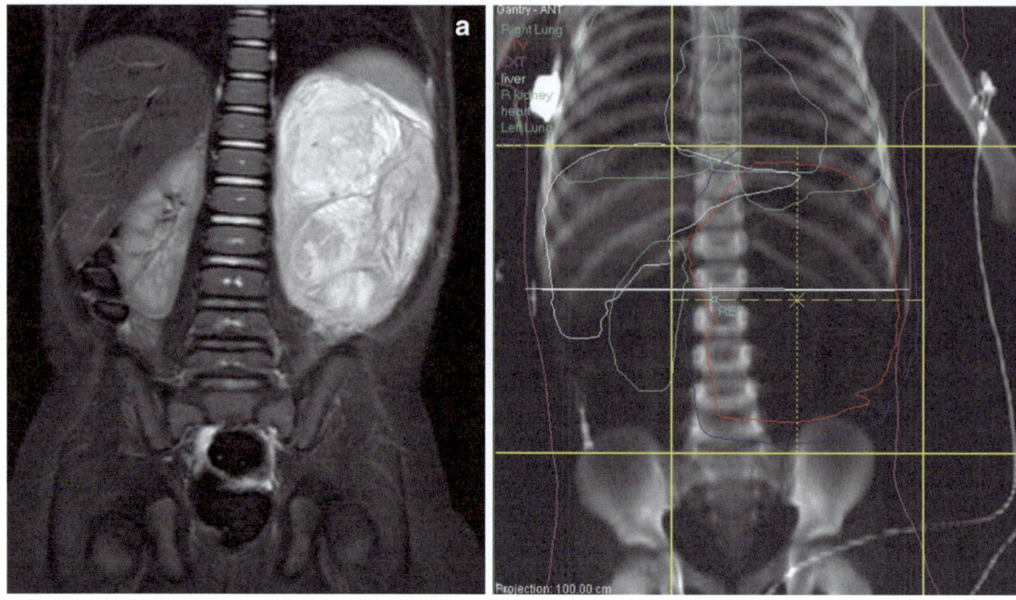

Fig. 13.1 (**a**) MRI right Wilms tumor. (**b**) Radiotherapy planning CT scan. *Red line* is outlining the gross renal tumor volume with heart, liver, left kidney and spleen demarcated. *Blue line* is the target planning volume and *yellow line* outlines the superior/inferior/medial and lateral margins of the radiation field

unfavourable or relapsed Wilms tumors and other renal tumors are treated with additional agents, including alkylating agents, topoisomerase II inhibitors (epipodophyllotoxins) and platinum compounds. High dose chemotherapy with peripheral stem cell/bone marrow rescue is administered for some cases.

Actinomycin D and vincristine have been in use since the 1960s and will be briefly mentioned here. The late effects due to other agents will be discussed in the relevant organ/system section.

Actinomycin D is known to cause acute hepatopathy with thrombocytopenia and histological manifestations of veno-occlusive disease (sinusoidal obstruction syndrome (SOS)) in a very low percentage of patients (Green et al. 1990). The first two UK studies reported an incidence of 1.4 % with single three weekly doses of 1.5 mg/m^2 with some early fatalities (Raine et al. 1991). Within the European studies, SOS was reported in 2.5 % of those treated with actinomycin D over 3–5 days compared to 0 % among those who received a lower weekly dose given over a single day, although a later publication of SIOP trials showed higher daily dose was detrimental compared with lower multiple doses of equivalent weekly dosages (Ludwig et al. 1999). Young age was also a risk factor and the majority of protocols now have an age-related sliding scale for actinomycin D doses. The Dutch group reported pathological changes in the liver which may be longstanding (Jagt et al. 2009). Usually there is complete recovery, but there are anecdotal reports of chronic hepatic disease with portal hypertension developing.

Vincristine may cause peripheral, autonomic or cranial neuropathy resulting in a loss of limb power, abnormal sensation, constipation and ptosis (Legha 1986). The recovery is usually complete after cessation of treatment. Very rarely vincristine can unmask peripheral neuropathy with increased severity of symptoms in patients with a family history of peripheral neuropathies particularly Charcot-Marie-Tooth (Graf et al. 1996).

13.4.4 Cardiovascular Toxicity

Both anthracyclines and cardiac radiation are responsible for the important cardiovascular toxicity seen in renal tumor survivors. Damage occurs at the time of the insult but may only be clinically apparent at a later date. Anthracycline-related injury is restricted to the myocytes, but radiation can cause damage to all layers of the heart including the major vessels.

The myocardium heals by replacing the myocytes by fibrosis and remodelling rather than regrowth. Previously it was thought that the total number of myocytes was static after birth but recent studies suggest there is a low rate of turnover decreasing with age. However, cardiac myocytes do not increase in overall numbers after the postnatal period and in fact there is a low level annual loss. Adaptation occurs in the young by remodelling using the capacity to increase myocyte volume.

13.4.4.1 Anthracyclines

There has been an appreciation of the risk of anthracycline-related preferential myocyte toxicity leading to cardiomyopathy since their introduction into the clinic. Pathologically they cause Z band disruption, vacuolation and myocyte death with replacement fibrosis but no inflammatory changes (Bristow et al. 1978).

The anticancer effects of anthracyclines are mediated primarily through inhibition of DNA synthesis, transcription and replication, but they also generate oxygen-derived free radicals using iron as a cofactor and the mitochondrial respiratory chain. These free radicals cause direct damage to proteins, lipids and DNA. The cardiac myocytes appear to have a poorly functioning oxygen free radical scavenging enzyme system compared with other tissues. This is felt to be the main cause for the preferential toxicity to cardiac muscle (Basser and Green 1993; Olson et al. 1981).

Since the 1970s the principal anthracycline used has been doxorubicin although the French group has used epirubicin (dose for dose epirubicin is thought to be less cardiotoxic in adults). Clinical heart failure which may occur acutely or many years from the completion of treatment is the commonest presentation. The cumulative risk of clinical congestive heart failure 20 years after diagnosis, a serious and potentially fatal late effect of anthracycline therapy, was reported to be 4.4 % in relapse-free Wilms tumor patients whose treatment included anthracyclines with or without whole lung irradiation and in 17.4 % in Wilms tumor patients whose treatment for initial and/or relapse therapy included anthracyclines with or without whole lung irradiation (Green et al. 2001, 2003). The relative risk (RR) of congestive heart failure increased by 4.5 (95 % confidence interval (CI) 1.6–12.6) for female sex, 3.2 (95 % CI 1.8–5.7) for every 100 mg/m^2 of anthracycline and 1.8 (95 % CI 1.2–2.8) for every 10 Gy of left abdominal irradiation (Green et al. 2003).

Sorensen et al. evaluated cardiac function 1.0–18.8 years (mean 7.1 years, standard deviation (SD) 3.9 years) after completion of treatment in 97 children whose therapy for Wilms tumor included an anthracycline (mean cumulative dose – 303 mg/m^2), in 39 children 0.5–20.0 years (mean, 8.9 years, SD, 5.0 years) after completion of treatment for Wilms tumor that had not included an anthracycline and 50 age-matched controls. Left ventricular afterload, measured as left ventricular end systolic wall stress (LVESWS), was significantly increased in the anthracycline-treated patients compared to those whose treatment had not included an anthracycline, but contractility, estimated by the stress velocity index (SVI) a measure controlled for afterload, was not significantly decreased among the anthracycline treated patients. Subclinical cardiac abnormalities were found in 25 % of the patients who received anthracyclines. In multivariate analysis that included cardiac radiation, only increasing cumulative dose and dose intensity were significant risk factors for impaired cardiac function (Sorensen et al. 1995). Serial evaluation of this cohort 4.4 ± 0.5 years after the initial evaluation demonstrated significant decreases in fractional shortening and left ventricular posterior wall thickness (Sorensen et al. 2003) and isovolumetric relaxation time (Dorup et al. 2004) in those who received anthracyclines in excess of 250 mg/m^2. These results contrasted with an analysis of cardiac function by echocardiogram and ECG in WT patients treated on SIOP 9/GPOH and SIOP 93-01/GPOH with a shorter mean follow-up of 2.9 years which demonstrated abnormalities in only 2.5 % of patients (Marx et al. 2002).

Studies have suggested that cardiac dysfunction is progressive, maybe as a result of myocyte loss and the inability to keep up with somatic growth after initial remodelling (Lipshultz et al. 2005; Pein et al. 2004). This is supported by long-term studies and a cardiac transplant survey. The survey reported what the age of cardiac transplantation was during pubertal development irrespective of age of anthracycline treatment (Levitt et al. 2009). It is anticipated that this may not be such a problem in survivors receiving a total dose of <250 mg/m^2 (Pein et al. 2004; Sorensen et al. 2003). Recent protocol design has reduced the total anthracycline dose to 250 mg/m^2.

Cumulative doxorubicin dose is the most important risk factor for the occurrence of subclinical abnormalities of cardiac function (Hausdorf et al. 1988; Kremer et al. 2002; Krischer et al. 1997; Lipshultz et al. 1995; Nysom et al. 1998; Sorensen et al. 1995, 2003). Bu'Lock et al. reported a shortening fraction of less than 30 % in 0 % (0 of 23 patients) of patients who received ≤100 mg/m^2 of anthracycline, compared with 4 % (2 of 48 patients) of patients who received 101–200 mg/m^2, 13 % (6 of 48 patients) of those who received 201–300 mg/m^2, 31 % (15 of 49 patients) of those who received 301–400 mg/m^2, 46 % (21 of 46 patients) of those who received 401–500 mg/m^2 and 58 % (7 of 12 patients) of those who received >500 mg/m^2 (Bu'Lock et al. 1995b). Hudson and colleagues reported that the odds ratio (OR) for decreased fractional shortening increased by 1.19 (95 % CI 1.01–1.39) ($p = 0.033$) for each increase in cumulative dose of 50 mg/m^2 (Hudson et al. 2007).

Females have been reported to have a greater risk of developing congestive heart failure (Green et al. 2001, 2003), a cardiac function test abnormality (gated nuclear angiocardiography and/or maximal cardiac index) (Silber et al. 1993) and/or decreased velocity of circumferential fibre shortening to end systolic wall stress ratio (Lipshultz et al. 1995; Postma et al. 2002) by most, but not all, authors (Bu'Lock et al. 1995a; Sorensen et al. 1995).

The treatment of clinical anthracycline cardiotoxicity is not in doubt and is similar to other causes of heart failure. However, there is controversy whether there is a benefit to starting treatment in patients with subclinical cardiotoxicity. Lipshultz suggested there was a short-term gain, but no long-term studies have been performed (Lipshultz et al. 2002).

13.4.4.2 Irradiation

Cardiac radiation occurs when the lungs and left flank receive radiation. Cardiac radiation potentiates the cardiotoxicity of anthracyclines and in its own right can cause damage to the different layers of the heart including the valves, myocardium and pericardium (Levitt and Saran 2004).

13.4.4.3 Aorta and Main Branches

There is a theoretical risk of long-term damage to arterial vessels although only a few cases have been reported. Damage is thought in part to be secondary to injury of the vasa vasorum (Foreman et al. 1995) with histopathological findings of lipid deposits and fibrosis similar to those of atheroma and therefore nonspecific (Fajardo 1999). Fewer than 30 cases have been cited in children treated for various solid tumors, although Ganry et al. suggested that some children may have undiagnosed asymptomatic stenosis (Ganry et al. 1993). They reported a cohort of 16 children treated between 1967 and 1993 which included 5 children treated for Wilms tumor with abdominal radiation of doses greater than 25 Gy between the ages of 14 and 36 months. Imaging identified aortic hypoplasia or stenosis and renal artery stenosis with a considerable latent period of 10–20 years from treatment to diagnosis (Ganry et al. 1993).

The other arteries of importance are the coronary arteries which are within the radiation field during lung radiation. There is little information regarding the risk of coronary artery disease in Wilms tumor survivors compared to many reports in survivors of Hodgkin lymphoma. The cardiac dose the Wilms tumor patients receive is significantly lower than that received during the treatment of Hodgkin lymphoma (Hancock et al. 1993).

13.4.5 Pulmonary Function

Pulmonary function may be impaired by radiation therapy, specific chemotherapeutic agents and/or chest wall surgery

Several groups of investigators reported studies of lung function in children treated with lung irradiation for metastatic Wilms tumor (Table 13.1). Wohl et al. evaluated 20 children, six of whom received a single course of whole lung radiation, six of whom received additional pulmonary radiation therapy and/or underwent thoracotomy and eight of whom received no whole lung radiation therapy. The total lung capacity (TLC) was 71 % and the vital capacity (VC) was 72 % of that predicted among children who received only bilateral whole lung irradiation. Those treated with a thoracotomy and/or additional pulmonary irradiation had a TLC which was 58 % and a VC which was 60 % of that predicted. The airways were relatively unaffected following lung irradiation, compared to the pulmonary parenchyma (Wohl et al. 1975).

Littman et al. evaluated lung function in ten patients who received whole lung radiation therapy for pulmonary metastases, five patients who received prophylactic whole lung radiation therapy and 18 patients who received no whole lung radiation therapy. They reported similar reductions in TLC and VC in patients treated for pulmonary metastases with whole lung irradiation doses of 1,200–1,370 cGy (Littman et al. 1976).

Benoist et al. studied 48 children following 2,000 cGy of whole lung irradiation for metastatic Wilms tumor. All patients received actinomycin D during pulmonary irradiation. These investigators found significant reductions in TLC and VC. They also demonstrated in 11 patients evaluated serially that the reduction in TLC and VC progressed between 18 and 48 months after therapy (Benoist et al. 1982).

Shaw et al. evaluated pulmonary function in 47 survivors of Wilms tumor, including three who received whole lung irradiation. The three had normal values for forced expiratory volume in 1 s (FEV_1) and TLC, but had decreased transfer factor for carbon monoxide (TCO) (Shaw et al. 1991).

Lung metastectomy may involve removal of normal lung tissue, but evidence below is reassuring. Pulmonary function was evaluated in 15 patients 3–30 years (median – 15 years) after undergoing lobectomy for congenital lobar emphysema at 1 week to 3 years of age (median – 3 months). Eight to 45 % (median – 22 %) of the total lung tissue by predicted weight was removed. Vital capacity (VC) was normal in 13 of 15 patients and total lung capacity (TLC) was normal in 14 of 14 patients, although the mean values for both VC (94 %) and TLC (93 %) were significantly decreased compared to normal values. Forced expiratory volume in 1 s (FEV_1) was below normal in 14 of 15 patients, with a mean predicted value of 73 % (McBride et al. 1980).

Table 13.1 Pulmonary function following whole lung irradiation for Wilms tumor

Author	Number of patients (number of eligible patients)	Radiation treatment dose (cGy) – range (median)	Thoracic surgery	Follow-up (years) range (mean ± SD)	VC (% predicted) (range)	FEV_1 (% of VC)	D_LCO (% predicted)
Wohl et al. (1975)	6	850–1,250	No	7–13 (10)	72 ± 8	90 ± 7.5	68 ± 14
	6	920–2,630	Yes	7–17 (11)	60 ± 22	88 ± 5.3	61 ± 16
Littman et al. (1976)	10 (metastases)	1,200–1,370	Yes[a]	4–12	65 (26–91)	61 (27–86)	
	5 (prophylaxis)	1,163–1,328	No	8–13	79 (73–84)	75 (66–75)	
Benoist et al. (1982)	48	2,000		2–17 (7 ± .25)	61 ± 13		
Shaw et al. (1991)	3	1,200	No			107	

[a]2 patients

13.4.6 Renal Function

Renal failure may occur in Wilms tumor patients as the result of genetic predisposition, surgical procedures, radiation therapy and/or chemotherapy.

Many survivors of Wilms tumor who develop chronic renal failure have syndromes associated with *WT1* mutations or deletions that predispose to renal disease. Breslow et al. reported that the risk of end-stage renal disease (ESRD) in Wilms tumor survivors 20 years after diagnosis was 1 % for those with unilateral tumor and 12 % for those with bilateral tumors. Patients with Denys-Drash syndrome, Wilms tumor, aniridia, genitourinary malformation, mental retardation (WAGR) syndrome or associated genitourinary anomalies had ESRD risks as high as 90 % (Breslow et al. 2005).

Survivors of childhood cancer who have undergone nephrectomy may be at risk for hyperfiltration injury and/or hypertension. Compensatory hypertrophy of the remaining kidney is a well-documented finding after nephrectomy (Bailey et al. 2002). Although this adaptation may initially increase glomerular filtration capacity, the later development of glomerulosclerosis (Gutierrez-Millet et al. 1986; Welch and McAdams 1986) and interstitial injury (Mitus et al. 1969) may ultimately lead to deterioration of renal function.

Clinically significant reductions in glomerular filtration rate after nephrectomy have been seen in a minority of survivors of Wilms tumor (Gutierrez-Millet et al. 1986; Mpofu and Mann 1992; Srinivas et al. 1998). One study reported no statistically significant differences in mean GFR between children who underwent nephrectomy for Wilms tumor or neuroblastoma (median follow-up after nephrectomy, 12 and 9 months, respectively) and children of comparable age who underwent nephrectomy for non-malignant disease (median follow-up after nephrectomy, 23 months) (Schell et al. 1995). However, 50 % of the childhood cancer survivors who underwent nephrectomy had chronic renal insufficiency (defined as GFR <90 mL/min/1.73 m^2). A comparison between children with Wilms tumor who did or did not receive whole abdominal irradiation demonstrated lower GFR in the irradiated group (73 % of normal) than in the nonirradiated group (95 % of normal) (de Graaf et al. 1996). In this study, the prevalence of chronic renal insufficiency was 34 %.

GFR and renal compensatory growth were assessed a minimum of 5 years after nephrectomy in 22 children with Wilms tumor who had received abdominal radiation and 15 children who underwent nephrectomy for congenital hydronephrosis. The estimated size of the remnant kidney was increased by 25–29 % in the Wilms tumor group compared to 42 % in the hydronephrosis group. Mean GFR was significantly lower in the Wilms tumor group than that of the hydronephrosis group (82 and 92 % of healthy controls, respectively) (Wikstad et al. 1986). Long-term follow-up of children (mean 12.9 ± 3 years after therapy) with Wilms tumor found a low GFR (less than 80 mL/min/1.73 m^2 as measured by ^{51}Cr EDTA clearance) in 19 % (Levitt et al. 1992). Children whose GFR measurements were decreased were more likely to have received higher doses of radiation to the kidney and demonstrated poorer renal growth as measured by renal ultrasound (Levitt et al. 1992).

The prevalence of microalbuminuria, which is indicative of glomerular hyperfiltration, following nephrectomy for Wilms tumor, is less clear and has been reported to range from 5 to 84 % (Finklestein et al. 1993; Srinivas et al. 1998). Diastolic hypertension may also be a late effect of treatment that includes nephrectomy. In an analysis of 1,171 children treated for Wilms tumor whose blood pressure was measured 5 years after diagnosis, 83 (7 %) had a diastolic blood pressure above the 95th percentile for age (Finklestein et al. 1993). The relative contribution of nephrectomy to this complication was unclear because a substantial proportion of patients with diastolic hypertension had also received abdominal radiotherapy.

Ifosfamide, carboplatin (CBDCA) and, rarely, cis-platinum (DDP) which are used in regimens for the treatment of children with high risk (e.g. diffuse anaplasia) or recurrent Wilms tumor, can adversely impact renal function.

The most frequent manifestation of ifosfamide-induced nephrotoxicity is proximal tubular dysfunction. A decrease in GFR occurs less often (Berrak et al. 2005; Fels et al. 1996; Ho et al. 1995; Loebstein et al. 1999; Prasad et al. 1996; Raney et al. 1994; Rossi et al. 1999; Skinner 2003; Stohr et al. 2007; Suarez et al. 1991). Acute renal tubular dysfunction often resolves prior to the next course of chemotherapy. However, permanent and potentially progressive kidney damage may occur (Skinner 2003).

Approximately 30 % of ifosfamide-treated children develop a persistent tubulopathy and 5 % have clinically significant Fanconi syndrome (Suarez et al. 1991). This syndrome is caused by a generalised dysfunction of renal proximal tubule cells and is defined by excessive urinary excretion of glucose, amino acids, phosphate, bicarbonate and other solutes handled by this nephron segment. In many cases, tubular dysfunction is asymptomatic. Although some children with ifosfamide-induced Fanconi syndrome recover sufficient renal tubular function, approximately one-third continue to have clinically significant renal tubular dysfunction (Skinner 2003).

A number of risk factors for chronic ifosfamide nephrotoxicity have been proposed, including cumulative dose (>60–100 g/m^2) (Fels et al. 1996; Ho et al. 1995; Loebstein et al. 1999; Skinner et al. 2000; Stohr et al. 2007), age <3–5 years at the time of treatment (Loebstein et al. 1999; Stohr et al. 2007), concurrent or previous platinum therapy (Loebstein et al. 1999; Marina et al. 2000), renal irradiation (Fels et al. 1996) and unilateral nephrectomy (Fels et al. 1996) or hydronephrosis (Raney et al. 1994).

The platinum-containing agents cisplatin and carboplatin (CBDCA) have a similar spectrum of activity. Cisplatin is more toxic to the kidney and is the major dose-limiting side effect causing an acute loss of renal function, which includes a magnesium-wasting tubulopathy. This effect may be long-standing (Skinner et al. 1998; Ariceta et al. 1997; Brock et al. 1991), hence Cisplatin is rarely used in the treatment of WT. Clinically important reductions in GFR and hypomagnesaemia are rare following CBDCA. The risk of renal insufficiency and tubulopathies may be higher with carboplatin/ifosfamide than with cisplatin/ifosfamide combination therapy (Hartmann et al. 2000; Marina et al. 2000). Daw et al. reported that, when CBDCA dosage was based on GFR to achieve targeted systemic exposure (6 mg/mL/min), no Wilms tumor patient developed clinically significant renal tubular dysfunction at the end of treatment with the combination of ifosfamide, CBDCA and etoposide (ICE) although urinary beta(2)-microglobulin excretion increased during therapy. Mean GFR (measured by ^{99m}Tc DTPA clearance) declined by 7 % after two cycles of ICE and by 38 % after nephrectomy; the mean carboplatin dose was reduced 32 % after nephrectomy. Mean GFR remained stable after the third ICE cycle. Treatment with ICE, nephrectomy and radiotherapy significantly reduced GFR, largely as the result of nephrectomy. They suggested that adjustment of carboplatin dosage on the basis of GFR and careful monitoring of renal function might alleviate nephrotoxicity related to ICE in patients who have previously undergone nephrectomy (Daw et al. 2009).

13.4.7 Musculoskeletal

Radiation treatment in young children is particularly detrimental to growth and development of normal tissues and the degree of damage is dependent on total dose, fractionation and field. The radiation fields most commonly used include the flank, whole abdomen and the chest wall including the spine. The musculoskeletal problems include loss of growth potential, spinal deformities and soft tissue hypoplasia.

Growth of the skeleton is affected with an impact on final height due to reduction in sitting height. The loss of height depends on the length of the spine radiated, age of the child and dose delivered. Wallace et al. studied 30 WT patients treated between 1945 and 1988 who received flank or whole abdominal radiation to a total dose of 20–30 Gy. The patients exhibited a decrease in sitting height of 2.4 standard deviation score (SDS), with a median final height of 1.0 SDS below the mean (Wallace et al. 1990). The degree of loss of height was related to the age at treatment. The estimated loss of height was 10 cm if treated at 1 year of age and 6 cm at 5 years of age. Megavoltage radiotherapy was more detrimental than orthovoltage. The later patients were also treated with actinomycin D, a radiation sensitizer (D'Angio et al. 1959), and this may have increased growth inhibition (Wallace and Shalet 1992).

Hogeboom et al. suggested with patient modelling using NWTS data that the threshold dose to effect spinal growth was 15 Gy with predictions of height deficit of 1.8 cm at final height for those receiving 10 Gy compared with 4 cm for those who receive 15–24 Gy during early childhood (Hogeboom et al. 2001). With modern protocols the loss of growth potential is probably not clinically significant. Lung function studies have shown some reduction in chest wall size.

In the pre-1960 era, irradiation of the flank including only part of the vertebral column (up to the midline) resulted in differential growth of the spine with the development of severe scoliosis. The treatment of the whole width of the vertebral body has prevented the severe deformities, but despite this, recent studies of patients treated between 1968 and 1994 quote incidence rates of spinal deformities between 10 and 70 % (Makipernaa et al. 1993; Paulino et al. 2000; Wallace et al. 1990). The variability in part is due to differences in the method of evaluation (clinical versus radiological), type of radiation (orthovoltage versus megavoltage), dose and length of follow-up. Two publications suggest a reduction in spinal problems occurs with doses below 24 Gy (Paulino et al. 2000; Rate et al. 1991). Other skeletal problems reported were kyphosis, hypoplasia of the iliac wing and leg length discrepancies (Paulino et al. 2000).

The soft tissues hypoplasia occurs after radiation but is usually not an important issue unless there is obvious truncal asymmetry when girls in particular comment on their poor body image. Breast hypoplasia has been highlighted but is not universal (Macklis et al. 1991; Rosenfield et al. 1989). Asymmetry may occur when the renal bed requires radiation for an upper pole tumor and there is unilateral field extension into the chest. Breast implants can be used for cosmetic purposes, but patients must be altered to the risk of radiation-induced breast cancer developing in the remaining breast tissue.

13.4.8 Fertility and Pregnancy Outcome

13.4.8.1 Ovarian Function

Depending on the extent of damage to the ovaries, two forms of premature ovarian failure can be distinguished (Chemaitilly et al. 2006). Survivors who lose ovarian function during cancer therapy or shortly after its completion are classified as having acute ovarian failure (AOF). Some survivors who retain ovarian function after the completion of cancer treatment will experience menopause prior to age 40 years and are classified as having premature menopause (Chemaitilly et al. 2006; Wallace et al. 2005). In general, older age at treatment; exposure to abdominal, pelvic and spinal radiotherapy; and certain chemotherapeutic drugs, especially alkylating agents, have been shown to increase the rate of ovarian failure in female cancer survivors (Chemaitilly et al. 2006; Sklar 1999).

Acute ovarian failure (loss ovarian function during cancer therapy or shortly after its completion) (AOF) occurred in 215 of 3,390 eligible participants in the Childhood Cancer Survivor Study (CCSS). Survivors with AOF were older at cancer diagnosis, more likely to have been diagnosed with Hodgkin lymphoma or to have received abdominal or pelvic radiotherapy than survivors without AOF (Chemaitilly et al. 2006). Of survivors who developed AOF, 75 % had received abdominal-pelvic irradiation. Radiation doses to the ovary ≥2,000 cGy were associated with the highest rate of AOF with over 70 % of such patients developing AOF (Chemaitilly et al. 2006).

The incidence of and risk factors for premature menopause (menopause prior to age 40 years) were evaluated in participants in the CCSS who were older than 18 years (Sklar et al. 2006). A total of 126 childhood cancer survivors and 33 control siblings developed premature menopause. The cumulative incidence of nonsurgical premature menopause was substantially higher among survivors than among siblings (8 % versus 0.8 %; RR = 13.21, 95 % CI = 3.26–53.51; p < .001), whereas the RR for surgically induced menopause (RR = 0.8, 95 % CI = 0.52–1.23) did not differ between the two groups (Sklar et al. 2006). A multiple Poisson regression model showed that risk factors for nonsurgical premature menopause included attained age, exposure to increasing doses of radiation to the ovaries, increasing alkylating agent score (based on number of alkylating agents and cumulative dose) and a diagnosis of Hodgkin lymphoma. For survivors who were treated with alkylating agents plus abdominal-pelvic radiation, the cumulative incidence of nonsurgical premature menopause approached 30 % (Sklar et al. 2006). The effect of abdominal radiation on ovarian function is born out by two studies performed on female WT survivors (Nussbaum Blask et al. 1999; Wallace et al. 1989).

Male fertility is not normally an issue unless moderate or high cumulative doses of alkylating agents are employed.

13.4.8.2 Uterine Function and Pregnancy Outcome

Several studies demonstrated that the offspring of women who received flank irradiation for Wilms tumor were more likely to have a birthweight of less than 2,500 g than were those born to women whose protocol treatment for Wilms tumor did not include flank irradiation (Byrne et al. 1988; Green et al. 1982; Li et al. 1987). Chiarelli et al. reported an increased relative risk of low-birthweight offspring among women treated for childhood cancer with greater than 25 Gy of abdominal-pelvic radiation (Chiarelli et al. 2000). Hawkins et al. reported that the mean birthweight of the offspring of women who received abdominal radiation for Wilms tumor, but not of those who received abdominal radiation for a malignancy other than Wilms tumor, was less than that of the offspring of unirradiated women or men (Hawkins and Smith 1989). The offspring of the female participants in the CCSS who received pelvic irradiation were more likely to weigh <2,500 g at birth than offspring of those who did not receive radiation to the pelvis (RR 1.85, 95 % CI 1.07–3.18, p = 0.03) (Green et al. 2002b). None of these studies reported the effect of the different radiation doses received by the musculoskeletal structures, uterus or ovaries from the various treatment volumes included in their analyses of low birth weight.

Green et al. reported that malposition of the foetus and early or threatened labour were more frequent among female Wilms tumor survivors who received abdominal irradiation than among those who did not, with the frequency increasing with increasing abdominal radiation dose. In addition, the frequency of both low birthweight <2,500 g and early gestational age <36 weeks increased with increasing abdominal radiation dose. No effect of abdominal irradiation on pregnancy outcome was observed in the partners of irradiated male Wilms tumor survivors or in their offspring (Green et al. 2002a).

Uterine function may be adversely impacted by both congenital malformation and treatment effects. Nicholson et al. reported uterine abnormalities in 8 % (2 of 24) of female Wilms tumor patients, one of whom had the WAGR syndrome (Nicholson et al. 1996). Critchley et al. suggested that damage to both the uterine vasculature and myometrium contributed to restricted foetal growth and early birth. They demonstrated that uterine length was significantly less in 10 women with ovarian failure who had been treated with whole abdomen irradiation. Endometrial thickness, based on weekly ultrasound examinations, did not increase in response to hormone replacement therapy in three women. No blood flow was detectable with Doppler ultrasound through either uterine artery of five women and through only one uterine artery in three additional women (Critchley et al. 1992; Critchley 1999). Others have confirmed the finding of reduced uterine volume despite sex steroid replacement therapy. In addition, uterine blood flow did not normalise in three of nine women, despite treatment with sex steroid replacement therapy (Holm et al. 1999).

13.4.9 Tumor Development

The occurrence of second tumors within the cancer population, either benign or malignant, is a well-recognised late sequelae of therapy and WT survivors are no exception. The less serious occurrence of osteochondromas, benign bone tumors, maybe associated with radiation of the epiphysis of growing bone. These tumors can cause pain, affect function and be unsightly requiring surgical intervention. Within the radiation field the incidence is between 6 and 20 % with only a rare report of malignant transformation (Jaffe et al. 1983; Libshitz and Cohen 1982; Tsuchiya et al. 1990). Interestingly, these tumors have been reported in unirradiated WT patients, some of whom had a family history of multiple exostosis (Walker et al. 1992). Hereditary multiple exostosis syndrome is associated with mutation on chromosome 11 short arm exostosin-1 (EXT1) or exostosin-2 (EXT2) (Jennes et al. 2009).

Patients exposed to radiotherapy and certain chemotherapy agents or with a known familial cancer predisposition syndrome have all been demonstrated to have an increased risk of second cancers. Studies across a number of countries have given a range of cumulative incidence of 0.65–0.8 % at 10 years increasing to 4.8–7.0 % at 30 years.

The National Wilms Tumor Study Group (NWTSG) in the USA reported 43 second cancers in a population of 5,278 patients diagnosed with WT between 1969 and 1991 giving a standardised incidence ratio (SIR) of 8.4 and a cumulative risk within 15 years of diagnosis of 1.6 % (Breslow et al. 1995).

A European study of WT survivors based on 1988 patients treated on the International Society of Paediatric Oncology WT Trials and Studies 1, 2, 5 and 6 described eight second cancers. The SIR was 4.15 and the cumulative risk of a second tumor within 15 years of diagnosis was 0.65 % (Carli et al. 1997).

In a German study of patients treated on SIOP protocols between 1989 and 2008, 0.6 % had developed an SMN after a mean follow-up 4.2 ± 3.7 years. Interestingly there was a high percentage of bone marrow malignancies with three acute lymphoblastic leukaemias, three acute myeloblastic leukaemias and one myelodysplasia out of a total 12 SMNs. This increase in bone marrow malignancies in the modern era of treatment is also highlighted in a large three country collaboration where it is postulated that intensive chemotherapy and reduced radiation doses may be the cause (Breslow et al. 2010). The follow-up period is too short to comment on the solid tumor development (Nourkami et al. 2009).

The British population based study on 1,400 WT survivors treated between 1940 and 1991 with a mean follow-up of 19 years reported the SIR for solid second primary neoplasms was 6.7 (95 % CI: 5.0–8.8) (Taylor et al. 2008). Within their cohort there were 81 second primary neoplasms, including 52 solid neoplasms, 3 acute myeloid leukaemias and 26 basal cell carcinomas. They noted that the cumulative incidence of solid tumor development increased with each decade of age from 2.3 % (1.4–3.5 %) at 30 years to 6.8 % (4.6–9.5 %) at 40 years and 12.2 % (7.3–18.4 %) at 50 years. No adjustment was made for the background population incidence of cancer increasing with age (Taylor et al. 2008).

The types of second cancers reported vary and include bone and soft tissue sarcomas, breast cancer, lymphoma, tumors of the digestive tract, melanoma, acute leukaemias and basal cell carcinomas (Garwicz et al. 2000; Hawkins et al. 1987, 1996; Taylor et al. 2008). Radiation therapy used to treat childhood cancer has been consistently shown to be an important contributory factor in the excess risk of subsequent cancers observed in long-term survivors of all childhood cancers (Neglia et al. 2001; Tucker et al. 1987). Within a cohort of WT survivors, Breslow reported that 73 % of second solid tumors occurred within the radiotherapy field and found clear evidence of an increase in the risk of second cancer with increasing dose of radiation (Breslow et al. 1995). This is supported by Taylor et al. who reported that 35 of 39 solid tumors were within the radiation field and the majority had an estimated radiation doses of >25 Gy (Taylor et al. 2008).

An interaction between radiotherapy and doxorubicin, a known radiation sensitizer, has been postulated and suggestive evidence of this interaction arises in a number of reports, although small numbers prevent solid statistical analysis to support this (Garwicz et al. 2000; Hawkins et al. 1996). In the NWTSG report, among 234 patients who received doxorubicin and greater than 35 Gy abdominal radiation, 8 second cancers were observed where only 2.22 were expected (SIR 36) (Breslow et al. 1995). The type and distribution of second cancers following WT would indicate that patients exposed to radiotherapy during their primary treatment are at the greatest risk of developing subsequent malignancies. These patients should be counselled appropriately and offered advice to minimise future carcinogenic risks such as smoking and sun exposure.

13.4.10 Quality of Life (QOL)

QOL is a holistic measure of an individual's perception of their position in life in relation to their culture/peers and their goals, expectations and concerns and changes over time. The WHO definition is multidimensional, bringing to together health status and the interaction of society, financial and economic issues. There are many studies reporting on QOL of cancer survivors either comparing the survivors with the population norms, siblings or between different cancer populations.

In general adult survivors of WT do not differ significantly compared with population norms on educational status or mental health assessments (Gurney et al. 2009; Lahteenmaki et al. 2008; Reulen et al. 2007) although Nathan noted that survivors' emotional status maybe compromised (Nathan et al. 2007). This finding was supported by a psychosocial outcomes study comparing WT and acute lymphoblastic leukaemia survivors and found love/sexual relationships, friendships, nonspecific social contacts and day-to-day coping were more difficult compared to the age-matched controls (Mackie et al. 2000). In the CCSS study, WT survivors were as likely to be employed as their siblings (Pang et al. 2008). Unfortunately health-related status is impaired, particularly if radiation is part of the treatment plan. The CCSS study highlighted that 12.7 % had limited performance which was the lowest rate of all cancer types (Ness et al. 2005). This is supported by other studies (Barr et al. 2000; Lahteenmaki et al. 2008; Speechley et al. 2006) although Nathan did not find a discrepancy in physical performance compared with normal controls (Nathan et al. 2007). However, in the BCCSS study, the physical component showed a normal result in the 16–19-year age group but worsened with age so that the survivors above 35 years of age showed a regression coefficient of –2.0 compared with population norms. Females performed consistently worse than males. Twenty-five percent stated they could not walk a mile with 9 % being unable to walk 100 yds (Reulen et al. 2007).

13.4.11 Follow-Up/Surveillance

Long-term survivors of childhood cancer are at risk for a variety of late effects from their successful cancer treatment as illustrated above. However, they may not be aware of their treatment exposures and thus may not be able to provide their health-care providers with critical information needed to guide surveillance. Kadan-Lottick reported that 91 % of CCSS participants reported their cancer diagnosis accurately, although 19 % could provide no detail regarding their diagnosis. Two percent did not report that they had a history of cancer. Twenty percent did not accurately report that they had been treated with doxorubicin and 8 % did not know they had been treated with radiation therapy (Kadan-Lottick et al. 2002). Despite their increased risk for late morbidity related to their treatment, 15.6 % of male and 6.7 % of female CCSS participants reported receiving no medical care during a 2 year period. Only 28.2 % of those at risk for anthracycline-related cardiomyopathy had received a screening echocardiogram and 40.8 % of those at risk for radiation-related breast cancer had undergone mammography (Nathan et al. 2008). Similar findings were noted in the UK with general practitioners reporting 65 % had no follow-up (Taylor et al. 2004).

The reasons for low rates of medical evaluation are varied and may include patient, physician and systemic factors (Landier et al. 2006). In an effort to increase rates of risk-based evaluation, several "Guidelines" have been published with the goal of shaping physician awareness and practice patterns (Children's Oncology Group 2009; Scottish Intercollegiate Guidelines Network 2004; Skinner et al. 2005). Within the guidelines is the requirement for treating oncologists to provide personalised treatment summaries. Unanswered still are many questions, including the cost-effectiveness of various screening strategies for the individual and society. The best venue for long-term follow-up and the correct medium should provide the survivor with the best combination of access to treatment data, up to date late effects information with effective patient pathways, and protection of confidentiality.

Conclusions

Wilms tumor is one of the success stories of paediatric oncology clinical research. The design of contemporary studies has been guided by the desire to maintain or improve survival rates for those currently known to have a good prognosis by developing treatment regimens with a lower likelihood of long-term morbidity. The data reviewed in this chapter have contributed to these innovative treatment strategies and will facilitate the survival of future patients with less long-term morbidity than is experienced by past and current patients.

References

Ariceta G, Rodriguez-Soriano J, Vallo A, Navajas A (1997) Acute and chronic effects of cisplatin therapy on renal magnesium homeostasis. Med Pediatr Oncol 28:35–40

Armstrong GT, Liu Q, Yasui Y, Neglia JP, Leisenring W, Robison LL, Mertens AC (2009) Late mortality among 5-year survivors of childhood cancer: a summary from the childhood cancer survivor study. J Clin Oncol 27:2328–2338

Bailey S, Roberts A, Brock C, Price L, Craft AW, Kilkarni R, Lee RE, Skillen AW, Skinner R (2002) Nephrotoxicity in survivors of Wilms' tumours in the North of England. Br J Cancer 87:1092–1098

Barr RD, Chalmers D, De Pauw S, Furlong W, Weitzman S, Feeny D (2000) Health-related quality of life in survivors of Wilms' tumor and advanced neuroblastoma: a cross-sectional study. J Clin Oncol 18:3280–3287

Basser RL, Green MD (1993) Strategies for prevention of anthracycline cardiotoxicity. Cancer Treat Rev 19:57–77

Benoist MR, Lemerle J, Jean R, Rufin P, Scheinmann P, Paupe J (1982) Effects on pulmonary function of whole lung irradiation for Wilms' tumour in children. Thorax 37:175–180

Berrak SG, Pearson M, Berberoglu S, Ilhan IE, Jaffe N (2005) High-dose ifosfamide in relapsed pediatric osteosarcoma: therapeutic effects and renal toxicity. Pediatr Blood Cancer 44:215–219

Breslow NE, Takashima JR, Whitton JA, Moksness J, D'Angio GJ, Green DM (1995) Second malignant neoplasms following treatment for Wilm's tumor: a report from the National Wilms' Tumor Study Group. J Clin Oncol 13:1851–1859

Breslow NE, Collins AJ, Ritchey ML, Grigoriev YA, Peterson SM, Green DM (2005) End stage renal disease in patients with Wilms tumor: results from the National Wilms Tumor Study Group and the United States Renal Data System. J Urol 174:1972–1975

Breslow NE, Lange JM, Friedman DL, Green DM, Hawkins MM, Murphy MFG, Neglia JP, Olsen JH, Peterson SM, Stiller CA, Robison LL (2010) Secondary malignant neoplasms following Wilms Tumor: an International Collaborative Study. Int J Cancer 127(3):657–666

Bristow MR, Mason JW, Billingham ME, Daniels JR (1978) Doxorubicin cardiomyopathy: evaluation by phonocardiograpy, endomyocardial biopsy and cardiac catheterization. Ann Intern Med 88:168–175

Brock PR, Koliouskas DE, Barratt TM, Yeomans E, Pritchard J (1991) Partial reversibility of cisplatin nephrotoxicity in children. J Pediatr 118:531–534

Bu'Lock FA, Martin RP, Mott MG (1995a) Increased risk of cardiac dysfunction after anthracyclines in girls. Med Pediatr Oncol 24:143–144

Bu'Lock FA, Mott MG, Oakhill A, Martin RP (1995b) Left ventricular diastolic function after anthracycline chemotherapy in childhood: relationship with systolic function, symptoms, and pathophysiology. Br Heart J 73:340–350

Byrne J, Mulvihill JJ, Connelly RR, Austin DA, Holmes GE, Holmes FF, Latourette HB, Meigs JW, Strong LC, Myers MH (1988) Reproductive problems and birth defects in survivors of Wilms' tumor and their relatives. Med Pediatr Oncol 16:233–240

Carli M, Frascella E, Tournade MF, de Kraker J, Rey A, Guzzinati S, Burgers JM, Delemarre JF, Masiero L, Simonato L (1997) Second malignant neoplasms in patients treated on SIOP Wilms Tumor Studies and Trials 1,2,5, and 6. Med Pediatr Oncol 29:239–244

Chemaitilly W, Mertens AC, Mitby P, Whitton J, Stovall M, Yasui Y, Robison LL, Sklar CA (2006) Acute ovarian failure in the Childhood Cancer Survivor Study. J Clin Endocrinol Metab 91:1723–1728

Chiarelli AM, Marrett LD, Darlington GA (2000) Pregnancy outcomes in females after treatment for childhood cancer. Epidemiology 11:161–166

Children's Oncology Group (2009) Long-term follow-up guidelines for survivors of childhood, adolescent, and young adult cancers. Children's Oncology Group. http://www.survivorshipguidelines.org/pdf/LTFUGuidelines.pdf

Cotton CA, Peterson S, Norkool PA, Takashima J, Grigoriev Y, Green DM, Breslow NE (2009) Early and late mortality after diagnosis of Wilms tumor. J Clin Oncol 27:1304–1309

Critchley HOD (1999) Factors of importance for implantation and problems after treatment for childhood cancer. Med Pediatr Oncol 33:9–14

Critchley HO, Wallace WH, Shalet SM, Mamtora H, Higginson J, Anderson DC (1992) Abdominal irradiation in childhood: the potential for pregnancy. Br J Obstet Gynecol 99:392–394

D'Angio GJ, Farber S, Maddock CL (1959) Potentiation of x ray effects by actinomycin D. Radiology 73:175–177

Daw NC, Gregornik D, Rodman J, Marina N, Wu J, Kun LE, Jenkins JJ, McPherson V, Wilimas J, Jones DP (2009) Renal function after ifosfamide, carboplatin and etoposide (ICE) chemotherapy, nephrectomy and radiotherapy in children with Wilms tumour. Eur J Cancer 45:99–106

de Graaf SS, van Gent H, Reitsma-Bierens WC, van Luyk WH, Dolsma WV, Postma A (1996) Renal function after unilateral nephrectomy for Wilms' tumour: the influence of radiation therapy. Eur J Cancer 32A:465–469

Dorup I, Levitt G, Sullivan I, Sorensen K (2004) Prospective longitudinal assessment of late anthracycline cardiotoxicity after childhood cancer: the role of diastolic function. Heart 90:1214–1216

Fajardo LF (1999) Is the pathology of radiation injury different in small vs large blood vessels? Cardiovasc Radiat Med 1:108–110

Fels LM, Bokemeyer C, van Rhee J, Schmoll HJ, Stolte H (1996) Evaluation of late nephrotoxicity in long-term survivors of Hodgkin's disease. Oncology 53:73–78

Finklestein JZ, Norkool P, Green DM, Breslow N, D'Angio GJ (1993) Diastolic hypertension in Wilms' tumor survivors: a late effect of treatment? A report from the National Wilms' Tumor Study Group. Am J Clin Oncol 16:201–205

Foreman NK, Laitt RD, Chambers EJ, Duncan AW, Cummins BH (1995) Intracranial large vessel vasculopathy and anaplastic meningioma 19 years after cranial irradiation for acute lymphoblastic leukaemia. Med Pediatr Oncol 24:265–268

Ganry O, Habrand JL, Lemerle J, Flamant F, Sarrazin D (1993) Arterial lesions after radiotherapy in children. Apropos of 16 cases. Arch Fr Pediatr 50:9–14

Garwicz S, Anderson H, Olsen J, Dollner H, Hertz H, Jonmundsson G, Langmark F, Lanning M, Moller T, Sankila R, Tulinius H (2000) Second malignant neoplasms after cancer in childhood and adolescence: a population-based case-control study in the 5 Nordic countries. The Nordic Society for Pediatric Hematology and Oncology. The Association of the Nordic Cancer Registries. Int J Cancer 88:672–678

Geenen MM, Cardous-Ubbink MC, Kremer LC, van den Bos C, van der Pal HJ, Heinen RC, Jaspers MW, Koning CC, Oldenburger F, Langeveld NE, Hart AA, Bakker PJ, Caron HN, van Leeuwen FE (2007) Medical assessment of adverse health outcomes in long-term survivors of childhood cancer. JAMA 297:2705–2715

Graf WD, Chance PF, Lensch MW, Eng LJ, Lipe HP, Bird TD (1996) Severe vincristine neuropathy in Charcot-Marie-Tooth disease type 1A. Cancer 77:1356–1362

Green DM, Fine WE, Li FP (1982) Offspring of patients treated for unilateral Wilms' tumor in childhood. Cancer 49:2285–2288

Green DM, Norkool P, Breslow NE, Finklestein JZ, D'Angio GJ (1990) Severe hepatic toxicity after treatment with vincristine and dactinomycin using single-dose or divided-dose schedules: a report from the National Wilms' Tumor Study. J Clin Oncol 8:1525–1530

Green DM, Grigoriev YA, Nan B, Takashima JR, Norkool PA, D'Angio GJ, Breslow NE (2001) Congestive heart failure after treatment for Wilms' tumor: a report from the National Wilms' Tumor Study Group. J Clin Oncol 19:1926–1934

Green DM, Peabody EM, Nan B, Peterson S, Kalapurakal JA, Breslow NE (2002a) Pregnancy outcome after treatment for Wilms tumor: a report from the National Wilms Tumor Study Group. J Clin Oncol 20:2506–2513

Green DM, Whitton JA, Stovall M, Mertens AC, Donaldson SS, Ruymann FB, Pendergrass TW, Robison LL (2002b) Pregnancy outcome of female survivors of childhood cancer: a report from the Childhood Cancer Survivor Study. Am J Obstet Gynecol 187:1070–1080

Green DM, Grigoriev YA, Nan B, Takashima JR, Norkool PA, D'Angio GJ, Breslow NE (2003) Correction to "Congestive heart failure after treatment for Wilms' tumor". J Clin Oncol 21:2447–2448

Gurney JG, Krull KR, Kadan-Lottick N, Nicholson HS, Nathan PC, Zebrack B, Tersak JM, Ness KK (2009) Social outcomes in the Childhood Cancer Survivor Study cohort. J Clin Oncol 27:2390–2395

Gutierrez-Millet V, Nieto J, Praga M, Usera G, Martinez MA, Morales JM (1986) Focal glomerulosclerosis and proteinuria in patients with solitary kidneys. Arch Intern Med 146:705–709

Hancock SL, Donaldson SS, Hoppe RT (1993) Cardiac disease following treatment of Hodgkin's disease in children and adolescents. J Clin Oncol 11:1208–1215

Hartmann JT, Fels LM, Franzke A, Knop S, Renn M, Maess B, Panagiotou P, Lampe H, Kanz L, Stolte H, Bokemeyer C (2000) Comparative study of the acute nephrotoxicity from standard dose cisplatin +/– ifosfamide and high-dose chemotherapy with carboplatin and ifosfamide. Anticancer Res 20:3767–3773

Hausdorf G, Morf G, Beron G, Erttmann R, Winkler K, Landbeck G, Keck EW (1988) Long term doxorubicin cardiotoxicity in childhood: non-invasive evaluation of the contractile state and diastolic filling. Br Heart J 60:309–315

Hawkins MM, Smith RA (1989) Pregnancy outcomes in childhood cancer survivors: probable effects of abdominal irradiation. Int J Cancer 43:399–402

Hawkins MM, Draper GJ, Kingston JE (1987) Incidence of second primary tumours among childhood cancer survivors. Br J Cancer 56:339–347

Hawkins MM, Wilson LM, Burton HS, Potok MH, Winter DL, Marsden HB, Stovall MA (1996) Radiotherapy, alkylating agents, and risk of bone cancer after childhood cancer. J Natl Cancer Inst 88:270–278

Ho PTC, Zimmerman K, Wexler LH, Blaney S, Jarosinski P, Weaver-McClure L, Izraeli S, Balis FM (1995) A prospective evaluation of ifosfamide-related nephrotoxicity in children and young adults. Cancer 76:2557–2564

Hogeboom CJ, Grosser SC, Guthrie KA, Thomas PR, D'Angio GJ, Breslow NE (2001) Stature loss following treatment for Wilms tumor. Med Pediatr Oncol 36:295–304

Holm K, Nysom K, Brocks V, Hertz H, Jacobsen N, Muller J (1999) Ultrasound B-mode changes in the uterus and ovaries and Doppler changes in the uterus after total body irradiation and allogeneic bone marrow transplantation in childhood. Bone Marrow Transplant 23:259–263

Hopewell JW (1980) The importance of vascular damage in the development of late radiation effects in normal tissues. In: Meyn RE, Withers HR (eds) Radiation biology in cancer research. Raven, New York, pp 449–459

Hudson MM, Rai SN, Nunez C, Merchant TE, Marina NM, Zalamea N, Cox C, Phipps S, Pompeu R, Rosenthal D (2007) Noninvasive evaluation of late anthracycline cardiac toxicity in childhood cancer survivors. J Clin Oncol 25:3635–3643

Jaffe N, Ried HL, Cohen M, McNeese MD, Sullivan MP (1983) Radiation induced osteochondroma in long-term survivors of childhood cancer. Int J Radiat Oncol Biol Phys 9:665–670

Jagt CT, Zuckermann M, Ten Kate F, Taminiau JAJM, Dijkgraaf MGW, Heij H, De Kraker J, Verschuur AC (2009) Veno-occlusive disease as a complication of preoperative chemotherapy for Wilms tumor: a clinico-pathological analysis. Pediatr Blood Cancer 53:1211–1215

Jennes I, Pedrini E, Zuntini M, Mordenti M, Balkassmi S, Asteggiano CG, Casey B, Bakker B, Sangiorgi L, Wuyts W (2009) Multiple osteochondromas: mutation update and description of the multiple osteochondromas mutation database (MOdb). Hum Mutat 30:1620–1627

Kadan-Lottick NS, Robison LL, Gurney JG, Neglia JP, Yasui Y, Hayashi R, Hudson M, Greenberg M, Mertens AC (2002) Childhood cancer survivors' knowledge about their past diagnosis and treatment: Childhood Cancer Survivor Study. JAMA 287:1832–1839

Kremer LC, van der Pal HJ, Offringa M, van Dalen EC, Voute PA (2002) Frequency and risk factors of subclinical cardiotoxicity after anthracycline therapy in children: a systematic review. Ann Oncol 13:819–829

Krischer JP, Epstein S, Cuthbertson DD, Goorin AM, Epstein ML, Lipshultz SE (1997) Clinical cardiotoxicity following anthracycline treatment for childhood cancer: the Pediatric Oncology Group experience. J Clin Oncol 15:1544–1552

Lahteenmaki PM, Sankila R, Pukkala E, Kyyronen P, Harila-Saari A (2008) Scholastic achievement of children with lymphoma or Wilms tumor at the end of comprehensive education—a nationwide, register-based study. Int J Cancer 123:2401–2405

Landier W, Wallace WH, Hudson MM (2006) Long-term follow-up of pediatric cancer survivors: education, surveillance, and screening. Pediatr Blood Cancer 46:149–158

Legha SS (1986) Vincristine neurotoxicity: pathophysiology and management. Med Toxicol 1:421–427

Levitt GA, Saran FH (2004) Cardiovascular complications. Radiation damage. In: Wallace WHB, Green DM (eds) Late effects of childhood cancer. Arnold Publishers, London, pp 101–113

Levitt GA, Yeomans E, Dicks Mireaux C, Breatnach F, Kingston J, Pritchard J (1992) Renal size and function after cure of Wilms' tumour. Br J Cancer 66:877–882

Levitt G, Anazodo A, Burch M, Bunch K (2009) Cardiac or cardiopulmonary transplantation in childhood cancer survivors: an increasing need? Eur J Cancer 45:3027–3034

Li FP, Gimbrere K, Gelber RD, Sallan SE, Flamant F, Green DM, Heyn RM, Meadows AT (1987) Outcome of pregnancy in survivors of Wilms' tumor. JAMA 257:216–219

Libshitz HI, Cohen MA (1982) Radiation induced osteochondromas. Radiology 142:643–647

Lipshultz SE, Lipsitz SR, Mone SM, Goorin AM, Sallan SE, Sanders SP, Orav EJ, Gelber RD, Colan SD (1995) Female sex and higher drug dose as risk factors for late cardiotoxic effects of doxorubicin therapy for childhood cancer. N Engl J Med 332:1738–1743

Lipshultz SE, Lipsitz SR, Sallan SE, Simbre VC II, Shaikh SL, Mone SM, Gelber RD, Colan SD (2002) Long-term Enalapril therapy for left ventricular dysfunction in doxorubicin-treated survivors of childhood cancer. J Clin Oncol 20:4517–4522

Lipshultz SE, Vlach SA, Lipsitz SR, Sallan SE, Schwartz ML, Colan SD (2005) Cardiac changes associated with growth hormone therapy among children treated with anthracyclines. Pediatrics 115:1613–1622

Littman P, Meadows AT, Polgar G, Borns PF, Rubin E (1976) Pulmonary function in survivors of Wilms' tumor. Cancer 37:2773–2776

Loebstein R, Atanackovic G, Bishai R, Wolpin J, Khattak S, Hashemi G, Gobrial M, Baruchel S, Ito S, Koren G (1999) Risk factors for long-term outcome of ifosfamide-induced nephrotoxicity in children. J Clin Pharmacol 39:454–461

Ludwig R, Weirich A, Abel A, Hofmann W, Graf N, Tournade M-F (1999) Hepatotoxicity in patients treated according to the nephroblastoma trial and study SIOP-9/GPOH. Med Pediatr Oncol 33:462–469

Mackie E, Hill J, Kondryn H, McNally R (2000) Adult psychosocial outcomes in long-term survivors of acute lymphoblastic leukaemia and Wilms' tumour: a controlled study. Lancet 355:1310–1314

Macklis RM, Oltikar A, Sallan SE (1991) Wilms' tumor patients with pulmonary metastases. Int J Radiat Oncol Biol Phys 21:1187–1193

Makipernaa A, Heikkila JT, Merikanto J, Marttinen E, Siimes MA (1993) Spinal deformity induced by radiotherapy for solid tumours in childhood: a long-term follow up study. Eur J Pediatr 152:197–200

Marina NM, Poquette CA, Cain AM, Jones D, Pratt CB, Meyer WH (2000) Comparative renal tubular toxicity of chemotherapy regimens including ifosfamide in patients with newly diagnosed sarcomas. J Pediatr Hematol Oncol 22:112–118

Marx M, Langer T, Graf N, Hausdorf G, Stöhr W, Ludwig R, Beck JD (2002) A multicentre analysis of anthracycline-induced cardiotoxicity in children following treatment according to the nephroblastoma studies SIOP 9/GPOH and SIOP 93-01/GPOH. Med Pediatr Oncol 39:18–24

McBride JT, Wohl ME, Strieder DJ, Jackson AC, Morton JR, Zwerdling RG, Griscom NT, Treves S, Williams AJ, Schuster S (1980) Lung growth and airway function after lobectomy in infancy for congenital lobar emphysema. J Clin Invest 66:962–970

Mitus A, Tefft M, Fellers FX (1969) Long term follow up of renal function of 108 children who underwent nephrectomy for malignant disease. Pediatrics 44:912–921

Mpofu C, Mann JR (1992) Urinary protein/creatinine index in follow up of patients with Wilms' tumour after nephrectomy. Arch Dis Child 67:1462–1466

Nathan PC, Ness KK, Greenberg ML, Hudson M, Wolden S, Davidoff A, Laverdiere C, Mertens A, Whitton J, Robison LL, Zeltzer L, Gurney JG (2007) Health-related quality of life in adult survivors of childhood Wilms tumor or neuroblastoma: a report from the Childhood Cancer Survivor Study. Pediatr Blood Cancer 49:704–715

Nathan PC, Greenberg ML, Ness KK, Hudson MM, Mertens AC, Mahoney MC, Gurney JG, Donaldson SS, Leisenring WM, Robison LL, Oeffinger KC (2008) Medical care in long-term survivors of childhood cancer: a report from the childhood cancer survivor study. J Clin Oncol 26:4401–4409

National Cancer Institute (2006) Common terminology criteria for adverse events v3.0 (CTCAE). Cancer Therapy Evaluation Program, Common Terminology Criteria for Adverse Events, Version 3.0, DCTD, NCI, NIH, DHHS; March 31, 2003. http://ctep.cancer.gov

Neglia JP, Friedman DL, Yasui Y, Mertens AC, Hammond S, Stovall M, Donaldson SS, Meadows AT, Robison LL (2001) Second malignant neoplasms in 5-year survivors of childhood cancer: Childhood Cancer Survivor Study. J Natl Cancer Inst 93:618–629

Ness KK, Mertens AC, Hudson MM, Wall MM, Leisenring WM, Oeffinger KC, Sklar CA, Robison LL, Gurney JG (2005) Limitations on physical performance and daily activities among long-term survivors of childhood cancer. Ann Intern Med 143:639–647

Nicholson HS, Blask AN, Markle BM, Reaman GH, Byrne J (1996) Uterine anomalies in Wilms' tumor survivors. Cancer 78:887–891

Nourkami N, Furtwangler R, Alkassar M, Graf N, SIOP/GPOH Neproblastoma Trials (2009) Secondary neoplasms after Wilms' tumor in Germany. Strahlenther Onkol 185:11–12

Nussbaum Blask AR, Nicholson HS, Markle BM, Wechsler-Jentzch K, O'Donnell RB, Byrne J (1999) Sonographic detection of uterine and ovarian abnormalities in female survivors of Wilms' tumor treated with radiotherapy. AJR Am J Roentgenol 172:759–763

Nysom K, Holm K, Lipsitz SR, Mone SM, Colan SD, Orav EJ, Sallan SE, Olsen JH, Hertz H, Jacobsen JR, Lipshultz SE (1998) Relationship between cumulative anthracycline dose and late cardiotoxicity in childhood acute lymphoblastic leukemia. J Clin Oncol 16:545–550

Oeffinger KC, Mertens AC, Sklar CA, Kawashima T, Hudson MM, Meadows AT, Friedman DL, Marina N, Hobbie W, Kadan-Lottick NS, Schwartz CL, Leisenring W, Robison LL (2006) Chronic health conditions in adult survivors of childhood cancer. N Engl J Med 355:1572–1582

Olson RD, Boerth RC, Gerber JG, Nies AS (1981) Mechanism of adriamycin cardiotoxicity: evidence for oxidative stress. Life Sci 29:1393–1401

Pang JW, Friedman DL, Whitton JA, Stovall M, Mertens AC, Robison LL, Weiss NS (2008) Employment status among adult survivors in the Childhood Cancer Survivor Study. Pediatr Blood Cancer 50:104–110

Paulino AC, Wen BC, Brown CK, Tannous R, Mayr NA, Zhen WK, Weidner GJ, Hussey DH (2000) Late effects in children treated with radiation therapy for Wilms' tumor. Int J Radiat Oncol Biol Phys 46:1239–1246

Pein F, Sakiroglu O, Dahan M, Lebidois J, Merlet P, Shamsaldin A, Villain E, de Vathaire F, Sidi D, Hartmann O (2004) Cardiac abnormalities 15 years and more after Adriamycin therapy in 229 childhood survivors of a solid tumour at the Institut Gustave Roussy. Br J Cancer 91:37–44

Postma A, Elzenga NJ, Haaksma J, Schasfoort-Van Leeuwen MJ, Kamps WA, Bink-Boelkens MT (2002) Cardiac status in bone tumor survivors up to nearly 19 years after treatment with doxorubicin: a longitudinal study. Med Pediatr Oncol 39:86–92

Prasad VK, Lewis IJ, Aparicio SR, Heney D, Hale JP, Bailey CC, Kinsey SE (1996) Progressive glomerular toxicity of ifosfamide in children. Med Pediatr Oncol 27:149–155

Raine J, Bowman A, Wallendszus K, Pritchard J (1991) Hepatopathy-thrombocytopenia syndrome–a complication of dactinomycin therapy for Wilms' tumor: a report from the United Kingdom Childrens Cancer Study Group. J Clin Oncol 9:268–273

Raney B, Ensign LG, Foreman J, Khan F, Newton W, Ortega J, Ragab A, Wharam M, Wiener E, Maurer H (1994) Renal toxicity of ifosfamide in pilot regimens of the Intergroup Rhabdomyosarcoma Study for patients with gross residual tumor. Am J Pediatr Hematol Oncol 16:286–295

Rate WR, Butler MS, Robertson WWJ, D'Angio GJ (1991) Late orthopedic effects in children with Wilms' tumor treated with abdominal irradiation. Med Pediatr Oncol 19:265–268

Reulen RC, Winter DL, Lancashire ER, Zeegers MP, Jenney ME, Walters SJ, Jenkinson C, Hawkins MM (2007) Health-status of adult survivors of childhood cancer: a large-scale population-based study from the British Childhood Cancer Survivor Study. Int J Cancer 121:633–640

Ries LAG, Melbert D, Krapcho M, Stinchcomb DG, Howlader N, Horner MJ, Mariotto A, Miller BA, Feuer EJ, Altekruse SF, Lewis DR, Clegg L, Eisner MP, Reichman M, Edwards BK (eds) (2008) SEER cancer statistics review, 1975–2005. National Cancer Institute, Bethesda

Ritchey ML, Kelalis PP, Breslow N, Etzioni R, Evans I, Haase GM, D'Angio GJ (1992) Surgical complications after nephrectomy for Wilms' tumor. Surg Gynecol Obstet 175:507–514

Rosenfield NS, Haller JO, Berdon WE (1989) Failure of development of the growing breast after radiation therapy. Pediatr Radiol 19:124–127

Rossi R, Pleyer J, Schafers P, Kuhn N, Kleta R, Deufel T, Jurgens H (1999) Development of ifosfamide-induced nephrotoxicity: prospective follow-up in 75 patients. Med Pediatr Oncol 32:177–182

Schell M, Cochat P, Hadj-Aissa A, Bouffet E, Dubourg L, Brunat-Mentigny M (1995) Renal function following unilateral nephrectomy for neuroblastoma and Wilms' tumour. Pediatr Nephrol 9:579–582

Scottish Intercollegiate Guidelines Network (2004) SIGN guideline 76: long-term follow of survivors of childhood cancer. A national clinical guideline. Royal College of Physicians, Edinburgh

Shaw NJ, Eden OB, Jenney ME, Stevens RF, Morris-Jones PH, Craft AW, Castillo L (1991) Pulmonary function in survivors of Wilms' tumor. Pediatr Hematol Oncol 8:131–137

Silber JH, Jakacki RI, Larsen RL, Goldwein JW, Barber G (1993) Increased risk of cardiac dysfunction after anthracyclines in girls. Med Pediatr Oncol 21:477–479

Skinner R (2003) Chronic ifosfamide nephrotoxicity in children. Med Pediatr Oncol 41:190–197

Skinner R, Pearson AD, English MW, Price L, Wyllie RA, Coulthard MG, Craft AW (1998) Cisplatin dose rate as a risk factor for nephrotoxicity in children. Br J Cancer 77:1677–1682

Skinner R, Cotterill SJ, Stevens MC (2000) Risk factors for nephrotoxicity after ifosfamide treatment in children: a UKCCSG Late Effects Group study. United Kingdom Children's Cancer Study Group. Br J Cancer 82:1636–1645

Skinner R, Wallace WHB, Levitt GA (2005) Therapy based long term follow up. Children's Cancer and Leukemia Group, Leicester

Sklar C (1999) Reproductive physiology and treatment-related loss of sex hormone production. Med Pediatr Oncol 33:2–8

Sklar CA, Mertens AC, Mitby P, Whitton J, Stovall M, Kasper C, Mulder J, Green D, Nicholson HS, Yasui Y, Robison LL (2006) Premature menopause in survivors of childhood cancer: a report from the Childhood Cancer Survivor Study. J Natl Cancer Inst 98:890–896

Sorensen K, Levitt G, Sebag-Montefiore D, Bull C, Sullivan I (1995) Cardiac function in Wilms' tumor survivors. J Clin Oncol 13:1546–1556

Sorensen K, Levitt GA, Bull C, Dorup I, Sullivan ID (2003) Late anthracycline cardiotoxicity after childhood cancer: a prospective longitudinal study. Cancer 97:1991–1998

Speechley KN, Barrera M, Shaw AK, Morrison HI, Maunsell E (2006) Health-related quality of life among child and adolescent survivors of childhood cancer. J Clin Oncol 24:2536–2543

Srinivas M, Agarwala S, Padhy AK, Gupta AK, Bajpai M, Bhatnagar V, Gupta DK, Mitra DK (1998) Somatic growth and renal function after unilateral nephrectomy for Wilms' tumor. Pediatr Surg Int 14:185–188

Stohr W, Paulides M, Bielack S, Jurgens H, Treuner J, Rossi R, Langer T, Beck JD (2007) Ifosfamide-induced nephrotoxicity in 593 sarcoma patients: a report from the Late Effects Surveillance System. Pediatr Blood Cancer 48:447–452

Suarez A, McDowell H, Niaudet P, Comoy E, Flamant F (1991) Long-term follow-up of ifosfamide renal toxicity in children treated for malignant mesenchymal tumors: an International Society of Pediatric Oncology report. J Clin Oncol 9:2177–2182

Taylor RE (1997) Morbidity from abdominal radiotherapy in the First United Kingdom Children's Cancer Study Group Wilms' Tumour Study. United Kingdom Children's Cancer Study Group. Clin Oncol (R Coll Radiol) 9:381–384

Taylor A, Hawkins M, Griffiths A, Davies H, Douglas C, Jenney M, Wallace WHB, Levitt G (2004) Long term follow-up of survivors of childhood cancer in the UK. Pediatr Blood Cancer 42:161–168

Taylor AJ, Winter DL, Pritchard-Jones K, Stiller CA, Frobisher C, Lancashire ER, Reulen RC, Hawkins MM, British Childhood Cancer Survivor Study (2008) Second primary neoplasms in survivors of Wilms' tumour-a population-based cohort study from the

British Childhood Cancer Survivor Study. Int J Cancer 122:2085–2093

Tsuchiya H, Morikawa S, Tomita K (1990) Osteosarcoma arising from a multiple exostosis lesion; case report. Jpn J Clin Oncol 20:296–298

Tucker MA, D'Angio GJ, Boice JD Jr, Strong LC, Li FP, Stovall M, Stone BJ, Green DM, Lombardi F, Newton W, Hoover RN, Faumeni JF Jr (1987) Bone sarcomas linked to radiotherapy and chemotherapy in children. N Engl J Med 317:588–593

Walker DA, Dillon M, Levitt G, Cervera A, Shaw D, Pritchard J (1992) Multiple exotosis (osteochondroma) and Wilms' tumour – a possible association. Med Pediatr Oncol 20:360–361

Wallace WH, Shalet SM (1992) Chemotherapy with actinomycin D influences the growth of the spine following abdominal irradiation. Med Pediatr Oncol 20:177

Wallace WHB, Shalet SM, Crowne EC, Morris-Jones PH, Gattamaneni HR (1989) Ovarian failure following abdominal irradiation in childhood: natural history and prognosis. Clin Oncol 1:75–79

Wallace WHB, Shalet SM, Morris-Jones PH, Swindell R, Gattamaneni HR (1990) Effect of abdominal irradiation on growth in boys treated for a Wilms' tumor. Med Pediatr Oncol 18:441–446

Wallace WH, Anderson RA, Irvine DS (2005) Fertility preservation for young patients with cancer: who is at risk and what can be offered? Lancet Oncol 6:209–218

Weirich A, Ludwig R, Graf N, Abel U, Leuschner I, Vujanic GM, Mehls O, Boos J, Beck J, Royer-Pokora B, Voute PA (2004) Survival in nephroblastoma treated according to the trial and study SIOP-9/GPOH with respect to relapse and morbidity. Ann Oncol 15:808–820

Welch TR, McAdams AJ (1986) Focal glomerulosclerosis as a late sequela of Wilms' tumor. J Pediatr 108:105–109

Wikstad I, Pettersson BA, Elinder G, Sokucu S, Aperia A (1986) A comparative study of size and function of the remnant kidney in patients nephrectomized in childhood for Wilms' tumor and hydronephrosis. Acta Paediatr Scand 75:408–414

Wohl MEB, Griscom NT, Traggis DG, Jaffe N (1975) Effects of therapeutic irradiation delivered in early childhood upon subsequent lung function. Pediatrics 55:507–516

Non-Wilms Pediatric Renal Tumors 14

Jeffrey S. Dome, Saskia L. Gooskens,
and M.M. van den Heuvel-Eibrink

Contents

J.S. Dome, MD, PhD (✉)
Divisions of Hematology and Oncology,
Children's National Medical Center,
111 Michigan Avenue NW,
Washington, 20010 DC, USA
e-mail: jdome@childrensnational.org

S.L. Gooskens, MD
M.M. van den Heuvel-Eibrink, MD, PhD
Department of Pediatric Hematology/Oncology,
ErasmusMC-Sophia Children's Hospital,
Dr Molewaterplein 60, Rotterdam, 3015 GJ,
The Netherlands
e-mail: s.gooskens@erasmusmc.nl;
m.vandenheuvel@erasmusmc.nl

Abstract

The vast majority of childhood renal tumors are Wilms tumors (nephroblastoma). All other pediatric kidney tumors comprise less than 15 % of childhood renal tumors and are therefore considered rare malignancies of childhood. The most frequently observed non-Wilms renal tumors include clear cell sarcoma of the kidney (CCSK), renal cell carcinoma (RCC), malignant rhabdoid tumor of the kidney (MRTK), and congenital mesoblastic nephroma (CMN). These tumor types are markedly heterogeneous in their clinical

K. Pritchard-Jones, J.S. Dome (eds.), *Renal Tumors of Childhood: Biology and Therapy*, Pediatric Oncology,
DOI 10.1007/978-3-662-44003-2_14, © Springer-Verlag Berlin Heidelberg 2014

characteristics. CMN occurs mainly in early infancy, MRTK occurs in infants and young toddlers, CCSK occurs in toddlers and young school-age children, and RCC is most common in adolescents. The outcome of CMN is excellent, with overall survival rates over 95 % without adjuvant chemotherapy. By contrast, patients with MRTK have overall survival rates of only 20–25 %, even with intensive multimodality treatment regimens. The outcomes of CCSK and RCC are intermediate between CMN and MRTK. The non-Wilms renal tumors also have markedly different biological characteristics, each bearing distinct genetic mutations and translocations. This chapter provides an overview of the major non-Wilms renal tumors of childhood, including the ultra-rare entities of renal medullary carcinoma, metanephric tumors, and renal sarcomas.

14.1 Introduction

The vast majority of childhood renal tumors are Wilms tumors (nephroblastoma). All other pediatric kidney tumors comprise less than 15 % of childhood renal tumors and are therefore considered rare malignancies of childhood. The most frequently observed non-Wilms renal tumors include clear cell sarcoma of the kidney (CCSK), renal cell carcinoma (RCC), malignant rhabdoid tumor of the kidney (MRTK), and congenital mesoblastic nephroma (CMN). These tumor types are markedly heterogeneous in their clinical characteristics. CMN occurs mainly in early infancy, MRT occurs in infants and young toddlers, CCSK occurs in toddlers and young school-age children, and RCC is most common in adolescents. The outcome of CMN is excellent, with overall survival rates over 95 % without adjuvant chemotherapy. By contrast, patients with MRTK have overall survival rates of only 20–25 %, even with intensive multimodality treatment regimens. The outcomes of CCSK and RCC are intermediate between CMN and MRTK. The non-Wilms renal tumors also have markedly different biological characteristics, each bearing distinct genetic mutations and translocations. This chapter provides an overview of the major non-Wilms renal tumors of childhood, including the ultra-rare entities of renal medullary carcinoma, metanephric tumors, and renal sarcomas.

14.2 Clear Cell Sarcoma of the Kidney

Clear cell sarcoma of the kidney (CCSK) was considered a Wilms tumor variant until 1970 when it was recognized as a separate clinicopathologic entity by Kidd (1970). The distinctive histopathologic features of CCSK were reported simultaneously in 1978 by Morgan and Kidd, Marsden and Lawler, and Beckwith and Palmer (Beckwith and Palmer 1978; Marsden and Lawler 1978; Morgan and Kidd 1978). Currently, it is obvious that on the basis of histologic, ultrastructural, molecular, and clinical manifestations, CCSK should no longer be considered a variant of Wilms tumor (Sotelo-Avila et al. 1985).

14.2.1 Epidemiology

CCSK comprises approximately 4 % of all primary renal tumors in children (Beckwith 1983; Sotelo-Avila et al. 1985; Green et al. 1994; Argani et al. 2000b; El Kababri et al. 2004). The median age at presentation is between 2 and 3 years, and there is a male predominance, with a male to female ratio of about 2 to 1 (Morgan and Kidd 1978; Sotelo-Avila et al. 1985; Green et al. 1994; Argani et al. 2000b; Seibel et al. 2004; Stoneham et al. 2009). The youngest patient with CCSK reported in the literature was a fetus (at 31 weeks gestation) and the oldest was 58 years of age (Hung 2005; Adnani et al. 2006). CCSK is rarely reported in the first 6 months of life and in adults, in whom it has been the subject of only isolated case reports (Suzuki et al. 1983; Mishra et al. 1993; Newbould and Kelsey 1993; Oda et al. 1993; Toyoda et al. 1998; Amin et al. 1999; Bhayani et al. 2001; Benchekroun et al. 2002; Mazzoleni et al. 2003; Rosso et al. 2003; Hung 2005; Adnani et al. 2006; Kural et al. 2006; van den Heuvel-Eibrink et al. 2008).

14.2.2 Clinical Features

Common clinical presenting symptoms of patients with CCSK are similar to those of patients with Wilms tumor, including abdominal distention and hematuria. However, most CCSK patients present with additional clinical signs, such as abdominal pain, vomiting, decreased oral intake, bone pain, hypertension, fever, and constipation (Kagan and Steckel 1986; Wood et al. 1990; Kusumakumary et al. 1997; Parikh et al. 1998; Yumura-Yagi et al. 1998; Sharma and Menon 2001; Taguchi et al. 2008). Some studies suggest a predilection for the involvement of the right kidney (Sotelo-Avila et al. 1985; Sandstedt et al. 1987; Parikh et al. 1998). Most patients with CCSK present with stage I, II, and III disease; stage IV is uncommon at diagnosis, and stage V (bilateral disease) is extremely rare in CCSK (Morgan and Kidd 1978; Sotelo-Avila et al. 1985; Green et al. 1994; Argani et al. 2000b; El Kababri et al. 2004; Seibel et al. 2004, 2006; van den Heuvel-Eibrink et al. 2008). About 5–10 % of the patients have distant metastatic disease at presentation (Sotelo-Avila et al. 1985; Green et al. 1994; Argani et al. 2000b; El Kababri et al. 2004; Seibel et al. 2004). The most frequent site of distant metastases is the bone, but the tumor also spreads to the lungs, liver, mediastinum, brain, orbit, and soft tissue (Green et al. 1994; Argani et al. 2000b; Seibel et al. 2006; Brownlee et al. 2007; Radulescu et al. 2008).

14.2.3 Pathology

There is a spectrum of histological appearances seen in CCSK, all of which show admixture of cord cells, septal cells, stromal fragments, myxoid material, and blood vessels in various proportions (Argani et al. 2000b; Iyer et al. 2005). Iyer et al. also found small, pyknotic cells (Iyer et al. 2005). In total, nine histological patterns are identified. The most common pattern is the classic pattern, whose features are seen at least focally in over 90 % of tumors (Akhtar et al. 1989; Newbould and Kelsey 1993; Yun 1993; Parikh et al. 1998; Amin et al. 1999; Argani et al. 2000b; Mazzoleni et al. 2003; Hung 2005; Iyer et al. 2005; Radhika et al. 2005; Kural et al. 2006). The classic subtype of CCSK is characterized by round to oval cells arranged perivascularly and also in sheets and clusters intimately associated with a metachromatic matrix mucopolysaccharide material. The cells may show nuclear grooves (Drut and Pomar 1991; Krishnamurthy and Bharadwaj 1998; Radhika et al. 2005). CCSK is easily confused with other neoplasms because the classic pattern is often modified and may mimic other neoplasms to a sometimes striking degree. The pathologist unaware of these variant patterns is likely to diagnose CCSK as another neoplasm with different therapeutic and prognostic implications. Other patterns are myxoid, sclerosing, cellular, epithelioid, palisading, spindle, storiform, and anaplastic (Sotelo-Avila et al. 1985; Punnett et al. 1989; Kusumakumary et al. 1997; Argani et al. 2000b; Iyer et al. 2003, 2005). Immunohistochemistry shows varying degrees of vimentin immunoreactivity in nearly all samples, but other markers are consistently negative (Park et al. 1997; Argani et al. 2000b; Rosso et al. 2003; Kural et al. 2006). These include stains for epithelial markers (cytokeratins and EMA), neural markers (S100 protein), neuroendocrine markers (chromogranin, synaptophysin), muscle markers (desmin), CD34, CD117 (c-kit), and CD99 (MIC2).

14.2.4 Genetics and Biology

In contrast to nephroblastoma, CCSK does not appear to be associated with genetic predisposition syndromes (i.e., WAGR, Beckwith-Wiedemann, and Denys-Drash syndromes), and familial CCSK cases have not been reported so far (Sotelo-Avila et al. 1985; Sohda et al. 1997; Argani et al. 2000b). Cytogenetic studies of CCSK have revealed a recurrent t(10;17)(q22;p13) clonal balanced translocation in some tumors (Punnett et al. 1989; Rakheja et al. 2004; Taguchi et al. 2008). The breakpoints of the translocation were recently mapped and found to involve the *YWHAE* gene on chromosome 17 and the *FAM22* gene on chromosome 10. The *YWHAE-FAM22* transcript was detected in six of 50 CCSKs tested, showing an overall incidence of 12 % (O'Meara et al. 2012). The *YWHAE* gene encodes the 14–3–3 epsilon protein, which modulates phosphoserine-containing proteins and plays a role in various signal transduction pathways, including Akt and MAPK (Muslin et al. 1996; Tzivion et al. 1998; Zuo et al. 2010). Comparative genomic hybridization (CGH) studies have found a high proportion of normal profiles in CCSK, with infrequent copy number variations. However, gain of chromosome 1q has been identified in several tumors, similar to findings in other malignancies (Barnard et al. 2000; Schuster et al. 2003). Other variations have been observed in chromosomes 4, 14, 10, and 19 (Barnard et al. 2000; Schuster et al. 2003).

The proto-oncogene *c-KIT* is overexpressed in CCSK but is not accompanied by gene amplification or activating mutations (Jones et al. 2007). In addition, dysregulation of the epidermal growth factor receptor (EGFR) pathway has been observed at multiple levels in clear cell sarcoma of the kidney (Little et al. 2007). Gene expression profiling studies have reported expression of neural markers (e.g., nerve growth factor receptor) and expression of member genes of the sonic hedgehog pathway and the phosphoinositide-3-kinase/Akt cell proliferation pathway in CCSK (Cutcliffe et al. 2005). Methylation analysis demonstrated loss of imprinting (LOI) of insulin-like growth factor-2 (IGF2) in 40–50 % of CCSKs, with retention of the normal somatic pattern at both the H19 and SNRPN loci (Sohda et al. 1997; Schuster et al. 2003). Consistent with LOI of IGF2, Yun et al. found high IGF2 expression (Yun 1993).

14.2.5 Treatment and Outcomes

The results of large cooperative group studies of CCSK are shown in Table 14.1. Historically, CCSK was treated using regimens used for nephroblastoma. Results from the first three National Wilms Tumor Studies (NWTS) suggested that the addition of doxorubicin to vincristine and dactinomycin improved the 6-year relapse-free survival (RFS) for patients with CCSK (Green et al. 1994). In NWTS-3, the addition of cyclophosphamide did not improve the 6-year RFS, but it should be emphasized that the cyclophosphamide dose and dose intensity were relatively low by today's standards (Green et al. 1994). Flank radiation therapy is considered part of standard therapy and has been used in the vast majority of NWTS patients.

In the fourth National Wilms Tumor Study (NWTS-4), patients with CCSK were randomized between 6 and 15 months of vincristine, doxorubicin, and dactinomycin chemotherapy. The results showed improved RFS with the longer course of therapy (8-year RFS of 87.8 % versus

Table 14.1 Treatment strategy and outcome of cooperative group studies of CCSK

Study	Chemotherapy (# patients)	Abdomen XRT	RFS (follow-up, years)	OS (follow-up, years)	Reference
NWTS 1-2	VA (8)	0 – >37.8 Gy (age based)	25 % (6 years)	25 % (6 years)	Green et al. (1994)
	VAD (58)		63.5 % (6 years)	71.9 % (6 years)	
NWTS 3	VAD (43)	0 – >37.8 Gy (age based)	64.4 % (6 years)	71.3 % (6 years)	Green et al. (1994)
	VADC (30)		58.2 % (6 years)	60.8 % (6 years)	
NWTS 4	VAD (6 months) (23)	10.8 Gy	60.6 % (8 years)	85.9 % (8 years)	Seibel et al. (2004)
	VAD (15 months) (17)		87.8 % (8 years)	87.5 % (8 years)	
NWTS 5	VDCE (110)	10.8 Gy	79 % (5 years)	89 % (5 years)	Seibel et al. (2006)
SIOP 9	VADI (10)	Stage II/III 30 Gy	75 % (2 years)	88 % (5 years)	Tournade et al. (2001)
SIOP 93-01	Stage I: VADI (27)	Stage II/III 30 Gy	–	91 % (5.9 years)	Furtwangler et al. (2005)
	Stage II-IV: IDECar (26)				
UKWT2	VAD (16)	Stage III 30 Gy	82 % (4 years)	88 % (4 years)	Stoneham et al. (2009)

Abbreviations: NWTS National Wilms Tumor Study Group, *SIOP* International Society of Pediatric Oncology, *UKWT* United Kingdom Wilms Tumor Study Group, *A* dactinomycin, *V* vincristine, *D* doxorubicin, *C* cyclophosphamide, *E* etoposide, *I* ifosfamide, *Car* carboplatin, *XRT* radiation therapy, *RFS* relapse-free survival, *OS* overall survival

60.6 %, $p=0.08$), but the overall survival (OS) was unchanged between the long and short chemotherapy regimens (8-year OS 87.5 % versus 85.9 %, $p=0.99$) (Seibel et al. 2004). NWTS-4 also compared the standard doxorubicin and dactinomycin administration schedules (doses divided over 3 days for doxorubicin and over 5 days for dactinomycin) with the "pulse-intensive" schedule (dose given on 1 day). The outcomes of the two schedules were equivalent, and patients experienced less severe hematologic toxicity and fewer physician and hospital encounters with the pulse-intensive schedule, which has now become the standard (Green et al. 1994; Seibel et al. 2004).

In the NWTS-5 protocol, patients with all stages of CCSK were treated with a radical nephrectomy followed by radiotherapy and chemotherapy with vincristine/doxorubicin/cyclophosphamide alternating with cyclophosphamide/etoposide for 24 weeks and flank radiation to a dose of 10.8 cGy (Seibel et al. 2006). Five-year event-free (EFS) and OS in NWTS-5 were 79 and 89 %, respectively. EFS by stage was 100 % (I), 87 % (II), 74 % (III), and 36 % (IV) (Seibel et al. 2006). The outstanding outcome for stage I disease confirms the previous review of 351 cases from NWTS 1-4, which showed a 98 % OS rate in patients with stage I disease, as defined by NWTS-5 staging definitions (Argani et al. 2000b). NWTS-5 updated stage I to designate tumors confined to the kidney, completely resected and without penetration of the renal capsule or involvement of the renal sinus vessels. Previously, stage I was defined by lack of tumor extension beyond the hilar plane, an imaginary line connecting the medial aspects of the upper and lower poles of the kidney. For CCSK, the updated definition identifies a group of patients with nearly 100 % survival (Kalapurakal et al. 2012).

In the SIOP-9 study, patients were treated with preoperative dactinomycin/vincristine and postoperative doxorubicin/dactinomycin/vincristine/ifosfamide. For local stage II or III disease, irradiation to the flank or abdomen was applied (Tournade et al. 2001; Furtwangler et al. 2005). With the SIOP-9 approach, the 2-year EFS was 75 % and 5-year OS was 88 % (Tournade et al. 2001). The SIOP 93-01/GPOH trial used a similar approach to SIOP-9, except that the postoperative chemotherapy regimen consisted of ifosfamide/etoposide/carboplatin/doxorubicin. On this study, the OS survival rate was 91 % (Furtwangler et al. 2005).

Treatment in the United Kingdom Children's Cancer Study Group 2 (UKCCSG-2) consisted of vincristine/dactinomycin/doxorubicin administered for 12 months. Patients with local stage I and II disease did not receive irradiation to the flank/abdomen, but patients with local stage III disease received 30 Gy (Mitchell et al. 2000). Four-year EFS and OS were 88 and 82 %, respectively. From the combined UKCCSG and French trials, 5-year EFS and OS were 63 and 75 %, respectively. Paradoxically, the OS for stage II disease (73 %) was inferior to the OS for stage III disease (86 %), suggesting the radiation therapy may be helpful for stage II (Stoneham et al. 2009).

14.2.6 Disease Recurrence in CCSK

Approximately 25 % of patients with CCSK will experience recurrence. Historically, late relapses were characteristic of CCSK, but in the NWTS-5 trial, only one of 21 relapses occurred beyond 3 years after diagnosis (Green et al. 1994; Charafe et al. 1997; Kusumakumary et al. 1997; Argani et al. 2000b; Seibel et al. 2006). Advanced stage, older age, lack of doxorubicin in upfront treatment, and absence of necrosis are important adverse prognostic factors for relapse (Argani et al. 2000b). The bone was historically the most frequent relapse site of CCSK (Morgan and Kidd 1978; Sotelo-Avila et al. 1985; Green et al. 1994; Argani et al. 2000b), but recent reports from the NWTSG and SIOP have indicated that the brain has surpassed the bone as the most common site of recurrence (Furtwangler et al. 2005; Seibel et al. 2006). The reason for the increase in central nervous system recurrences is unclear, but it is possible that the brain is a sanctuary site that allows tumor cells to avoid exposure to modern intensive chemotherapy. It is important to include the brain in imaging surveillance for patients who are off-therapy for CCSK. Notably, a case series of patients with recurrent CCSK with brain metastases showed that six of eight patients had durable survival with a combination of ifosfamide/carboplatin/etoposide chemotherapy, surgery, and radiation therapy (Radulescu et al. 2008).

14.3 Malignant Rhabdoid Tumor of the Kidney

Malignant rhabdoid tumor of the kidney (MRTK) is a rare, highly aggressive type of cancer occurring in early childhood associated with rapid progression and a very poor prognosis. In the past, MRTK was classified as a subtype of Wilms tumor but in the early 1980s it was recognized as a distinct tumor type. To date, the exact cell origin of the MRTK has not been elucidated. Although MRTK was first described in the kidney, it is recognized to occur in many organs and soft tissues. MRTK arising in the brain is referred to as "atypical teratoid-rhabdoid tumor."

14.3.1 Epidemiology

The true incidence of MRTK is not known, but European data suggest that less than 0.5 per million children per year will suffer from MRTK, underscoring the rarity of the disease (Haas et al. 1981). The median age at presentation has been reported to vary between 10 and 18 months, and males and females are equally affected (Brennan et al. 2004; Tomlinson et al. 2005; Reinhard et al. 2008; van den Heuvel-Eibrink et al. 2011).

14.3.2 Clinical Characteristics

Patients with MRTK generally present with a palpable abdominal mass and have other symptoms such as hematuria (gross or microscopic), fever, infection, hypertension, and anemia (Amar et al. 2001). Hypercalcemia, caused by increased parathormone levels, is associated with MRTK, but is a nonspecific finding because hypercalcemia is seen in other non-Wilms renal tumors including congenital mesoblastic nephroma (Amar et al. 2001; Tomlinson et al. 2005). Most MRT cases present with a high tumor stage. Series of renal MRT consistently show that more than two-thirds of children have stage III or IV disease (Brennan et al. 2004; Tomlinson et al. 2005; Reinhard et al. 2008; van den Heuvel-Eibrink et al. 2011). By contrast, in Wilms tumor, only 33 % of children have stage III or IV (Amar et al. 2001). Common metastatic sites are regional lymph nodes, lungs, liver, bone, and brain.

It is difficult to discriminate MRTK from Wilms tumor based on imaging alone. Both tumors can present as a large intrarenal mass involving the renal hilum with invasion of the renal vein and inferior vena cava (Graf et al. 2000). MRTK on ultrasound appears as a large, heterogeneously, lobulated mass, due to hemorrhage, fat, necrosis, or calcification (Ahmed et al. 2007). Several CT findings are suggestive of MRT, including calcifications, subcapsular hematoma, and subcapsular fluid collections (Mitchell et al. 2006). However, these findings are also found in children with other renal tumors.

14.3.3 Histology

"Rhabdoid" tumor got its name based on its resemblance to rhabdomyoblasts, though it does not demonstrate muscle differentiation. On histology, MRTK is characterized by solid proliferations of monotone tumor cells with vesicular nuclei and prominent nucleoli, abundant eosinophilic cytoplasm, and intracytoplasmic inclusions (Vujanic et al. 1996; Biegel et al. 2002). Immunohistochemical analysis shows monophenotypic tumor cells, positive for vimentin and negative for actin, myosin, desmin, PAS, and cytokeratin (Graf et al. 2000; Kinoshita et al. 2001). The histological diagnosis can further be confirmed by INI1 (encoded by *SMARCB1*) staining, which is absent in cases of MRTK in contrast to other renal tumors and rhabdomyosarcoma (Hoot et al. 2004). Other tumors that may lack INI1 staining include renal medullary carcinoma, some liver tumors (there is debate as to whether these are rhabdoid tumors), epithelioid sarcomas, and schwannomas.

14.3.4 Genetics and Biology

It had long been debated whether renal, CNS, and extrarenal rhabdoid tumors are distinct cancers that possess similar histologic appearances or whether they are the same cancer in different anatomic locations. This issue was largely put to rest when the majority of rhabdoid tumors, regardless of anatomic site, were found to have biallelic inactivating mutations in *SMARCB1* (also known as *INI1*, *BAF47*, and *hSNF5*), located at chromosome 22q11.2 (Versteege et al. 1998; Biegel et al. 1999). Whereas previous studies showed that inactivating mutations in both copies of *SMARCB1* occur in about 75 % of malignant rhabdoid tumors, comprehensive analysis of the 22q11.1 locus has revealed that more than 95 % of tumors have detectable mutations (Jackson et al. 2009). Remarkably, up to 35 % of patients with seemingly sporadic rhabdoid tumor have a germline mutation in one allele of *SMARCB1* (Bourdeaut et al. 2011; Eaton et al. 2011). Carriers can present with more than one primary tumor.

SMARCB1 encodes a member of the SWI/SNF chromatin remodeling complex, which regulates transcription of specific targets by mobilizing nucleosomes and controlling access of the transcriptional machinery to promoters. Mice heterozygous for *Smarcb1* are predisposed to rhabdoid tumors that display a histological appearance identical to human rhabdoid tumor (Klochendler-Yeivin et al. 2000; Roberts et al. 2000; Guidi et al. 2001). While loss of *SMARCB1* occurs in the vast majority of human rhabdoid tumors, mutations of *SMARCA4* (*BRG1*), another member of the SWI/SNF complex, have been described in patients lacking *SMARCB1* mutations (Hasselblatt et al. 2011). Gene expression studies of rhabdoid tumor have identified multiple other genes/pathways with altered expression (Gadd et al. 2010).

14.3.5 Treatment

Historically, patients with MRTK were treated as Wilms tumor, using vincristine-/dactinomycin-/doxorubicin-based therapy. In more recent years, additional agents (cyclophosphamide, etoposide, carboplatin, ifosfamide) have been added, but the outcomes have remained poor, with overall survival rates not exceeding 30 %. Tomlinson et al. reviewed the outcomes of patients treated on NWTS 1–5 and found the overall survival rate to be only 23 % (Tomlinson et al. 2005). Patients with lower-stage disease fared better than those with advanced stage and age was an important prognostic factor. The 4-year overall survival rate was only 9 % in infants aged 0–5 months, compared to an overall survival rate of 41 % in children older than 2 years at diagnosis ($p<.0001$). Remarkably, patients treated on NWTS-5 fared no better than patients treated on the earlier studies, indicating the lack of progress achieved for this tumor (Tomlinson et al. 2005). Unlike CCSK, where the use of doxorubicin markedly improved outcome, this drug had no discernible effect for MRTK (Tomlinson et al. 2005).

Similar results were observed in the SIOP trials 93-01 and 2001 (van den Heuvel-Eibrink et al. 2011). Most patients received preoperative therapy with vincristine/dactinomycin followed by postoperative chemotherapy consisting of etoposide, carboplatin, ifosfamide, doxorubicin, and radiotherapy. Although responses to vincristine/dactinomycin were observed, response to preoperative therapy did not translate to improved overall survival. Despite this multi-agent treatment regimen, outcome was poor and the disease progressed early, underscoring the biological aggressiveness.

Despite the generally poor results with conventional cytotoxic therapies, there have been case reports of patients with advanced-stage disease who responded to chemotherapy and have had durable survival. Regimens containing ifosfamide/carboplatin/etoposide alternating with vincristine/doxorubicin/cyclophosphamide have been effective (Waldron et al. 1999; Wagner et al. 2002; Yamamoto et al. 2006). Some centers have advocated high-dose therapy with stem-cell rescue for extrarenal MRTK based on a few successfully treated cases (Madigan et al. 2007). There has also been some success with intensive chemotherapy for central nervous system (CNS) atypical teratoid/rhabdoid tumors (Chi et al. 2009). It should be noted that although the genetics of CNS malignant rhabdoid tumor is similar to extra-CNS malignant rhabdoid tumor, the clinical picture differs. CNS malignant rhabdoid tumor rarely disseminates beyond the neuraxis, whereas extra-CNS malignant rhabdoid tumor is frequently diffusely metastatic.

Even if there are occasional patients who benefit from conventional cytotoxic agents, it has become clear that novel therapeutic approaches are urgently required to improve outcomes. The mechanism by which the SWI/SNF complex inactivation leads to rhabdoid tumor is multifactorial, but may provide clues regarding potential therapeutic targets. Accumulating evidence suggests that in its native form, the SWI/SNF complex inhibits cell cycle progression by transcriptionally repressing *CCND1* (encodes cyclin D1) and activating $p16^{INK4A}$ and $p21^{CIP}$ (Betz et al. 2002; Versteege et al. 2002; Isakoff et al. 2005). Based on this observation, therapies targeting cyclin D1 and CDK4 have been tested in preclinical models of MRT with some evidence of activity (Katsumi et al. 2011; Smith et al. 2011). Loss of *SMARCB1* has also been shown to activate expression of the mitotic regulator Aurora A kinase and the sonic hedgehog pathway (Jagani et al. 2010; Lee et al. 2011). Targets such as CXCR4, IGF2, and the INI1 pathway should be considered for future treatment strategies (Koga et al. 2009; Yanagisawa et al. 2009).

14.4 Renal Cell Carcinoma

Pediatric renal cell carcinoma (RCC) is an understudied tumor. Although the US Surveillance, Epidemiology, and End Results (SEER) program indicates that RCC is the second most common renal malignancy in children and adolescents (Howlader et al. 2011), most of the knowledge about childhood RCC comes from relatively small retrospective reviews and case series. The major cooperative groups for pediatric kidney tumors, the National Wilms Tumor Study Group (NWTSG), and the International Society of Pediatric Oncology (SIOP), historically did not focus on RCC. Until the current Children's Oncology Group (COG) AREN0321 study opened in 2006, there has not been a prospective analysis on the biology and treatment of RCC.

14.4.1 Epidemiology

The SEER program reports an age-adjusted incidence of RCC of 0.5 cases per million people under the age of 19 years (Howlader et al. 2011). Wilms tumor is more prevalent until the 15–19-year age group, at which point the incidence of RCC surpasses that of Wilms tumor. A German population-based study of childhood RCC showed the median age at diagnosis was 10.6 years, with a male to female ratio of 1 to 1.1 (Selle et al. 2006).

14.4.2 Clinical Features and Staging

The most common symptoms at diagnosis are pain (30–40 %), gross hematuria (30–40 %), and abdominal mass (20–25 %). Nonspecific constitutional symptoms such as fever, weight loss, and lethargy are seen in 15–40 % of children (Castellanos et al. 1974; Indolfi et al. 2003). Modern studies of pediatric RCC use the American Joint Committee on Cancer (AJCC) tumor/node/metastasis (TNM) staging system, which was last updated in 2010 (Edge et al. 2010), but the historical literature reported results based on the modified Robson classification (Table 14.2) (Carcao et al. 1998). Using the Robson system, more than half of pediatric RCC patients present with advanced-stage (III or IV) disease (Table 14.3) (Geller and Dome 2004). The most common sites of metastasis are lymph nodes, lung, bone, and brain.

14.4.3 Pathology

The histology of pediatric RCC is distinct from that of adult RCC. In the older literature, many cases of pediatric RCC were described as having clear cells with a papillary pattern (Dehner et al.

Table 14.2 Staging systems for pediatric RCC

Stage	Modified Robson	AJCC (2010)
I	Localized disease confined by the renal capsule	T1 N0 M0
II	Localized disease invading the renal capsule but confined by Gerota's fascia	T2 N0 M0
III	A. Involvement of renal vein or inferior vena cava	T1 N1 M0 or
		T2 N1 M0 or
	B. Regional lymph node involvement	T3 N0 M0 or
		T3 N1 M0
IV	Distant metastatic disease	T4 N0 M0 or
		T4 N1 M0 or
		Any T any N M1

AJCC American Joint Cancer Committee on Cancer
T primary tumor
TX primary tumor cannot be assessed
T0 no evidence of primary tumor
T1 tumor 7 cm or less in greatest dimension, limited to the kidney
T1a tumor 4 cm or less
T1b tumor more than 4 cm, but not more than 7 cm
T2 tumor more than 7 cm in greatest dimension, limited to the kidney
T2a tumor more than 7 cm but less than or equal to 10 cm
T2b Tumor more than 10 cm
T3 tumor extends into major veins or perinephric tissues but not into the ipsilateral adrenal gland and not beyond Gerota's fascia
T3a tumor grossly extends into the renal vein or its segmental (muscle containing branches), or tumor invades perirenal and/or renal sinus fat but not beyond Gerota's fascia
T3b tumor extends into the vena cava below the diaphragm
T3c tumor grossly extends into vena cava above the diaphragm or invades the wall of the vena cava
T4 tumor invades beyond Gerota's fascia including continuous extension into the ipsilateral adrenal gland
N regional lymph nodes (Hilar, abdominal para-aortic, and paracaval nodes):
NX regional lymph nodes cannot be assessed
N0 no regional lymph node metastasis
N1 metastasis to regional lymph nodes
M distant metastasis
MX distant metastasis cannot be assessed
M0 no distant metastasis
M1 distant metastasis

1970; Lack et al. 1985). Renshaw described tumors with distinctive voluminous clear cytoplasm, which he proposed were a newly recognized type of RCC involving translocations of Xp11 (Renshaw 1999). In 2004, the World Health Organization officially recognized translocation RCC, which is associated with a family of translocations involving the *TFE3* or *TFEB* genes, as a distinct class of RCC (Eble et al. 2004). It is now estimated that translocation RCC accounts for 50–70 % of pediatric and young adult RCC (Ramphal et al. 2006; Geller et al. 2008). Other histologic types of RCC described in children include papillary RCC, chromophobe RCC, sarcomatoid RCC, collecting duct carcinoma, RCC arising from Wilms tumor, renal medullary carcinoma, RCC after neuroblastoma, and RCC not otherwise specified (Medeiros et al. 1999; Bruder et al. 2004; Ramphal et al. 2006; Geller et al. 2008). The clear cell (conventional) subtype, by far the most common type of RCC in adults, is uncommonly observed in children. A careful morphological and molecular analysis by Bruder included 6 pediatric patients with the histologic appearance of clear cell RCC (Bruder et al. 2004). However, none of these cases had LOH at chromosome 3p, the site of the *VHL* gene, or mutations of *VHL*, indicating that the clear cell RCC in children is distinct from adult clear cell RCC.

14.4.4 Genetics and Biology

Several genetic syndromes are associated with predisposition to RCC (Linehan et al. 2010). The best described is von Hippel-Lindau (VHL) syndrome (retinal angiomas, cerebellar and spinal hemangioblastoma, hemangiomas of various organs, clear cell RCC, pheochromocytoma, and pancreatic tumors), caused by mutations in the *VHL* gene at chromosome 3p25. *VHL* encodes a protein that regulates the level of the hypoxia-inducible factor (HIF) family of transcription factors. VHL is a component of a protein complex that promotes the ubiquitin-mediated degradation of HIF, which binds to promoters of genes involved in angiogenesis, erythropoiesis, energy metabolism, iron metabolism, cell proliferation, apoptosis, and other processes that are dysregulated in human cancer (Linehan et al. 2010). Tuberous sclerosis (skin lesions, seizures, mental retardation, multiorgan hamartomatous lesions)

Table 14.3 Recent series of pediatric RCC >10 patients

	Stage[a]				
	I	II	III	IV	Reference
% alive and relapse free (# of patients)	94 % (18)	100 % (2)	42 % (12)	0 % (9)	Indolfi et al. (2003)
	100 % (3)	50 % (2)	100 % (5)	0 % (3)	Geller and Dome (2004)
	91 % (11)	100 % (7)	75 % (4)	50 % (8)	Selle et al. (2006)†
	100 % (5)	100 % (3)	100 % (1)	75 % (4)	Ramphal et al. (2006)†
	100 % (3)	100 % (1)	33 % (3)	25 % (4)	Varan (2007)
	100 % (3)	100 % (1)	75 % (4)	33 % (3)	Geller et al. (2008)
Total	95 % (43)	94 % (16)	62 % (29)	29 % (31)	–

[a]Modified Robson stage except for studies marked with†, which used the American Joint Committee on Cancer (AJCC) staging system. With the AJCC system, not all patients with stage IV disease had distant metastatic disease; more than 1 positive regional lymph node constituted stage IV in previous versions of the AJCC classification system. This may explain the better outcomes for stage IV disease in the series using the AJCC system instead of the Robson system

is caused by mutations in the *TSC1* and *TSC2* genes, which encode the hamartin and tuberin proteins, central regulators of the mammalian target of rapamycin (mTOR) pathway. The most common renal tumor in individuals with tuberous sclerosis is angiomyolipoma, but affected individuals are also susceptible to RCC with clear cell morphology (Bjornsson et al. 1996). Hereditary papillary RCC is caused by mutations in the *MET* oncogene, which encodes the hepatocyte growth factor receptor, which signals through the phosphatidylinositol 3-kinase (PI3K) pathway (Schmidt et al. 1997). The Birt-Hogg-Dubé syndrome (skin fibrofolliculomas, lung cysts, chromophobe RCC) is caused by mutations in *FLCN*, which encodes the protein folliculin, which interacts with the mTOR pathway (Nickerson et al. 2002). Individuals with germline mutations of two tricarboxylic acid (Krebs) cycle genes, fumarate hydratase (*FH*), and succinate dehydrogenase (*SDH*) are also susceptible to RCC. *FH* is the gene responsible for hereditary leiomyomatosis, a cancer predisposition syndrome in which patients develop uterine and cutaneous leiomyomas as well as papillary RCC (Tomlinson et al. 2002). Germline mutations of the *SDHB*, *SDHC*, and *SDHD* genes are responsible for familial paraganglioma and pheochromocytoma. Individuals with *SDHB* mutations are also at risk for early onset RCC (Neumann et al. 2004; Vanharanta et al. 2004). Mutations of the *FH* and *SDH* genes impair progression through the tricarboxylic acid cycle, thereby diminishing oxidative phosphorylation and leading cells to rely on glycolysis for energy metabolism even in normoxic conditions (Linehan et al. 2010).

Translocation RCC is associated with translocations involving genes that encode members of the microphthalmia (MiTF) family of transcription factors. The most commonly involved gene is *TFE3* on chromosome Xp11, which can fuse to several partners including *ASPL* (17q25), *PRCC* (1q21), *PSF* (1p34), *NonO* (Xq12), and *CLTC* (17q23) (Argani and Ladanyi 2005). The TFE3-ASPL translocation is the same translocation seen in alveolar soft part sarcoma (Argani et al. 2001a). A recent gene expression study has identified several novel genes that are differentially expressed between the Xp11 translocation carcinomas and conventional renal carcinomas and has shown that Xp11 translocation carcinomas may be more similar to alveolar soft part sarcoma than to conventional renal carcinomas (Tsuda et al. 2007). Additionally, gene expression profiling has identified potential therapeutic targets in the Xp11 translocation RCC. For example, the ASPL-TFE3 fusion protein transactivates the promoter of the MET receptor tyrosine kinase, leading to MET protein overexpression. Inhibition of the MET receptor tyrosine kinase may therefore be a potential avenue of targeted therapy for these RCC (Tsuda et al. 2007). Translocation RCC also express high levels of phosphorylated S6, a measure of mTOR pathway activation, which suggests that mTOR inhibition may be effective in this tumor type (Argani et al. 2010).

A less common type of translocation RCC involves a fusion of the untranslated *alpha* gene (11q12) to the *TFEB* gene (6p21) (Argani et al. 2001b; Davis et al. 2003). Interestingly, 15 % of translocation RCC occurs in individuals who were previously treated with chemotherapy for a variety of pediatric malignancies and nonmalignant conditions (Argani et al. 2006).

14.4.5 Treatment and Outcomes

Tumor resection is the mainstay of therapy for pediatric RCC. Most patients are presumed to have Wilms tumor and undergo radical nephrectomy and lymph node sampling according to Wilms tumor surgical guidelines. A role for radical lymph node dissection remains to be determined (Geller and Dome 2009).

Many patients with localized disease have fared well without adjuvant therapy. Among adults and children with translocation RCC, age ≥25 years, lymph node involvement, high Fuhrman grade, and presence of distant metastatic disease were associated with poor survival (Malouf et al. 2011). In pure pediatric series, however, local lymph node involvement was not associated with unfavorable outcome, even among patients who did not receive adjuvant therapy (Geller et al. 2008). The Children's Oncology Group AREN0321 study is prospectively evaluating the need for adjuvant therapy in children, adolescents, and young adults with RCC without distant metastatic disease. Patient outcomes reported in the large recent series of pediatric RCC are listed in Table 14.3.

Children with metastatic RCC have a poor prognosis (Table 14.3). Although successes with high-dose interleukin-2 have been reported (MacArthur et al. 1994), it is recognized in that non-clear cell renal cell carcinomas do not typically respond well to immunotherapy (Upton et al. 2005; Malouf et al. 2010). Emerging data on translocation RCC suggests that some tumors respond to vascular endothelial growth factor receptor (VEGF)-targeted therapy (sunitinib, sorafenib, ramucirumab) (Choueiri et al. 2010; Malouf et al. 2010). Among the agents reported, sunitinib seems to be most active. In one series, 7 of 14 patients (50 %) treated with sunitinib as either first- or second-line therapy for translocation RCC had partial or complete response (Malouf et al. 2010). Seven of 7 patients who had progressive disease on VEGF-directed therapy and switched to mTOR inhibitors showed at least transient disease stabilization, including one with a partial response. Responses to gemcitabine/doxorubicin alternating with gemcitabine/oxaliplatin have also been observed (Geller et al. 2008). Prospective studies to evaluate therapies for metastatic and recurrent childhood RCC are warranted.

14.5 Renal Medullary Carcinoma

Renal medullary carcinoma (RMC) is a renal epithelial neoplasm that has been described as the "7th sickle cell nephropathy" (Davis et al. 1995). It is an aggressive cancer that occurs in adolescent and young adult patients with sickle-cell trait or hemoglobin SC disease (Davis et al. 1995). The mean age of presentation is 19 years, with a reported range from 5 to 40 years. There is a male predominance, with a male to female ratio of 2 to 1 (Simpson et al. 2005). There is no single pathognomonic genetic abnormality seen in RMC, but *BCR-ABL* translocations or *ABL* gene amplification has been described in rare cases, as have *ALK* gene rearrangements (Stahlschmidt et al. 1999; Simpson et al. 2005; Marino-Enriquez et al. 2011). Absence of SMARCB1 (INI1/hSNF5) protein staining by immunohistochemistry has been observed in RMC, suggesting that rhabdoid tumor of the kidney and RMC may have common biological, as well as clinical, features (Cheng et al. 2008). Both are characterized by an aggressive metastatic pattern and relative chemotherapy resistance.

Patients with RMC almost always present with metastatic disease and have fatal outcomes (Davis et al. 1995; Simpson et al. 2005). Transient responses have been observed after treatment with methotrexate/vinblastine/doxorubicin/cisplatin (MVAC) or platinum/gemcitabine/taxane (Pirich et al. 1999; Simpson et al. 2005; Strouse et al. 2005; Bell 2006; Walsh et al. 2010). A patient with RMC was shown to have a complete tumor response after treatment with the proteosome inhibitor bortezomib (Ronnen et al. 2006).

14.6 Congenital Mesoblastic Nephroma

14.6.1 Epidemiology

Congenital mesoblastic nephroma (CMN) is a rare tumor that accounts for about 3 % of pediatric renal tumors (Howell et al. 1982). The mean age at presentation is 3.4 months, but rare cases have been diagnosed in children up to 9 years of age (Howell et al. 1982). CMN is the most common renal neoplasm in the first month of infancy (van den Heuvel-Eibrink et al. 2008). Most large series show a predominance in boys, with a male to female ratio of about 2 to 1 (Howell et al. 1982; Furtwaengler et al. 2006). In the series from the National Wilms Tumor Study Group, 14 % of CMN were associated with congenital malformations including genitourinary and gastrointestinal anomalies, polydactyly, and hydrocephalus (Howell et al. 1982).

14.6.2 Clinical Features and Staging

Common presenting signs include abdominal mass, hypertension, and hematuria (Howell et al. 1982). Patients are usually asymptomatic and the mass is detected as an incidental finding. In some patients, the tumor is diagnosed on prenatal ultrasound (Furtwaengler et al. 2006). Approximately 12 % of patients present with hypercalcemia (Chan et al. 1987; Furtwaengler et al. 2006). Metastatic disease at the time of initial presentation is practically unheard of; among 101 patients in two of the largest series, there were no cases of lymph node involvement or distant metastatic disease (Howell et al. 1982; Furtwaengler et al. 2006). However, cases of metastasis to the brain and lung have been documented at the time of recurrence (Joshi et al. 1986; Heidelberger et al. 1993; Ali et al. 1994). The staging systems used for CMN are the same as those used for Wilms tumor, typically the NWTS/COG system or the SIOP system (Metzger and Dome 2005).

14.6.3 Pathology, Genetics, and Biology

There are two main histologic subtypes of CMN: classic (or conventional) and cellular (or atypical) (Joshi et al. 1986; Pettinato et al. 1989). It has been proposed that the term "atypical" is misnomer, because the majority of CMN have the cellular histology. Some CMN have a mixed pattern with features of both subtypes. Classic CMN tends to present in very young infants and neonates, whereas cellular CMN is seen in older infants (Furtwaengler et al. 2006).

Cellular CMN is morphologically similar to infantile fibrosarcoma (IFS), and both have the chromosomal translocation t(12;15)(p13;q25), which results in a fusion of the *ETV6 (TEL)* gene with the *NTRK3* gene (Knezevich et al. 1998a, b; Rubin et al. 1998). *ETV6* encodes a transcription factor with a helix-loop-helix protein dimerization domain and *NTRK3* encodes a receptor tyrosine kinase. The chimeric ETV6-NTRK3 protein is postulated to have constitutively active tyrosine kinase growth pathway signaling (Wai et al. 2000). A recent gene expression analysis of infantile fibrosarcoma/CMN showed that these tumors have a distinct gene expression profile compared to other pediatric renal tumors (Gadd et al. 2012). The expression pattern was consistent with receptor tyrosine kinase activation, with evidence of PI3-AKT, SRC, and MAPK activation. Interestingly, 4/14 cellular CMN manifested the gene expression pattern of CMN, but did not have detectable *ETV6-NTRK6* transcript, indicating that molecular mechanisms other than the *ETV6-NTRK6* fusion are responsible for the development of some cellular CMN (Gadd et al. 2012).

14.6.4 Treatment and Outcomes

Outcomes for patients with CMN are generally excellent when treated with nephrectomy only, with overall survival rates of 95 % (Howell et al. 1982; Chan et al. 1987; Furtwaengler et al. 2006). The few tumors that recur are almost exclusively the cellular subtype. It remains to be established whether patients with stage III cellular CMN benefit from adjuvant chemotherapy. In a series published by the German Pediatric Oncology Group (GPOH), two of five patients with stage III cellular CMN developed recurrent disease, whereas only one of the remaining 45 patients had recurrence (Furtwaengler et al. 2006).

Studies of cellular CMN have shown that these tumors respond to regimens containing different combinations of vincristine, dactinomycin, doxorubicin, and cyclophosphamide (Loeb et al. 2002; Furtwaengler et al. 2006). This is not unexpected based on the sensitivity of infantile fibrosarcoma to similar sarcoma-directed therapy (Grier et al. 1985; Kurkchubasche et al. 2000; Orbach et al. 2010). Responses to ifosfamide/carboplatin/etoposide (ICE) have also been noted in patients with tumors refractory to the other agents (Loeb et al. 2002).

14.7 Metanephric Neoplasms

Metanephric tumors comprise a rare group of renal tumors that include a purely epithelial lesion (metanephric adenoma), a purely stromal lesion (metanephric stromal tumor), and a mixed stromal-epithelial lesion (metanephric adenofibroma) (Argani 2005). Metanephric tumors are thought to be related to Wilms tumor and some consider them to represent the most well-differentiated form of Wilms tumor. Patients with metanephric adenoma have ranged from 5 to 83 years of age, but typically occur in the fifth to sixth decades of life. They are often discovered incidentally, but can present with pain and hematuria. About 10 % of patients had polycythemia, which resolves once the tumor is resected. The differential diagnosis is epithelial-predominant Wilms tumor and the solid variant of papillary RCC. The tumors are benign and do not require adjuvant therapy. Metanephric stromal tumor (MST) presents at a median age of 13 months (range, newborn to 13 years). The lesion resembles the spindle cell stroma of classic congenital mesoblastic nephroma but is a distinct entity (Argani and Beckwith 2000). No cases of recurrence have been described, but three cases were associated with vascular abnormalities such as aneurysms and angiodysplasia (Argani and Beckwith 2000). Metanephric adenofibroma (MAF) has a median age of 30 months (range, 5–36 years) (Arroyo et al. 2001). MAF has been subclassified into a usual type, MAF with mitoses, MAF in the setting of Wilms tumor and MAF in the setting of papillary renal cell carcinoma. Most patients with MAF were treated with chemotherapy for Wilms tumor, so it is difficult to say how patients would fare without chemotherapy, though the histology suggests a benign behavior. In a series of 25 patients, no recurrences were observed (Arroyo et al. 2001).

14.8 Renal Sarcomas

Renal sarcomas are rare malignancies that comprise less than 1 % of all malignant renal tumors (Vogelzang et al. 1993; Lalwani et al. 2011). True sarcomas of the kidney are unusual at any age (Raney et al. 2008). According to the 2004 World Health Organization (WHO) classification, primary renal sarcomas are classified based on histopathology into three categories: mesenchymal neoplasms (clear cell sarcoma of the kidney, rhabdomyosarcoma, extra-skeletal Ewing's sarcoma, anaplastic sarcoma of the kidney), mixed mesenchymal and epithelial tumors (primary renal synovial sarcoma), and neuroendocrine tumors (primitive neuroectodermal tumor/Ewing sarcoma) (Lalwani et al. 2011; Eble et al. 2004 #1854).

14.8.1 Rhabdomyosarcoma (RMS)

The most frequent variety of soft-tissue sarcoma in children is RMS. Primary renal RMSs are extremely rare (Raney et al. 2008; Lalwani et al. 2011). The median age of pediatric RMS patients is 6.35 years (range, 2.6–17.8 years) (Raney et al. 2008). Usually, children with this disease present with large tumors and may have metastases (Raney et al. 2008). The histological subtypes of RMS include embryonal, alveolar, and pleomorphic variants. Due to its origin, immunohistochemical stains are positive for desmin, myoglobin, and myogenin (Eble et al. 2004; Lalwani et al. 2011). Radical nephrectomy is the treatment of choice (Lalwani et al. 2011). Patients with localized renal RMS should be treated as having a form of unfavorable-site RMS and classified in Stage 2 or 3 (depending on diameter and regional lymph node involvement). Patients with metastatic disease should be treated on Stage 4 RMS protocols (Raney et al. 2008). Renal RMS is an aggressive neoplasm with unfavorable prognosis; in a series of 10 pediatric renal RMS patients, 4 patients died after a median of 0.57 years (Dalfior et al. 2008).

14.8.2 Anaplastic Sarcoma of the Kidney (ASK)

ASK is an exceptionally rare tumor (0.15 % of all pediatric renal tumors). The clinical features include a large renal mass and a female predominance. The age distribution is broad, ranging from infancy (10 months) to 41 years (Vujanic et al. 2007). Histologically, ASK shows a polyphenotypic mesenchymal pattern with both cystic and solid areas. Immunohistochemistry shows positivity for desmin. In the differential diagnosis, the most important tumor to be considered is anaplastic Wilms tumor (Vujanic et al. 2007). Although patients with ASK are treated according to different therapeutic protocols, the overall outcome is reasonably good (77 % 8-year overall survival). Previously, patients have responded well to treatment given to anaplastic Wilms tumors. Therefore, it is sensible to keep treating them the same way until more is known about the tumor's origin and pathogenesis (Vujanic et al. 2007).

14.8.3 Primary Renal Synovial Sarcoma

Primary synovial sarcoma (SS) of the kidney is very rare. Since its description in 1999, fewer than 70 cases have been reported in literature (Iacovelli et al. 2012). SSs affect patients between 17 and 61 years with a slight male predominance (Chen et al. 2001). Renal SS is characterized by a specific translocation t(X;18) (p11.2;q11.2), resulting in the fusion of SYT gene on chromosome 18 with an SSX family gene on chromosome X (Dassi et al. 2009; Iacovelli et al. 2012). Histologically, two different forms of SSs are seen: monophasic (only spindle cells) and biphasic (glandular elements and spindle epithelial cells). Spindle cells are immunoreactive for vimentin, CD99, and bcl2 (Argani et al. 2000a). Radical nephrectomy is the first approach for patients with metastatic and nonmetastatic disease. Response to chemotherapy (anthracyclines combined with ifosfamide) has been reported in patients with metastatic disease; however, the value of chemotherapy in the adjuvant setting has yet to be proven. About 35 % of the patients have local relapse or abdominal lymph node metastases after surgery, and the 5-year overall survival is 42–89 % (Lalwani et al. 2011; Iacovelli et al. 2012).

14.8.4 Primitive Neuroectodermal Tumor (PNET)/Ewing Sarcoma

PNET of the kidney is a rare tumor, with about 50 cases reported in literature (Pomara et al. 2004). PNETs are commonly seen in childhood or adolescence (median age 20 years) (Maccioni et al. 2000). It is very difficult to differentiate PNET and extraosseous Ewing sarcoma as separate entities. Both share common stem-cell precursor and unique chromosomal abnormality t(11;22) (q24;q12). However, the stages of differentiation in which the stem-cell precursor are blocked are different in both the tumors, explaining their different biological behavior and prognosis (Pomara et al. 2004). Diffuse CD99 positivity and strong membrane positivity for MIC2 are characteristic (Pomara et al. 2004). Renal PNET is more aggressive than in the other sites; it often recurs locally and metastasizes early to regional lymph nodes, lungs, liver, bone, and bone marrow, resulting in a poor prognosis (5-year overall survival 45–55 %) (Pomara et al. 2004). PNETs demonstrate a high response to a combination of surgery, irradiation, and chemotherapy (Miser et al. 1987).

14.9 Late Breaking Updates

Since this chapter was submitted, several new developments have occurred in the field of non-Wilms pediatric renal tumors. A large series of patients with CCSK ($n = 191$) treated on the SIOP 9301 and 2001 studies was reported. Five-year event-free survival (EFS) and overall survival (OS) were 79 % and 86 %, respectively. Stage IV disease and young age were significant adverse prognostic factors for EFS (Furtwangler et al. 2013). The SIOP and Associazione Italiana Ematologia Oncologia Pediatrica groups reported a series of 37 patients with relapsed CCSK. The most common sites of relapse were the brain ($n = 13$), lungs ($n = 7$) and bone ($n = 5$). Treatment of relapse consisted of chemotherapy ($n = 30$), surgery ($n = 19$) and/or radiotherapy ($n = 19$). High-dose therapy with autologous stem cell transplant was used in 14 patients. Five-year EFS and OS after relapse were 18 % and 26 %, respectively (Gooskens et al. 2014). Ueno et al published a study on DNA methylation that resulted in a methylation profile that distinguishes CCSK from other pediatric renal tumors. A combination of four genes was sufficient to distinguish Wilms tumor, CCSK, CMN, MRTK and Ewing sarcoma. The methylation status of *THBS1* alone was sufficient to distinguish CCSK from other pediatric renal tumors (Ueno et al. 2013). Karlsson et al published a study reporting that CCSK demonstrates an embryonic signature indicative of a primitive nephrogenic origin and found remarkably few genetic imbalances (Karlsson et al. 2014). Next generation sequencing efforts are ongoing and may provide novel insight into clinically relevant prognostic markers and molecular targets.

Venkatramani et al reported a series of 21 patients with renal and extrarenal non-central nervous system malignant rhabdoid tumor who were treated at a single institution between 1983 and 2012 (Venkatramani et al. 2014). Starting in 2002, patients received a treatment regimen consisting of vincristine, doxorubicin and high-dose cyclophosphamide. The 5-year OS of patients treated before and after 2002 was 20 % and 54 %, respectively. Four patients who received high-dose therapy with autologous stem cell rescue were alive at last follow-up. The authors conclude that high-dose alkylator therapy followed by high-dose therapy/stem cell rescue is a promising treatment for malignant rhabdoid tumor. A caveat to concluding that there is benefit to autologous stem cell rescue is that there is likely a selection bias favoring those patients. In this series, the median time to progression was only 4 months; patients who were doing well long enough to get to stem cell transplant were likely an inherently more favorable group. Preclinical rhabdoid tumor models have provided leads to promising new biological agents, including an inhibitor of EZH2, a histone methyltransferase that is thought to be essential for viability in rhabdoid cells with *SMARCB1* mutations (Knutson et al. 2013). MRTK xenografts treated with an EZH2 inhibitor showed durable regression, even after cessation of drug administration.

References

Adnani A, Latib R, Bouklata S et al (2006) [Clear cell sarcoma of the kidney in an adult: a case report] Sarcome a cellules claires du rein chez l'adulte: a propos d'un cas. J Radiol 87:136–138

Ahmed HU, Arya M, Levitt G et al (2007) Part I: Primary malignant non-Wilms' renal tumours in children. Lancet 8:730–737

Akhtar M, Ali MA, Sackey K et al (1989) Fine-needle aspiration biopsy of clear-cell sarcoma of the kidney: light and electron microscopic features. Diagn Cytopathol 5:181–187

Ali AA, Finlay JL, Gerald WL et al (1994) Congenital mesoblastic nephroma with metastasis to the brain: a case report. Am J Pediatr Hematol Oncol 16: 361–364

Amar AM, Tomlinson G, Green DM et al (2001) Clinical presentation of rhabdoid tumors of the kidney. J Pediatr Hematol Oncol 23:105–108

Amin MB, de Peralta-Venturina MN, Ro JY et al (1999) Clear cell sarcoma of kidney in an adolescent and in young adults: a report of four cases with ultrastructural, immunohistochemical, and DNA flow cytometric analysis. Am J Surg Pathol 23:1455–1463

Argani P (2005) Metanephric neoplasms: the hyperdifferentiated, benign end of the Wilms tumor spectrum? Clin Lab Med 25:379–392

Argani P, Beckwith JB (2000) Metanephric stromal tumor: report of 31 cases of a distinctive pediatric renal neoplasm. Am J Surg Pathol 24:917–926

Argani P, Ladanyi M (2005) Translocation carcinomas of the kidney. Clin Lab Med 25:363–378

Argani P, Faria PA, Epstein JI et al (2000a) Primary renal synovial sarcoma: molecular and morphologic delineation of an entity previously included among embryonal sarcomas of the kidney. Am J Surg Pathol 24:1087–1096

Argani P, Perlman EJ, Breslow NE et al (2000b) Clear cell sarcoma of the kidney: a review of 351 cases from the National Wilms Tumor Study Group Pathology Center. Am J Surg Pathol 24:4–18

Argani P, Antonescu CR, Illei PB et al (2001a) Primary renal neoplasms with the ASPL-TFE3 gene fusion of alveolar soft part sarcoma: a distinctive tumor entity previously included among renal cell carcinomas of children and adolescents. Am J Pathol 159:179–192

Argani P, Hawkins A, Griffin CA et al (2001b) A distinctive pediatric renal neoplasm characterized by epithelioid morphology, basement membrane production, focal HMB45 immunoreactivity, and t(6;11)(p21.1;q12) chromosome translocation. Am J Pathol 158:2089–2096

Argani P, Lae M, Ballard ET et al (2006) Translocation carcinomas of the kidney after chemotherapy in childhood. J Clin Oncol 24:1529–1534

Argani P, Hicks J, De Marzo AM et al (2010) Xp11 translocation renal cell carcinoma (RCC): extended immunohistochemical profile emphasizing novel RCC markers. Am J Surg Pathol 34:1295–1303

Arroyo MR, Green DM, Perlman EJ et al (2001) The spectrum of metanephric adenofibroma and related lesions: clinicopathologic study of 25 cases from the National Wilms Tumor Study Group Pathology Center. Am J Surg Pathol 25:433–444

Barnard M, Bayani J, Grant R et al (2000) Comparative genomic hybridization analysis of clear cell sarcoma of the kidney. Med Pediatr Oncol 34:113–116

Beckwith JB (1983) Wilms' tumor and other renal tumors of childhood: a selective review from the National Wilms' Tumor Study Pathology Center. Hum Pathol 14:481–492

Beckwith JB, Palmer NF (1978) Histopathology and prognosis of Wilms tumors: results from the First National Wilms' Tumor Study. Cancer 41:1937–1948

Bell MD (2006) Response to paclitaxel, gemcitabine, and cisplatin in renal medullary carcinoma. Pediatr Blood Cancer 47:228

Benchekroun A, Ghadouane M, Zannoud M et al (2002) Clear cell sarcoma of the kidney in an adult. A case report. Ann Urol (Paris) 36:33–35

Betz BL, Strobeck MW, Reisman DN et al (2002) Re-expression of hSNF5/INI1/BAF47 in pediatric tumor cells leads to G1 arrest associated with induction of p16ink4a and activation of RB. Oncogene 21:5193–5203

Bhayani SB, Liapis H, Kibel AS (2001) Adult clear cell sarcoma of the kidney with atrial tumor thrombus. J Urol 165:896–897

Biegel JA, Zhou JY, Rorke LB et al (1999) Germ-line and acquired mutations of INI1 in atypical teratoid and rhabdoid tumors. Cancer Res 59:74–79

Biegel JA, Tan L, Zhang F et al (2002) Alterations of the hSNF5/INI1 gene in central nervous system atypical teratoid/rhabdoid tumors and renal and extrarenal rhabdoid tumors. Clin Cancer Res 8:3461–3467

Bjornsson J, Short MP, Kwiatkowski DJ et al (1996) Tuberous sclerosis-associated renal cell carcinoma. Clinical, pathological, and genetic features. Am J Pathol 149:1201–1208

Bourdeaut F, Lequin D, Brugieres L et al (2011) Frequent hSNF5/INI1 germline mutations in patients with rhabdoid tumor. Clin Cancer Res 17:31–38

Brennan BM, Foot AB, Stiller C et al (2004) Where to next with extracranial rhabdoid tumours in children. Eur J Cancer 40:624–626

Brownlee NA, Perkins LA, Stewart W et al (2007) Recurring translocation (10;17) and deletion (14q) in clear cell sarcoma of the kidney. Arch Pathol Lab Med 131:446–451

Bruder E, Passera O, Harms D et al (2004) Morphologic and molecular characterization of renal cell carcinoma in children and young adults. Am J Surg Pathol 28:1117–1132

Carcao MD, Taylor GP, Greenberg ML et al (1998) Renal-cell carcinoma in children: a different disorder from its adult counterpart. Med Pediatr Oncol 31:153–158

Castellanos RD, Aron BS, Evans AT (1974) Renal adenocarcinoma in children: incidence, therapy and prognosis. J Urol 111:534–537

Chan HS, Cheng MY, Mancer K et al (1987) Congenital mesoblastic nephroma: a clinicoradiologic study of 17 cases representing the pathologic spectrum of the disease. J Pediatr 111:64–70

Charafe E, Penault-Llorca F, Mathoulin-Portier MP et al (1997) [Clear cell sarcoma of the kidney relapsing after 10 years of asymptomatic evolution] Sarcome a cellules claires du rein recidivant apres 10 ans d'evolution asymptomatique. Ann Pathol 17:400–402

Chen S, Bhuiya T, Liatsikos EN et al (2001) Primary synovial sarcoma of the kidney: a case report with literature review. Int J Surg Pathol 9:335–339

Cheng JX, Tretiakova M, Gong C et al (2008) Renal medullary carcinoma: rhabdoid features and the absence of INI1 expression as markers of aggressive behavior. Mod Pathol 21:647–652

Chi SN, Zimmerman MA, Yao X et al (2009) Intensive multimodality treatment for children with newly diagnosed CNS atypical teratoid rhabdoid tumor. J Clin Oncol 27:385–389

Choueiri TK, Lim ZD, Hirsch MS et al (2010) Vascular endothelial growth factor-targeted therapy for the treatment of adult metastatic Xp11.2 translocation renal cell carcinoma. Cancer 116:5219–5225

Cutcliffe C, Kersey D, Huang CC et al (2005) Clear cell sarcoma of the kidney: up-regulation of neural markers with activation of the sonic hedgehog and Akt pathways. Clin Cancer Res 11:7986–7994

Dalfior D, Eccher A, Gobbo S et al (2008) Primary pleomorphic rhabdomyosarcoma of the kidney in an adult. Ann Diagn Pathol 12:301–303

Dassi V, Das K, Singh BP et al (2009) Primary synovial sarcoma of kidney: a rare tumor with an atypical presentation. Indian J Urol 25:269–271

Davis CJ Jr, Mostofi FK, Sesterhenn IA (1995) Renal medullary carcinoma. The seventh sickle cell nephropathy. Am J Surg Pathol 19:1–11

Davis IJ, His BL, Arroyo JD et al (2003) Cloning of a novel Alpha-TFEB fusion in renal tumors harboring the t(6;11)(p21;q12) chromosome translocation. Proc Natl Acad Sci U S A 100:6051–6056

Dehner LP, Leestma JE, Price EB Jr (1970) Renal cell carcinoma in children: a clinicopathologic study of 15 cases and review of the literature. J Pediatr 76:358–368

Drut R, Pomar M (1991) Cytologic characteristics of clear-cell sarcoma of the kidney (CCSK) in fine-needle aspiration biopsy (FNAB): a report of 4 cases. Diagn Cytopathol 7:611–614

Eaton KW, Tooke LS, Wainwright LM et al (2011) Spectrum of SMARCB1/INI1 mutations in familial and sporadic rhabdoid tumors. Pediatr Blood Cancer 56:7–15

Eble JN, Sauter G, Epstein JI, Sesternhenn IA (2004) World Health Organization Classification of Tumours. Pathology and genetics of tumours of the urinary system and male genital organs. IARC Press, Lyon

Edge S, Byrd D, Compton C et al (2010) AJCC cancer staging handbook, 7th edn. Springer, New York

El Kababri M, Khattab M, El Khorassani M et al (2004) [Clear cell sarcoma of the kidney. A study of 13 cases] Sarcome renal a cellules claires. A propos d'une serie de 13 cas. Arch Pediatr 11:794–799

Furtwaengler R, Reinhard H, Leuschner I et al (2006) Mesoblastic nephroma–a report from the Gesellschaft fur Padiatrische Onkologie und Hamatologie (GPOH). Cancer 106:2275–2283

Furtwangler R, Reinhard H, Beier R et al (2005) Clear-cell sarcoma (CCSK) of the kidney – results of the SIOP 93-01/GPOH trial. Pediatr Blood Cancer 45:423

Furtwangler R, Gooskens SL, van Tinteren H, et al (2013) Clear cell sarcomas of the kidney registered on International Society of Pediatric Oncology (SIOP) 93-01 and 2001 protocols: a report of the SIOP Renal Tumour Study Group. Eur J Cancer 49:3497–3506

Gadd S, Sredni ST, Huang CC et al (2010) Rhabdoid tumor: gene expression clues to pathogenesis and potential therapeutic targets. Lab Invest 90:724–738

Gadd S, Beezhold P, Jennings L et al (2012) Mediators of Receptor Tyrosine Kinase activation in infantile fibrosarcoma: a Children's Oncology Group study. J Pathol 228:119–130

Geller JI, Dome JS (2004) Local lymph node involvement does not predict poor outcome in pediatric renal cell carcinoma. Cancer 101:1575–1583

Geller JI, Dome JS (2009) Retroperitoneal lymph node dissection for pediatric renal cell carcinoma. Pediatr Blood Cancer 52:430

Geller JI, Argani P, Adeniran A et al (2008) Translocation renal cell carcinoma: lack of negative impact due to lymph node spread. Cancer 112:1607–1616

Gooskens SL, Furtwangler R, Spreafico et al (2014) Treatment and outcome of patients with relapsed clear cell sarcoma of the kidney: a combined SIOP and AIEOP study. Br J Cancer 111:227–233

Graf N, Tournade MF, de Kraker J (2000) The role of preoperative chemotherapy in the management of Wilms' tumor. The SIOP studies. International Society of Pediatric Oncology. Urol Clin North Am 27:443–454

Green DM, Beckwith JB, Breslow NE et al (1994) Treatment of children with stages II to IV anaplastic Wilms' tumor: a report from the National Wilms' Tumor Study Group. J Clin Oncol 12:2126–2131

Grier HE, Perez-Atayde AR, Weinstein HJ (1985) Chemotherapy for inoperable infantile fibrosarcoma. Cancer 56:1507–1510

Guidi CJ, Sands AT, Zambrowicz BP et al (2001) Disruption of Ini1 leads to peri-implantation lethality and tumorigenesis in mice. Mol Cell Biol 21:3598–3603

Haas JE, Palmer NF, Weinberg AG et al (1981) Ultrastructure of malignant rhabdoid tumor of the kidney. A distinctive renal tumor of children. Hum Pathol 12:646–657

Hasselblatt M, Gesk S, Oyen F et al (2011) Nonsense mutation and inactivation of SMARCA4 (BRG1) in an atypical teratoid/rhabdoid tumor showing retained SMARCB1 (INI1) expression. Am J Surg Pathol 35:933–935

Heidelberger KP, Ritchey ML, Dauser RC et al (1993) Congenital mesoblastic nephroma metastatic to the brain. Cancer 72:2499–2502

Hoot AC, Russo P, Judkins AR et al (2004) Immunohistochemical analysis of hSNF5/INI1 distinguishes renal and extra-renal malignant rhabdoid tumors from other pediatric soft tissue tumors. Am J Surg Pathol 28:1485–1491

Howell CG, Othersen HB, Kiviat NE et al (1982) Therapy and outcome in 51 children with mesoblastic nephroma: a report of the National Wilms' Tumor Study. J Pediatr Surg 17:826–831

Howlader N, Noone AM, Krapcho M, Neyman N, Aminou R, Waldron W, Altekruse SF, Kosary CL, Ruhl J, Tatalovich Z, Cho H, Mariotto A, Eisner MP, Lewis DR, Chen HS, Feuer EJ, Cronin KA, Edwards BK (2011) SEER cancer statistics review, 1975–2008. National Cancer Institute, Bethesda, http://seer.cancer.gov/csr/1975_2008/</csr/1975_2008/>

Hung NA (2005) Congenital "clear cell sarcoma of the kidney". Virchows Arch 446:566–568

Iacovelli R, Altavilla A, Ciardi A et al (2012) Clinical and pathological features of primary renal synovial sarcoma: analysis of 64 cases from 11 years of medical literature. BJU Int 110(10):1449–54

Indolfi P, Terenziani M, Casale F et al (2003) Renal cell carcinoma in children: a clinicopathologic study. J Clin Oncol 21:530–535

Isakoff MS, Sansam CG, Tamayo P et al (2005) Inactivation of the Snf5 tumor suppressor stimulates cell cycle progression and cooperates with p53 loss in oncogenic transformation. Proc Natl Acad Sci U S A 102:17745–17750

Iyer VK, Kapila K, Verma K (2003) Fine needle aspiration cytology of clear cell sarcoma of the kidney with spindle cell pattern. Cytopathology 14:160–164

Iyer VK, Agarwala S, Verma K (2005) Fine-needle aspiration cytology of clear-cell sarcoma of the kidney: study of eight cases. Diagn Cytopathol 33:83–89

Jackson EM, Sievert AJ, Gai X et al (2009) Genomic analysis using high-density single nucleotide polymorphism-based oligonucleotide arrays and multiplex ligation-dependent probe amplification provides a comprehensive analysis of INI1/SMARCB1 in malignant rhabdoid tumors. Clin Cancer Res 15:1923–1930

Jagani Z, Mora-Blanco EL, Sansam CG et al (2010) Loss of the tumor suppressor Snf5 leads to aberrant activation of the Hedgehog-Gli pathway. Nat Med 16:1429–1433

Jones C, Rodriguez-Pinilla M, Lambros M et al (2007) c-KIT overexpression, without gene amplification and mutation, in paediatric renal tumours. J Clin Pathol 60:1226–1231

Joshi VV, Kasznica J, Walters TR (1986) Atypical mesoblastic nephroma. Pathologic characterization of a potentially aggressive variant of conventional congenital mesoblastic nephroma. Arch Pathol Lab Med 110:100–106

Kagan AR, Steckel RJ (1986) Clear cell sarcoma of the kidney: a renal tumor of childhood that metastasized to bone. AJR Am J Roentgenol 146:64–66

Kalapurakal JA, Perlman EJ, Seibel NL et al (2012) Outcomes of patients with revised stage I clear cell sarcoma of kidney treated in National Wilms Tumor Studies 1-5. Int J Radiat Oncol Biol Phys 85(2):428–31

Karlsson J, Holmquist Mengelbier L et al (2014). Clear cell sarcoma of the kidney demonstrates an embryonic signature indicative of a primitive nephrogenic origin. Genes Chromosomes Cancer 53(5):381–391

Katsumi Y, Iehara T, Miyachi M et al (2011) Sensitivity of malignant rhabdoid tumor cell lines to PD 0332991 is inversely correlated with p16 expression. Biochem Biophys Res Commun 413:62–68

Kidd JM (1970) Exclusion of certain renal neoplasms from the category of Wilms tumor. Am J Pathol 59:16a

Kinoshita Y, Tamiya S, Oda Y et al (2001) Establishment and characterization of malignant rhabdoid tumor of the kidney. Oncol Rep 8:43–48

Klochendler-Yeivin A, Fiette L, Barra J et al (2000) The murine SNF5/INI1 chromatin remodeling factor is essential for embryonic development and tumor suppression. EMBO Rep 1:500–506

Knezevich SR, Garnett MJ, Pysher TJ et al (1998a) ETV6-NTRK3 gene fusions and trisomy 11 establish a histogenetic link between mesoblastic nephroma and congenital fibrosarcoma. Cancer Res 58:5046–5048

Knezevich SR, McFadden DE, Tao W et al (1998b) A novel ETV6-NTRK3 gene fusion in congenital fibrosarcoma. Nat Genet 18:184–187

Knutson SK, Warholic NM, Wigle TJ et al (2013) Durabloe tumor regression in genetically altered malignant rhabdoid tumors by inhibition of methyltransferase EZH2. Proc Natl Acad Scie USA 100: 7922–7927

Koga Y, Matsuzaki A, Suminoe A et al (2009) Long-term survival after autologous peripheral blood stem cell transplantation in two patients with malignant rhabdoid tumor of the kidney. Pediatr Blood Cancer 52:888–890

Krishnamurthy S, Bharadwaj R (1998) Fine needle aspiration cytology of clear cell sarcoma of the kidney. A case report. Acta Cytol 42:1444–1446

Kural AR, Onal B, Ozkara H et al (2006) Adult clear cell sarcoma of the kidney: a case report. BMC Urol 6:11

Kurkchubasche AG, Halvorson EG, Forman EN et al (2000) The role of preoperative chemotherapy in the treatment of infantile fibrosarcoma. J Pediatr Surg 35:880–883

Kusumakumary P, Chellam VG, Rojymon J et al (1997) Late recurrence of clear cell sarcoma of the kidney. Med Pediatr Oncol 28:355–357

Lack EE, Cassady JR, Sallan SE (1985) Renal cell carcinoma in childhood and adolescence: a clinical and pathological study of 17 cases. J Urol 133:822–828

Lalwani N, Prasad SR, Vikram R et al (2011) Pediatric and adult primary sarcomas of the kidney: a cross-sectional imaging review. Acta Radiol 52:448–457

Lee S, Cimica V, Ramachandra N et al (2011) Aurora A is a repressed effector target of the chromatin remodeling protein INI1/hSNF5 required for rhabdoid tumor cell survival. Cancer Res 71:3225–3235

Linehan WM, Srinivasan R, Schmidt LS (2010) The genetic basis of kidney cancer: a metabolic disease. Nat Rev Urol 7:277–285

Little SE, Bax DA, Rodriguez-Pinilla M et al (2007) Multifaceted dysregulation of the epidermal growth factor receptor pathway in clear cell sarcoma of the kidney. Clin Cancer Res 13:4360–4364

Loeb DM, Hill DA, Dome JS (2002) Complete response of recurrent cellular congenital mesoblastic nephroma to chemotherapy. J Pediatr Hematol Oncol 24:478–481

MacArthur CA, Isaacs H Jr, Miller JH et al (1994) Pediatric renal cell carcinoma: a complete response to recombinant interleukin-2 in a child with metastatic disease at diagnosis. Med Pediatr Oncol 23:365–371

Maccioni F, Della Rocca C, Salvi PF et al (2000) Malignant peripheral neuroectodermal tumor (MPNET) of the kidney. Abdom Imaging 25:103–106

Madigan CE, Armenian SH, Malogolowkin MH et al (2007) Extracranial malignant rhabdoid tumors in childhood: the Childrens Hospital Los Angeles experience. Cancer 110:2061–2066

Malouf GG, Camparo P, Oudard S et al (2010) Targeted agents in metastatic Xp11 translocation/TFE3 gene fusion renal cell carcinoma (RCC): a report from the Juvenile RCC Network. Ann Oncol 21:1834–1838

Malouf GG, Camparo P, Molinie V et al (2011) Transcription factor E3 and transcription factor EB renal cell carcinomas: clinical features, biological behavior and prognostic factors. J Urol 185:24–29

Marino-Enriquez A, Ou WB, Weldon CB et al (2011) ALK rearrangement in sickle cell trait-associated renal medullary carcinoma. Genes Chromosomes Cancer 50:146–153

Marsden HB, Lawler W (1978) Bone-metastasizing renal tumour of childhood. Br J Cancer 38:437–441

Mazzoleni S, Vecchiato L, Alaggio R et al (2003) Clear cell sarcoma of the kidney in a newborn. Med Pediatr Oncol 41:153–155

Medeiros LJ, Palmedo G, Krigman HR et al (1999) Oncocytoid renal cell carcinoma after neuroblastoma: a report of four cases of a distinct clinicopathologic entity. Am J Surg Pathol 23:772–780

Metzger ML, Dome JS (2005) Current therapy for Wilms' tumor. Oncologist 10:815–826

Miser JS, Kinsella TJ, Triche TJ et al (1987) Treatment of peripheral neuroepithelioma in children and young adults. J Clin Oncol 5:1752–1758

Mishra VK, Krishnani N, Bhandari M (1993) Clear cell sarcoma of kidney in an adult. Br J Urol 72:118

Mitchell C, Jones PM, Kelsey A et al (2000) The treatment of Wilms' tumour: results of the United Kingdom Children's cancer study group (UKCCSG) second Wilms' tumour study. Br J Cancer 83:602–608

Mitchell C, Pritchard-Jones K, Shannon R et al (2006) Immediate nephrectomy versus preoperative chemotherapy in the management of non-metastatic Wilms' tumour: results of a randomised trial (UKW3) by the UK Children's Cancer Study Group. Eur J Cancer 42:2554–2562

Morgan E, Kidd JM (1978) Undifferentiated sarcoma of the kidney: a tumor of childhood with histopathologic and clinical characteristics distinct from Wilms' tumor. Cancer 42:1916–1921

Muslin AJ, Tanner JW, Allen PM et al (1996) Interaction of 14-3-3 with signaling proteins is mediated by the recognition of phosphoserine. Cell 84:889–897

Neumann HP, Pawlu C, Peczkowska M et al (2004) Distinct clinical features of paraganglioma syndromes associated with SDHB and SDHD gene mutations. JAMA 292:943–951

Newbould MJ, Kelsey AM (1993) Clear cell sarcoma of the kidney in a 4-month-old infant: a case report. Med Pediatr Oncol 21:525–528

Nickerson ML, Warren MB, Toro JR et al (2002) Mutations in a novel gene lead to kidney tumors, lung wall defects, and benign tumors of the hair follicle in patients with the Birt-Hogg-Dube syndrome. Cancer Cell 2:157–164

O'Meara E, Stack D, Lee CH et al (2012) Characterization of the chromosomal translocation t(10;17)(q22;p13) in clear cell sarcoma of kidney. J Pathol 227:72–80

Oda H, Shiga J, Machinami R (1993) Clear cell sarcoma of kidney. Two cases in adults. Cancer 71:2286–2291

Orbach D, Rey A, Cecchetto G et al (2010) Infantile fibrosarcoma: management based on the European experience. J Clin Oncol 28:318–323

Parikh SH, Chintagumpala M, Hicks MJ et al (1998) Clear cell sarcoma of the kidney: an unusual presentation and review of the literature. J Pediatr Hematol Oncol 20:165–168

Park DY, Kim YM, Chi JG (1997) Intracranial metastasis from clear cell sarcoma of the kidney–a case report. J Korean Med Sci 12:473–476

Pettinato G, Manivel JC, Wick MR et al (1989) Classical and cellular (atypical) congenital mesoblastic nephroma: a clinicopathologic, ultrastructural, immunohistochemical, and flow cytometric study. Hum Pathol 20:682–690

Pirich LM, Chou P, Walterhouse DO (1999) Prolonged survival of a patient with sickle cell trait and metastatic renal medullary carcinoma. J Pediatr Hematol Oncol 21:67–69

Pomara G, Cappello F, Cuttano MG et al (2004) Primitive Neuroectodermal Tumor (PNET) of the kidney: a case report. BMC Cancer 4:3

Punnett HH, Halligan GE, Zaeri N et al (1989) Translocation 10;17 in clear cell sarcoma of the kidney. A first report. Cancer Genet Cytogenet 41: 123–128

Radhika S, Bakshi A, Rajwanshi A et al (2005) Cytopathology of uncommon malignant renal neoplasms in the pediatric age group. Diagn Cytopathol 32:281–286

Radulescu VC, Gerrard M, Moertel C et al (2008) Treatment of recurrent clear cell sarcoma of the kidney with brain metastasis. Pediatr Blood Cancer 50:246–249

Rakheja D, Weinberg AG, Tomlinson GE et al (2004) Translocation (10;17)(q22;p13): a recurring translocation in clear cell sarcoma of kidney. Cancer Genet Cytogenet 154:175–179

Ramphal R, Pappo A, Zielenska M et al (2006) Pediatric renal cell carcinoma: clinical, pathologic, and molecular abnormalities associated with the members of the mit transcription factor family. Am J Clin Pathol 126:349–364

Raney B, Anderson J, Arndt C et al (2008) Primary renal sarcomas in the Intergroup Rhabdomyosarcoma Study Group (IRSG) experience, 1972-2005: a report from the Children's Oncology Group. Pediatr Blood Cancer 51:339–343

Reinhard H, Reinert J, Beier R et al (2008) Rhabdoid tumors in children: prognostic factors in 70 patients diagnosed in Germany. Oncol Rep 19:819–823

Renshaw AA (1999) Renal cell carcinomas in children and young adults: Increased incidence of papillary architecture and unique subtypes. Am J Surg Pathol 23:795–802

Roberts CW, Galusha SA, McMenamin ME et al (2000) Haploinsufficiency of Snf5 (integrase interactor 1) predisposes to malignant rhabdoid tumors in mice. Proc Natl Acad Sci U S A 97:13796–13800

Ronnen EA, Kondagunta GV, Motzer RJ (2006) Medullary renal cell carcinoma and response to therapy with bortezomib. J Clin Oncol 24:e14

Rosso D, Ghignone GP, Bernardi D et al (2003) Clear cell sarcoma of the kidney with invasion of the inferior vena cava. Urol Int 70:251–252

Rubin BP, Chen CJ, Morgan TW et al (1998) Congenital mesoblastic nephroma t(12;15) is associated with ETV6-NTRK3 gene fusion: cytogenetic and molecular relationship to congenital (infantile) fibrosarcoma. Am J Pathol 153:1451–1458

Sandstedt BE, Delemarre JF, Harms D et al (1987) Sarcomatous Wilms' tumour with clear cells and hyalinization. A study of 38 tumours in children from the SIOP nephroblastoma file. Histopathology 11:273–285

Schmidt L, Duh FM, Chen F et al (1997) Germline and somatic mutations in the tyrosine kinase domain of the MET proto-oncogene in papillary renal carcinomas. Nat Genet 16:68–73

Schuster AE, Schneider DT, Fritsch MK et al (2003) Genetic and genetic expression analyses of clear cell sarcoma of the kidney. Lab Invest 83:1293–1299

Seibel NL, Li S, Breslow NE et al (2004) Effect of duration of treatment on treatment outcome for patients with clear-cell sarcoma of the kidney: a report from the National Wilms' Tumor Study Group. J Clin Oncol 22:468–473

Seibel NL, Sun J, Anderson JR et al (2006) Outcome of clear cell sarcoma of the kidney (CCSK) treated on the National Wilms Tumor Study-5 (NWTS). J Clin Oncol 24:A9000

Selle B, Furtwangler R, Graf N et al (2006) Population-based study of renal cell carcinoma in children in Germany, 1980-2005: more frequently localized tumors and underlying disorders compared with adult counterparts. Cancer 107:2906–2914

Sharma SC, Menon PA (2001) Clear cell sarcoma of the kidney. J Postgrad Med 47:206–207

Simpson L, He X, Pins M et al (2005) Renal medullary carcinoma and ABL gene amplification. J Urol 173:1883–1888

Smith ME, Cimica V, Chinni S et al (2011) Therapeutically targeting cyclin D1 in primary tumors arising from loss of Ini1. Proc Natl Acad Sci U S A 108:319–324

Sohda T, Soejima H, Matsumoto T et al (1997) Insulin-like growth factor 2 gene imprinting in clear cell sarcoma of the kidney. Hum Pathol 28:1315–1318

Sotelo-Avila C, Gonzalez-Crussi F, Sadowinski S et al (1985) Clear cell sarcoma of the kidney: a clinicopathologic study of 21 patients with long-term follow-up evaluation. Hum Pathol 16:1219–1230

Stahlschmidt J, Cullinane C, Roberts P et al (1999) Renal medullary carcinoma: prolonged remission with chemotherapy, immunohistochemical characterisation and evidence of bcr/abl rearrangement. Med Pediatr Oncol 33:551–557

Stoneham S, Kheder M, Moroz V et al (2009) Clear Cell Sarcoma of the Kidney (CCSK) – combined 20 year experience of therapeutic outcomes from United Kingdom (UK) and France. Pediatr Blood Cancer 53:753

Strouse JJ, Spevak M, Mack AK et al (2005) Significant responses to platinum-based chemotherapy in renal medullary carcinoma. Pediatr Blood Cancer 44: 407–411

Suzuki H, Honzumi M, Itoh Y et al (1983) Clear-cell sarcoma of the kidney seen in a 3-day-old newborn. Z Kinderchir 38:422–424

Taguchi K, Okada A, Kamiya H et al (2008) Clear cell sarcoma of the kidney: a case-report of an 11-year-old boy and a review of 11 cases in Japan. J Rural Med 3:19–22

Tomlinson IP, Alam NA, Rowan AJ et al (2002) Germline mutations in FH predispose to dominantly inherited uterine fibroids, skin leiomyomata and papillary renal cell cancer. Nat Genet 30:406–410

Tomlinson GE, Breslow NE, Dome J et al (2005) Rhabdoid tumor of the kidney in the National Wilms' Tumor Study: age at diagnosis as a prognostic factor. J Clin Oncol 23:7641–7645

Tournade MF, Com-Nougue C, de Kraker J et al (2001) Optimal duration of preoperative therapy in unilateral and nonmetastatic Wilms' tumor in children older than 6 months: results of the Ninth International Society of Pediatric Oncology Wilms' Tumor Trial and Study. J Clin Oncol 19:488–500

Toyoda Y, Yamashita C, Sugimoto T et al (1998) Clear cell sarcoma of kidney with tumor extension into the right atrium. J Cardiovasc Surg (Torino) 39: 489–491

Tsuda M, Davis IJ, Argani P et al (2007) TFE3 fusions activate MET signaling by transcriptional up-regulation, defining another class of tumors as candidates for therapeutic MET inhibition. Cancer Res 67:919–929

Tzivion G, Luo Z, Avruch J (1998) A dimeric 14-3-3 protein is an essential cofactor for Raf kinase activity. Nature 394:88–92

Ueno H, Okita H, Akimoto S, et al (2013) DNA methylation profile distinguishes clear cell sarcoma of the kidney from other pediatric renal tumors. PLoS One 8:e62233

Upton MP, Parker RA, Youmans A et al (2005) Histologic predictors of renal cell carcinoma response to interleukin-2-based therapy. J Immunother 28:488–495

van den Heuvel-Eibrink MM, Grundy P, Graf N et al (2008) Characteristics and survival of 750 children diagnosed with a renal tumor in the first seven months of life: a collaborative study by the SIOP/GPOH/SFOP, NWTSG, and UKCCSG Wilms tumor study groups. Pediatr Blood Cancer 50: 1130–1134

van den Heuvel-Eibrink MM, van Tinteren H, Rehorst H et al (2011) Malignant rhabdoid tumours of the kidney (MRTKs), registered on recent SIOP protocols from 1993 to 2005: a report of the SIOP renal tumour study group. Pediatr Blood Cancer 56:733–737

Vanharanta S, Buchta M, McWhinney SR et al (2004) Early-onset renal cell carcinoma as a novel extraparaganglial component of SDHB-associated heritable paraganglioma. Am J Hum Genet 74:153–159

Varan A, Akyuz C, Sari N et al (2007) Renal cell carcinoma in children: experience of a single center. Nephron Clin Pract 105:c58–61

Venkatramani R, Shoureshi P, Malvar J, et al (2014) High dose alkylator therapy for extracranial malignant rhabdoid tumors in children. Pediatr Blood Cancer 61:1357–1361

Versteege I, Sevenet N, Lange J et al (1998) Truncating mutations of hSNF5/INI1 in aggressive paediatric cancer. Nature 394:203–206

Versteege I, Medjkane S, Rouillard D et al (2002) A key role of the hSNF5/INI1 tumour suppressor in the control of the G1-S transition of the cell cycle. Oncogene 21:6403–6412

Vogelzang NJ, Fremgen AM, Guinan PD et al (1993) Primary renal sarcoma in adults. A natural history and management study by the American Cancer Society, Illinois Division. Cancer 71:804–810

Vujanic GM, Sandstedt B, Harms D et al (1996) Rhabdoid tumour of the kidney: a clinicopathological study of 22 patients from the International Society of Paediatric Oncology (SIOP) nephroblastoma file. Histopathology 28:333–340

Vujanic GM, Kelsey A, Perlman EJ et al (2007) Anaplastic sarcoma of the kidney: a clinicopathologic study of 20 cases of a new entity with polyphenotypic features. Am J Surg Pathol 31:1459–1468

Wagner L, Hill DA, Fuller C et al (2002) Treatment of metastatic rhabdoid tumor of the kidney. J Pediatr Hematol Oncol 24:385–388

Wai DH, Knezevich SR, Lucas T et al (2000) The ETV6-NTRK3 gene fusion encodes a chimeric protein tyrosine kinase that transforms NIH3T3 cells. Oncogene 19:906–915

Waldron PE, Rodgers BM, Kelly MD et al (1999) Successful treatment of a patient with stage IV rhabdoid tumor of the kidney: case report and review. J Pediatr Hematol Oncol 21:53–57

Walsh A, Kelly DR, Vaid YN et al (2010) Complete response to carboplatin, gemcitabine, and paclitaxel in a patient with advanced metastatic renal medullary carcinoma. Pediatr Blood Cancer 55:1217–1220

Wood DP Jr, Kay R, Norris D (1990) Renal sarcomas of childhood. Urology 36:73–78

Yamamoto M, Suzuki N, Hatakeyama N et al (2006) Treatment of stage IV malignant rhabdoid tumor of the kidney (MRTK) with ICE and VDCy: a case report. J Pediatr Hematol Oncol 28:286–289

Yanagisawa S, Kadouchi I, Yokomori K et al (2009) Identification and metastatic potential of tumor-initiating cells in malignant rhabdoid tumor of the kidney. Clin Cancer Res 15:3014–3022

Yumura-Yagi K, Inoue M, Wakabayashi R et al (1998) Successful double autografts for patients with relapsed clear cell sarcoma of the kidney. Bone Marrow Transplant 22:381–383

Yun K (1993) Clear cell sarcoma of the kidney expresses insulin-like growth factor-II but not WT1 transcripts. Am J Pathol 142:39–47

Zuo S, Xue Y, Tang S et al (2010) 14-3-3 epsilon dynamically interacts with key components of mitogen-activated protein kinase signal module for selective modulation of the TNF-alpha-induced time course-dependent NF-kappaB activity. J Proteome Res 9:3465–3478

15 Wilms Tumor in Countries with Limited Resources

Monika Metzger, Judith A. Wilimas, Mhamed Harif, and Trijn Israels

Contents

M. Metzger, MD (✉) • J.A. Wilimas, MD
Department of Oncology, St Jude Children's Research Hospital, 262 Danny Thomas Pl, Memphis, TN 38105, USA
e-mail: monika.metzger@stjude.org; judith.wilimas@stjude.org

M. Harif, MD
Department of Hematology/Oncology, Mohammed VI University Hospital, 6 Rue Ibn Sina, Hay Amarchich, Marrakech, Morocco

T. Israels, MD, PhD
Department of Pediatric Oncology, VU University Medical Center, De Boelelaan 1117, 1081 HV, Amsterdam, The Netherlands

Abstract

In this chapter we summarize the status of Wilms tumor therapy in countries with limited resources, as well as the challenges faced in those settings. There is a complicated interrelationship of different factors that contribute to delayed diagnosis leading to advanced disease at presentation, inadequate therapy and often 'abandonment' of therapy. For many countries with limited resources cancer is not a priority unlike infections. Political instability in times of civil unrest can lead to lack of adequate healthcare facilities, or hamper access to facilities. Cultural and religious beliefs sometimes also play a role in refusal or abandonment of therapy. Alternative medicine is sometimes perceived as a gentler alternative and less expensive. Lack of parental education has been recognized as an important factor leading to abandonment of therapy. However, not only limited education of the parents is an obstacle for care, lack of community awareness among the population and community health care workers plays a role in delayed diagnosis as well. Once a patient comes to medical attention with advanced disease and in poor general condition, lack of qualified caregivers, medications and supportive care further compromise outcome. Children diagnosed with cancer in these countries are commonly malnourished resulting in an increased risk of infection, post-surgical complications and mortality, and are often unable to tolerate

K. Pritchard-Jones, J.S. Dome (eds.), *Renal Tumors of Childhood: Biology and Therapy*, Pediatric Oncology, DOI 10.1007/978-3-662-44003-2_15, © Springer-Verlag Berlin Heidelberg 2014

chemotherapy. Adequate treatment is best provided in paediatric centres where basic imaging, chemotherapy, physicians and nurses trained to give the drugs, and a skilled surgeon and appropriate surgical facilities are available. Survival rates in countries with limited resources range from 38 – 81%. Improvements in survival from this point will require stepwise institution of protocols asking specific questions, including socio-economic queries, similar to the approach in the early days of NWTS and SIOP. Fortunately, the infrastructure exists in many areas to ask and answer these questions.

Key Points

1. Cure rates in high-income countries are excellent with either preoperative chemotherapy or surgery followed by chemotherapy and radiotherapy if necessary.
2. Optimal treatment requires a written protocol designed for local conditions that clearly describes diagnostic approach and therapy.
3. Staging can be accomplished cost-effectively using history, physical examination, ultrasound, chest roentgenogram and surgery in most patients.
4. Other renal tumors can be mistaken for Wilms tumor; therefore careful attention to clinical presentation and pathology is crucial.
5. Free medical treatment and social support to enable poor parents to complete treatment are effective interventions to improve results.

15.1 Introduction

The purpose of this chapter is to briefly summarize the status of Wilms tumor therapy in countries with limited resources. Previous chapters in this book clearly document the clinical presentation of this tumor and the remarkable improvements in therapy mediated by the carefully designed and implemented studies of the SIOP and NWTS groups (Green 2004). Efforts to translate high cure rates to countries with limited resources have met with variable success. We will discuss these efforts and examine the reasons for success and failure.

The NWTS and SIOP studies have achieved remarkably similar results using primary surgery followed by chemotherapy (NWTS) or preoperative chemotherapy followed by surgery (SIOP). Cure rates have improved so dramatically that more recent studies have concentrated on decreasing therapy, particularly radiation therapy, to avoid late effects of treatment and to identify prognostic biologic markers that may allow tailoring of therapy (Green 2004). These studies have spanned more than four decades, and it is important to realize that other factors have contributed significantly to the improvements in survival. A well-organized multidisciplinary approach with advances in surgical technique, anaesthesia, diagnostic imaging, nursing and supportive care has had a considerable impact, but socioeconomic changes may be even more important. Education, nutrition, access to medical care and alleviation of poverty have resulted in earlier diagnosis, lack of comorbidities such as infection and malnutrition and markedly decreased abandonment of therapy in higher-income countries.

15.2 Obstacles to care of Children with Cancer in Countries with Limited Resources

Figure 15.1 illustrates the complicated interrelationship of different factors that contribute to delayed diagnosis leading to advanced disease at

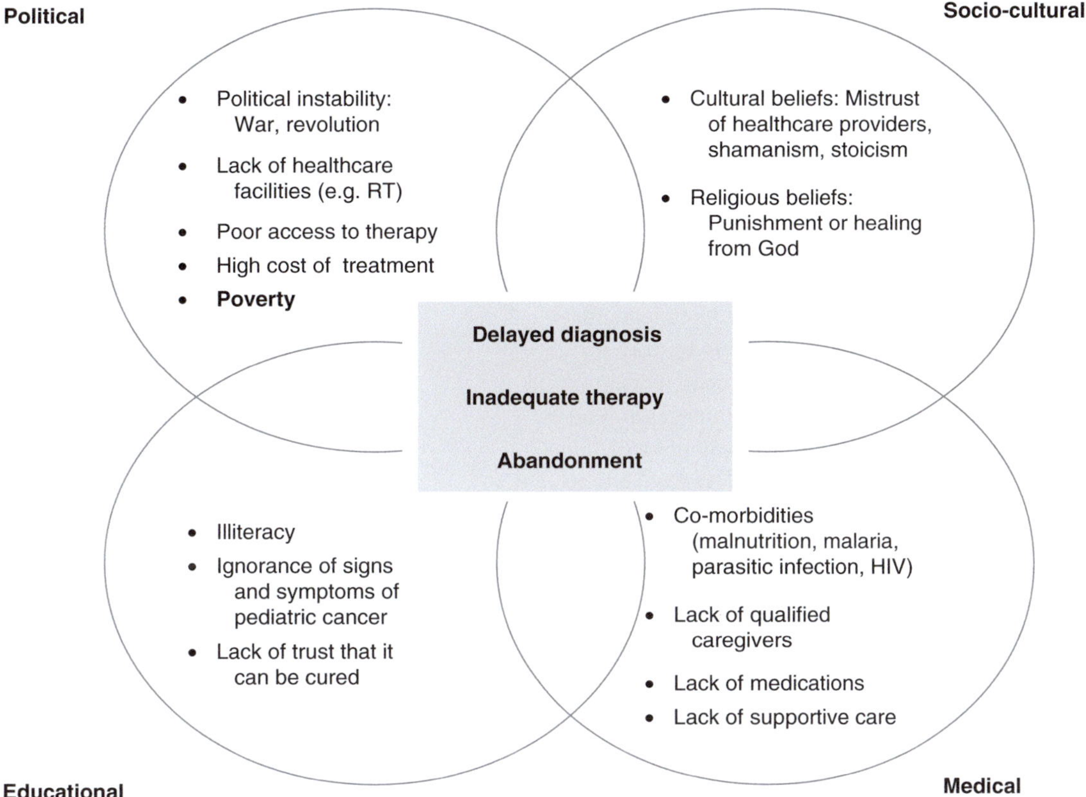

Fig. 15.1 Illustration showing the interrelationship of different factors that contribute to delayed diagnosis, inadequate therapy and abandonment of therapy for children with Wilms tumors in countries with limited resources

presentation, inadequate therapy and often 'abandonment' of therapy. 'Abandonment' of therapy, defined as failure to complete paediatric cancer treatment, is a common problem in low-income countries (Arora et al. 2007). Several studies have identified related factors and effective interventions. In Recife, Brazil, abandonment of treatment for acute lymphoblastic leukaemia (ALL) was reduced from 16 to 1.5 % by social support that included housing, travel expenses, family education and job training. For many low-income countries, cancer is not part of the health-care agenda; priority is given to infections, like diarrhoea and malaria control. Political instability in times of war and revolution can lead to lack of adequate health-care facilities or hamper access to facilities which may be far away and difficult or unsafe to reach. Furthermore, time away from home, leaving the rest of the family behind often places an even greater emotional and financial burden on parents who depend on daily wages and cannot afford the cost of treatment. Most families in sub-Saharan Africa are unable to pay for their child's cancer treatment (Howard et al. 2004). Even if the child receives free hospitalization and treatment, it is difficult for many to pay for the additional costs of a treatment that often takes weeks or months. In Malawi, the child and one family member usually stay in the hospital during this time. Interviews have shown that absence from home (work on the field, loss of income) and extra costs during the stay in the hospital (food) are important concerns for parents (Israels et al. 2008). Financial issues related to the treatment are major concerns for the guardians, and poverty as the greatest obstacle in providing adequate care of children with cancer in resource-limited countries cannot be overemphasized. It is necessary to provide not only medical treatment but also travel allowances and adequate nutritional support when offering prolonged treatment that needs several journeys and long hospital stays in resource poor settings like Malawi. Cultural and religious beliefs sometimes also play a role in refusal or abandonment of therapy. Alternative medicine (Fig. 15.2) and herbal medicine are sometimes perceived as a gentler alternative and less expensive (Sachdeva et al. 2005). In cases of extreme religiosity, parents may believe the disease is punishment from God or they may trust in being able to pray for a miraculous healing. Lack of parental education has been recognized as an important factor leading to abandonment of therapy (Sweet-Cordero et al. 1999). However, not only limited education of the parents is an obstacle for care, lack of community awareness among the population and community health-care workers plays a role in delayed diagnosis (Workman et al. 2007). Once a patient comes to medical attention with advanced disease (Fig. 15.3) and in poor general condition, lack of qualified caregivers, medications and supportive care further compromise outcome. Children diagnosed with cancer in low-income countries are commonly malnourished (Fig. 15.4), resulting in an increased risk of infection with a variety of bacterial, viral, fungal and parasitic pathogens, post-surgical complications and mortality (Sala et al. 2004), and are often unable to tolerate chemotherapy (Israels et al. 2009a). In Malawi, more than half of the children with Wilms tumor were severely and acutely malnourished at diagnosis (Israels et al. 2009a). Adequate nutritional support is essential.

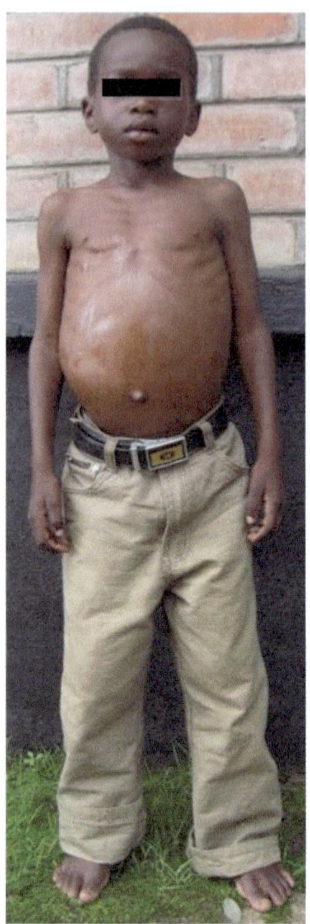

Fig. 15.2 Malawian child with a Wilms tumo(u)r

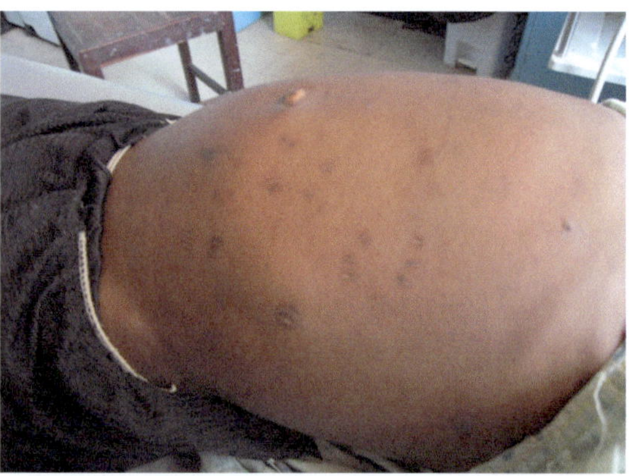

Fig. 15.3 Scratches placed on the mass by a traditional healer in Malawi

15.3 Epidemiological Features

Few reliable population-based cancer registries exist in countries with limited resources. It is however estimated that 160,000–200,000 children are diagnosed with cancer worldwide each year. Only 20–30 % have access to appropriate treatment (Parkin et al. 2005; Howard et al. 2008).

The incidence of Wilms tumor is 6–9 per million children younger than 15 years of age and accounts for 5–7 % of all childhood cancers. It is reported to be higher among the black population in Africa and the United States compared to other ethnic groups (Stiller and Parkin 1990, 1996). Hospital-based registries reflect a high prevalence of Wilms tumors. In Malawi,

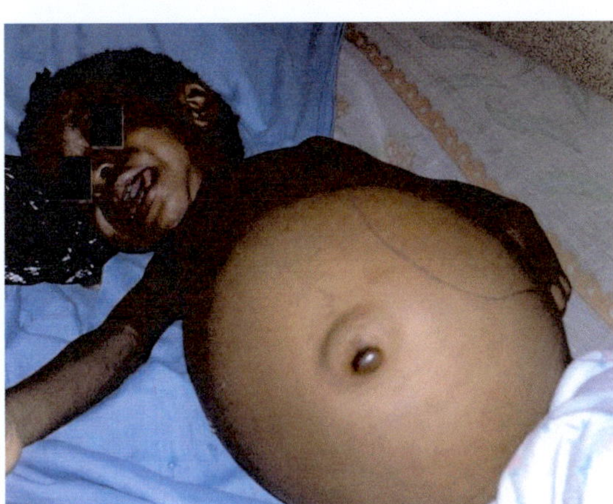

Fig. 15.4 Patient with advanced Wilms tumor from Mali

Wilms tumor is the second most commonly diagnosed malignant abdominal tumor after Burkitt lymphoma (Israels et al. 2010). In Sudan, Wilms tumor is reported to be the most frequent solid tumor in children less than 4 years of age (Abuidris et al. 2008a).

Cancer registries and data management programs are essential in low-income countries to better assess the needs, so as to be able to negotiate governmental and non-governmental support, but also for quality improvement initiatives (Ayoub et al. 2007). As treatment programs for paediatric oncology are developed, Wilms tumors should be one of the first tumors to be treated because of its frequency and curability. Treatment also requires development of multidisciplinary capacities that may benefit other children and programs across the hospital. Careful clinical research is essential to develop protocols appropriate for local conditions (Ribeiro and Pui 2005; Yaris et al. 2004).

15.4 Levels of Oncology Care

Adequate treatment is best provided in paediatric centres where basic imaging, chemotherapy, physicians and nurses trained to give the drugs and a skilled surgeon and appropriate surgical facilities are available (Corrigan and Feig 2004). With the lack of oncologists in sub-Saharan Africa, astute general practitioners and general surgeons at times will fill the void by learning to apply a handful of chemotherapeutic agents necessary to treat Wilms tumors (Hadley 2010). Table 15.1 defines the different levels of facilities and resources that may be available to treat patients with Wilms tumors in different settings. The diagnosis can be based on a careful history and physical exam with clinical symptoms (generally a large abdominal mass – Fig. 15.5). The basic workup should include a complete blood count, urinalysis, chest roentgenogram and ultrasound of the abdomen. Additional testing depends on the findings of the basic studies and available tests which will vary depending upon the resources of the treating centre. Some paediatric oncology centres even in developing countries have the capability of doing a workup equivalent to that in the United States or Europe. Confirmation of the diagnosis ultimately depends upon pathologic review after surgery which is frequently delayed until preoperative chemotherapy has shrunk the tumor. Needle biopsies have been reported to be useful in some centres, but they can increase the stage, may result in bleeding or infection and may be difficult for the pathologist to interpret (Vujanic et al. 2003). Unfortunately, pathologic diagnosis of Wilms tumor may be difficult even after removal of the tumor bearing kidney. There are very few paediatric pathologists in developing countries; specimens are often not processed appropriately; interpretation of histology may be difficult after pretreatment, special stains and immunohistochemistry are unavailable; and misdiagnosis of unfavourable histology and clear cell sarcoma is common. Central pathology review would be helpful but is difficult to arrange and costly (Vujanic et al. 2009). One alternative is telepathology; however, the necessary infrastructure cannot always be implemented in some resource poor countries that do not have reliable internet access or electricity.

While radiotherapy improves prognosis for a subgroup of patients, patients in a Level 1 facility will not have access to it. Even when radiation oncology is available, resources are often scarce and overbooked with adults, radiotherapists often not comfortable treating children and frequently the unit is not operational. Supportive care including the availability of morphine and antibi-

Table 15.1 Levels of paediatric oncology centres

Level	Medical facilities	Specialists	Drugs	Supportive care	Diagnosis
1 Pilot program	General paediatric ward	Paediatrician Nurses General surgeon Twinning relationship	Vincristine Actinomycin (Adriamycin)	Antibiotics Morphine Financial support for transportation and meals	Physical exam CBC Urinalysis Chest XR Ultrasound
2 Paediatric oncology unit	Paediatric oncology ward Radiotherapy	Pathologist Paediatric oncologist Paediatric surgeon Radiation oncologist Oncology Nurses	Adriamycin Cyclophosphamide Etoposide Ifosfamide Carboplatin	Blood products Central venous access	CT scan of chest and abdomen Multidisciplinary organization of care
3 Centre of excellence	Intensive care unit	Paediatric pathologist Paediatric radiation oncologist Pharmacists (oncology) Intensivist		Mechanical ventilation Haemodyalisis Pressure support End-of-life care	Special stains and immuno-histochemistry Cytogenetics

Adapted from Howard et al. (2005)

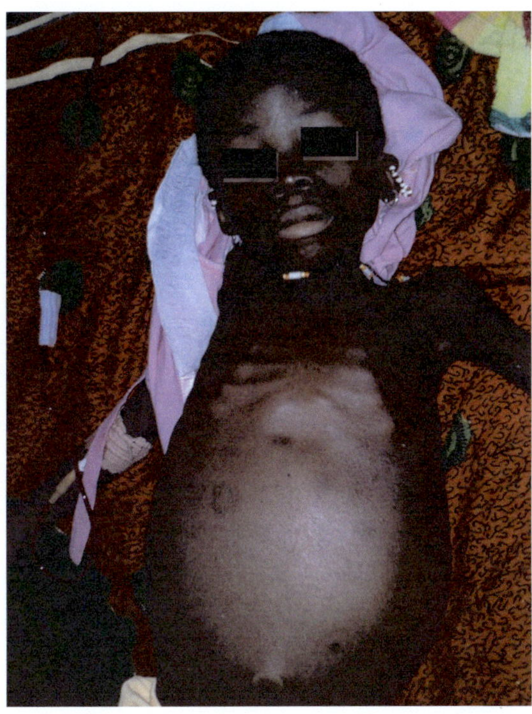

Fig. 15.5 Malnourished child with advanced Wilms tumor from Mali

otics is essential, and blood transfusion facilities are of great value whenever possible; however, safety is often an issue. Furthermore, food for a parent and siblings, money for transportation and time for education are very important in order to increase the likelihood of success (Howard et al. 2004). Palliative care is often not available, and, tragically, dying children are often denied narcotic analgesics because of concerns of parents and caregivers about addiction and short-sighted government policies. Many pilot programs in resource-limited countries have started with a twinning relationship that provides not only financial support for the basic medical requirements but also capacity training and ongoing intellectual support (Howard et al. 2005).

In Europe (SIOP studies), preoperative chemotherapy is given to shrink the tumor, reduce the risk of surgical complications such as tumor rupture during surgery and induce a more favourable tumor stage at the time of surgery. SIOP studies have shown that equivalent cure rates can be achieved with a less intensive postoperative chemotherapy schedule with fewer patients requiring irradiation (Reinhard et al. 2004). This would seem to be a useful strategy for patients in developing countries where tumors at presentation are often large, supportive care limited and radiotherapy not often available. While there are potential problems with this approach, given the dismal prognosis of other renal tumors in resource-limited countries, this should not be an obstacle. In the SIOP studies, up to 5 % of tumors were not Wilms tumor and occasionally were benign. The 4 weeks of preoperative chemotherapy advocated by SIOP may not always seem sufficient to shrink a tumor that can occupy more than 50 % of the abdominal cavity (Fig. 15.6). However, a prospective study from Malawi looking at tumor shrinkage after 4 weeks in localized disease and 6 weeks in metastatic disease showed a mean tumor volume reduction of 40 and 60 %, respectively (Israels et al. 2009b). Some groups, like AHOPCA (Asociacion de Hemato-Oncología Pediátrica de Centro America), now advocate for preoperative chemotherapy whenever the tumor crosses the midline, and the patient is malnourished or in poor general condition to tolerate anaesthesia

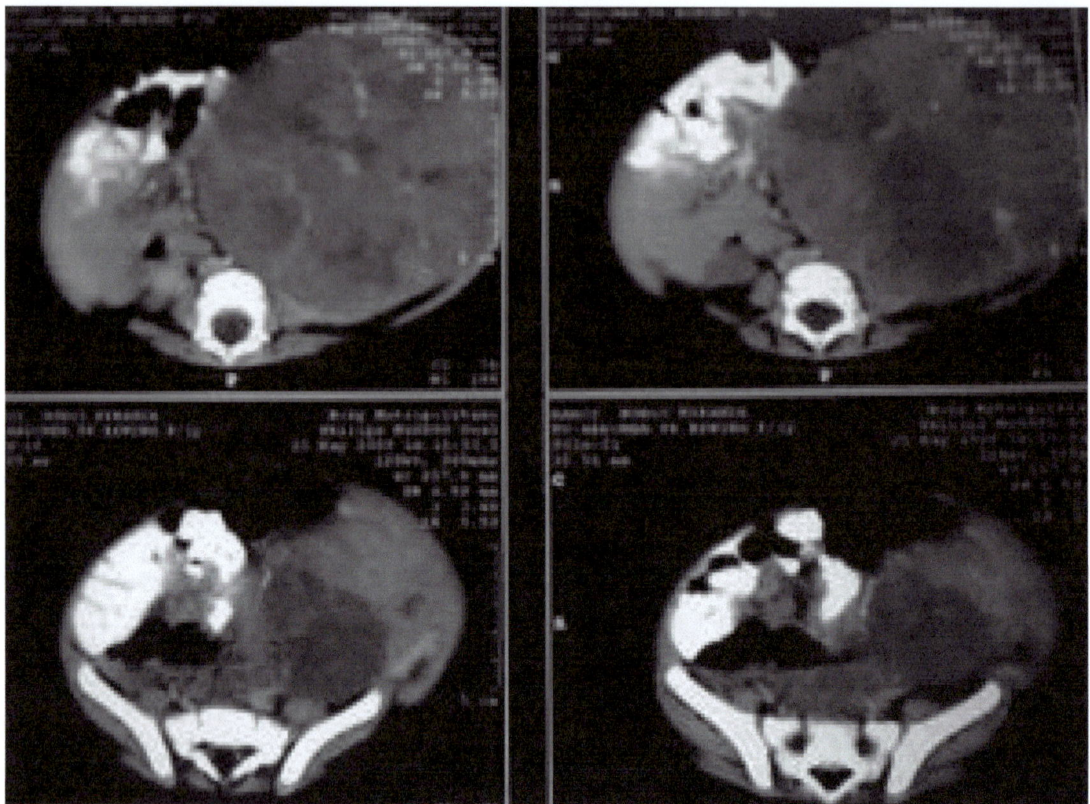

Fig. 15.6 Computer tomography of a 13 month old patient with Wilms tumor in Central America

or has probable stage III disease by imaging. Preoperative therapy in these cases is used to shrink the size of the tumor and provide a window of time to treat comorbid conditions like malnutrition and bacterial or parasitic infection.

15.5 Therapy

Appropriate therapy of Wilms tumor includes surgery, chemotherapy, and supportive care. Radiotherapy is used in patients with advanced stage or unfavourable histology disease in centres with advanced capabilities. Unfortunately, safe radiotherapy for children is often unavailable in developing countries. Recent NWTS and SIOP studies have shown that omitting or decreasing radiation therapy may not compromise cure rates, but these studies have not been done in children with very advanced disease or huge tumors. Studies from Nicaragua (Baez et al. 2002) and Morocco (Madani et al. 2006) have demonstrated that cure can be achieved in some patients with advanced disease without radiotherapy, but higher cure rates in these patients may require radiotherapy.

Supportive care must include postoperative care, treatment of infections, nutritional support (sometimes of the entire family to prevent abandonment), housing, education, transportation and pain medication.

Treatment must be administered according to a written protocol designed for local capabilities and conditions. Collection of data is crucial to adjust the protocol to provide adequate intensity of therapy and avoid morbidity and mortality.

15.6 Results of Therapy in Countries with Limited Resources

Table 15.2 shows the therapies as well as the results of a selected number of countries with limited resources. Survival rates range from 38 to 81 % and numbers of patients from 21 to 327. Obviously, there is a great deal of variability in both the reports and capabilities of the various centres. In general, results are better in centres that have the capability of administering radiation therapy. Whether this is a reflection of a contribution of radiation therapy to survival or the fact that centres that have radiotherapy available are generally in areas with more resources and less advanced disease, fewer comorbidities and less abandonment is not clear. Treatment in all cases was according to a protocol although, with a few exceptions, not all children with Wilms tumor received treatment. Our experience in Central America where protocol therapy was available to all children; experienced physicians, surgeons and nurses administered therapy; and radiation therapy was available suggests that overall survival rates are in the range of 60 %. Improvements in survival from this point will require stepwise institution of protocols asking specific questions, including socio-economic queries, similar to the approach in the early days of NWTS and SIOP. Fortunately, the infrastructure exists in many areas to ask and answer these questions.

Table 15.2 Outcome of patients treated in various low-income countries

Treatment approach	Total patients	Preoperative chemotherapy (*n*)	Postoperative chemotherapy [stage, histology] (*n*)	Radiotherapy in Gy (stage)	EFS (years)	OS (years)
Upfront surgery						
Egypt (Abd El-Aal et al. 2005)	62	–	VA × 24 weeks [I]	1,080 cGy tumor bed (III and II–IV, UH)	58 % (4)	70 % (4)
			VA × 52 weeks [II, FH]	1,080 cGy abdomen (spill)		
			VAD × 52 weeks [III and IV, FH]	1,200 cGy pulmonary metastases		
			VADC × 52 weeks [II, III, and IV, UH]	1,800 cGy hepatic metastases		
AHOPCA (Valverde et al. 2008)	223	–	NWTS-4	NWTS-4	54 % (3)	76 % (3)
Preoperative chemotherapy						
Malawi (Israels et al. 2009b)	21	VA × 4 weeks [I, II, and III]	VA × 4 weeks [I, IR]	None	5/21 [24 %] refractory	8/21 [38 %] are alive
		VAD × 6–9 weeks [IV]	VA × 26 weeks [I, HR and II, IR]		2/21 [10 %] relapsed	
			VAD × 26 weeks [II, HR and III]		4/21 [20 %] abandoned	
					2/21 [10 %] died	
Morocco (Madani et al. 2006)	86	VA × 4 weeks [I, II, and III]	VA × 18 weeks[I]	1,500 cGy abdomen [II and III, or II, UH]	77 % (5)	79 % (5)
		VAD × 6 weeks [IV]	VA × 28 weeks [II and III, FH]	3,000 cGy abdomen [UH]		
			VADI × 37 weeks [II and III UH]			

(continued)

Table 15.2 (continued)

Treatment approach	Total patients	Preoperative chemotherapy (*n*)	Postoperative chemotherapy [stage, histology] (*n*)	Radiotherapy in Gy (stage)	EFS (years)	OS (years)
Mixed						
Asia (Sen et al. 1998)	62	VA×4 weeks (15)	VA×60 weeks [I and II, FH] VAD×60 weeks [III-V, any UH]	Doses and fields not described (18)	*Did not relapse* Stages: I – 81 % II – 75 % III – 42 % IV – 14 % V – 50 %	*Are alive* 69 % favourable histology 50 % unfavourable histology
South Africa (Davidson et al. 2006)	188	VA (41)	VA VAD VADC VADCE	2,000 cGy tumor bed (I-IV early era) 1,080 cGy tumor bed (III) 1,200 cGy pulmonary metastases	75 % (5)	81 % (5)
Turkey (Kutluk et al. 2006)	327	VA and epirubicin (23)	A (27) VA (264) VADC (22) As per SIOP-9 (14)	1,800–4,000 cGy	56 % (10)	61 % (10)
Sudan (Abuidris et al. 2008b)	37	Not described (13)	As per NWTS-5	Doses and fields not described	4/37 (11 %) completed therapy and are alive 4 months to 4 years	
Turkey (Yildiz et al. 2000)	106	SIOP (8)	NWTS-4 (98)	According to NWTS-4	72 % (5)	77 % (5)

15.7 Late Breaking Updates

As mentioned in the concluding remarks, the International Society of Pediatric Oncology – Pediatric Oncology in Developing Countries (SIOP PODC) produced and published an adapted treatment guideline for the management of children with Wilms tumor in low-income countries. An adapted guideline for concomitant supportive care has also been published (Israels et al. 2013a, b). The SIOP Africa/PODC Collaborative Wilms Tumor Project started in 2013 and comprises nine treatment centers in six countries in sub-Saharan Africa. The project is implementing the SIOP PODC consensus adapted treatment guidelines as a prospective clinical trial with uniform outcome evaluation. The project aims to improve care and survival, strengthen local multidisciplinary teams and facilitate the establishment of an active regional childhood cancer network (Israels et al. 2013a, b).

References

Abd El-Aal HH, Habib EE, Mishrif MM (2005) Wilms' tumor: the experience of the pediatric unit of Kasr El-Aini center of radiation oncology and nuclear medicine (NEMROCK). J Egypt Natl Canc Inst 17:308–314

Abuidris DO, Ahmed ME, Elgaili EM, Arora RS (2008a) Childhood cancer in Sudan: 1999–2007. Trop Doct 38:208–210

Abuidris DO, Elimam ME, Nugud FM, Elgaili EM, Ahmed ME, Arora RS (2008b) Wilms tumour in Sudan. Pediatr Blood Cancer 50:1135–1137

Arora RS, Eden T, Pizer B (2007) The problem of treatment abandonment in children from developing countries with cancer. Pediatr Blood Cancer 49:941–946

Ayoub L, Fu L, Pena A et al (2007) Implementation of a data management program in a pediatric cancer unit in a low income country. Pediatr Blood Cancer 49:23–27

Baez F, Fossati BF, Ocampo E et al (2002) Treatment of childhood Wilms' tumor without radiotherapy in Nicaragua. Ann Oncol 13:944–948

Corrigan JJ, Feig SA (2004) Guidelines for pediatric cancer centers. Pediatrics 113:1833–1835

Davidson A, Hartley P, Desai F, Daubenton J, Rode H, Millar A (2006) Wilms tumour experience in a South African centre. Pediatr Blood Cancer 46:465–471

Green DM (2004) The treatment of stages I-IV favorable histology Wilms' tumor. J Clin Oncol 22:1366–1372

Hadley GP (2010) Can surgeons fill the void in the management of children with solid tumours in not-developing countries? Pediatr Blood Cancer 55:16–17

Howard SC, Pedrosa M, Lins M et al (2004) Establishment of a pediatric oncology program and outcomes of childhood acute lymphoblastic leukemia in a resource-poor area. JAMA 291:2471–2475

Howard SC, Ribeiro RC, Pui CH (2005) Strategies to improve outcomes of children with cancer in low-income countries. Eur J Cancer 41:1584–1587

Howard SC, Metzger ML, Wilimas JA et al (2008) Childhood cancer epidemiology in low-income countries. Cancer 112:461–472

Israels T, Chirambo C, Caron H, de Kraker J, Molyneux E, Reis R (2008) The guardians' perspective on paediatric cancer treatment in Malawi and factors affecting adherence. Pediatr Blood Cancer 51:639–642

Israels T, van de Wetering MD, Hesseling P, van Geloven N, Caron HN, Molyneux EM (2009a) Malnutrition and neutropenia in children treated for Burkitt lymphoma in Malawi. Pediatr Blood Cancer 53:47–52

Israels T, Kambugu J, Kouya F, El-Mallawany NK, Hesseling PB, Kaspers GJ, Eden T, Renner L, Molyneux EM (2013b) Clinical trials to improve childhood cancer care and survival in sub-Saharan Africa. Nat Rev Clin Oncol 10(10):599–604

Israels T, Molyneux EM, Caron HN et al (2009b) Preoperative chemotherapy for patients with Wilms tumor in Malawi is feasible and efficacious. Pediatr Blood Cancer 53:584–589

Israels T, Renner L, Hendricks M, Hesseling P, Howard S, Molyneux E (2013a) SIOP PODC: recommendations for supportive care of children with cancer in a low-income setting. Pediatr Blood Cancer 60(6):899–904

Israels T, Ribeiro RC, Molyneux EM (2010) Strategies to improve care for children with cancer in Sub-Saharan Africa. Eur J Cancer 46(11):1960–1966

Kutluk T, Varan A, Buyukpamukcu N et al (2006) Improved survival of children with wilms tumor. J Pediatr Hematol Oncol 28:423–426

Madani A, Zafad S, Harif M et al (2006) Treatment of Wilms tumor according to SIOP 9 protocol in Casablanca, Morocco. Pediatr Blood Cancer 46:472–475

Parkin DM, Bray F, Ferlay J, Pisani P (2005) Global cancer statistics, 2002. CA Cancer J Clin 55:74–108

Reinhard H, Semler O, Burger D et al (2004) Results of the SIOP 93-01/GPOH trial and study for the treatment of patients with unilateral nonmetastatic Wilms Tumor. Klin Padiatr 216:132–140

Ribeiro RC, Pui CH (2005) Saving the children–improving childhood cancer treatment in developing countries. N Engl J Med 352:2158–2160

Sachdeva A, Jain V, Jadav, SP (2005) Move to alternative medicine why? and when? the Indian scneario. Pediatr Blood Cancer 45:578, Ref type: abstract

Sala A, Pencharz P, Barr RD (2004) Children, cancer, and nutrition–a dynamic triangle in review. Cancer 100:677–687

Sen S, Kadamba P, Al-AbdulAaly M, Mammen KE, Ahmed S (1998) Results of Wilms' tumour management in two tertiary-care hospitals in Asia. Pediatr Surg Int 13:42–44

Stiller CA, Parkin DM (1990) International variations in the incidence of childhood renal tumours. Br J Cancer 62:1026–1030

Stiller CA, Parkin DM (1996) Geographic and ethnic variations in the incidence of childhood cancer. Br Med Bull 52:682–703

Sweet-Cordero A, Antillon F, Baez F (1999) Factors that influence abandonment of care among children with cancer in Guatemala. Med Peidatr Oncol 33(151), Ref type: abstract

Valverde P, Luna-Fineman S, Ortiz R, Peña A, Bonilla M, Metzger ML, Wilimas J (2008) Treatment of Wilms Tumor in Central America: results of the first Collaborative AHOPCA Protocol. SIOP Brazil, Ref type: abstract

Vujanic GM, Kelsey A, Mitchell C, Shannon RS, Gornall P (2003) The role of biopsy in the diagnosis of renal tumors of childhood: results of the UKCCSG Wilms tumor study 3. Med Pediatr Oncol 40:18–22

Vujanic GM, Sandstedt B, Kelsey A, Sebire NJ (2009) Central pathology review in multicenter trials and studies: lessons from the nephroblastoma trials. Cancer 115:1977–1983

Workman GM, Ribeiro RC, Rai SN, Pedrosa A, Workman DE, Pedrosa F (2007) Pediatric cancer knowledge: assessment of knowledge of warning signs and symptoms for pediatric cancer among Brazilian community health workers. J Cancer Educ 22:181–185

Yaris N, Mandiracioglu A, Buyukpamukcu M (2004) Childhood cancer in developing countries. Pediatr Hematol Oncol 21:237–253

Yildiz I, Yuksel L, Ozkan A et al (2000) Multidisciplinary approach to Wilms' tumor: 18 years of experience. Jpn J Clin Oncol 30:17–20

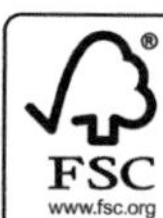

MIX
Papier aus verantwortungsvollen Quellen
Paper from responsible sources
FSC® C105338

If you have any concerns about our products,
you can contact us on
ProductSafety@springernature.com

In case Publisher is established outside the EU,
the EU authorized representative is:
Springer Nature Customer Service Center GmbH
Europaplatz 3, 69115 Heidelberg, Germany

Printed by Libri Plureos GmbH
in Hamburg, Germany